Two week loan

Please return on or before the last date stamped below.
Charges are made for late return.

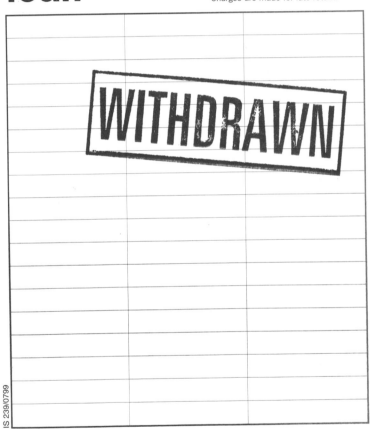

IS 239/0799

INFORMATION SERVICES PO BOX 430, CARDIFF CF10 3XT

CLINICAL RETINA

David A. Quillen, MD
Barbara A. Blodi, MD

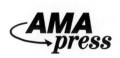
AMA press

American Medical Association

Physicians dedicated to the health of America

AMA Press

Vice President, Business Products: Anthony J. Frankos
Publisher: Michael Desposito
Editorial Director: Mary Lou White
Director, Production and Manufacturing: Jean Roberts
Senior Acquisitions Editor: Barry Bowlus
Developmental Editor: Katharine Dvorak
Copy Editor: Maxine Gere
Director, Marketing: J. D. Kinney
Marketing Manager: Reg Schmidt
Senior Production Coordinator: Rosalyn Carlton
Senior Print Coordinator: Ronnie Summers

Internet address: www.ama-assn.org

Additional copies of this book may be ordered by calling 800 621-8335. Mention product number OP856902.

ISBN 1-57947-284-2

The authors, editors, and publisher of this work have checked with sources believed to be reliable in their efforts to confirm the accuracy and completeness of the information presented herein and that the information is in accordance with the standard practices accepted at the time of publication. However, neither the authors, editors, and publisher, nor any party involved in the creation and publication of this work warrant that the information is in every respect accurate and complete, and they are not responsible for any errors or omissions or for any consequences from application of the information in this book.

In light of ongoing research and changes in clinical experience and in governmental regulations, readers are encouraged to confirm the information contained herein with additional sources, in particular as it pertains to drug dosage and usage. Readers are urged to check the package insert for each drug they plan to administer for any change in indications and dosage and for additional warnings and precautions, especially for new or infrequently used drugs.

Library of Congress Cataloging-in-Publication Data

Clinical retina / edited by David A. Quillen, Barbara A. Blodi.
    p. ; cm.
Includes bibliographical references and index.
   ISBN 1-57947-284-2
1. Retina--Diseases. 2. Retina--Diseases--Atlases.
   [DNLM: 1. Retinal Diseases--physiopathology. 2. Retina--physiology.
3. Retinal Diseases--diagnosis. 4. Retinal Diseases--therapy. WW 270
C6146 2002] I. Quillen, David A., 1964- II. Blodi, Barbara A.
   RE551 .C575 2002
   617.7'35—dc21
                    2002009372

BP90:02-P-052:10/02

To Betsy and our children, Erin, Matthew, and Jack. —DQ

To Justin, Jeremy, and Andrea. —BB

CONTENTS

PREFACE

As we began our careers in ophthalmology, we were charged with the daunting task of teaching retina to ophthalmology residents. *Clinical Retina* evolved out of our efforts to provide residents the essential information about a given retinal condition in an organized, clinically relevant manner. Our goal was not to create another comprehensive, multi-volume reference book. There are several outstanding references currently available. Instead, we have attempted to develop a textbook-atlas that provides the reader a summary of the information on common and unusual retinal diseases. The use of high-quality color figures was a must.

Contributing authors from the United States, Canada, and England have joined together to produce *Clinical Retina.* The textbook is organized using the traditional classification of retinal diseases. Within each chapter, conditions are presented in alphabetic order using a two-page format: text on the left page, figures on the right. Therefore, in two pages, the reader can review the essential material about a given retinal condition. The text is organized into sections: general information; symptoms; clinical features; ancillary testing; pathology/pathogenesis; treatment/prognosis; and systemic evaluation. A list of selected references is provided for those readers who desire more information.

Chapter 1 provides a review of the retinal anatomy and physiology and highlights important structures using ample clinical examples. Chapter 2 reviews commonly used ancillary studies including fluorescein angiography, electrophysiology, and ultrasonography.

Chapter 3, Clinical Features of Retinal Disease, describes a variety of ophthalmoscopic findings and provides a differential diagnosis of the most common conditions likely to manifest a particular feature. Photographic examples are provided. This chapter provides a more "problem-based" approach to learning retina. If readers do not immediately recognize the diagnosis, they can identify significant clinical features and review the most common associations. Then, they can refer to the specific condition in the body of the textbook for more detailed information.

Chapters 4 through 12 cover the spectrum of retinal disease: Macular Diseases; Retinal Vascular Diseases; Hereditary Retinal Disorders; Drug Toxicities; Intraocular Tumors; Inflammatory Diseases; Trauma; Peripheral Retinal Diseases; and Diseases of the Vitreous. Chapter 13 reviews the histopathology of selected retinal diseases.

The major clinical trials for retinal diseases are summarized in Chapter 14, Clinical Trials in Retina. The reviews highlight the study objectives, treatment groups and trial design, summary of results, and implications for clinical practice. Chapter 15, Laser Photocoagulation and Photodynamic Therapy for Retinal and Choroidal Disease, provides information on the indications, treatment techniques, complications, and follow-up considerations of laser photocoagulation for a variety of conditions and photodynamic therapy for age-related macular degeneration.

Clinical Retina contains over 800 color and black and white photographs, one of the largest collections of retinal images in any ophthalmology textbook. The CD-ROM contains all of the figures displayed in the book as well as 50 additional images provided in a self-assessment program. Every attempt was made to ensure that the images used were of high quality and representative of the condition featured.

ACKNOWLEDGMENTS

I am thankful to God for the opportunity to prepare this book. The entire process has been a tremendous life experience and I am grateful for the chance to participate. I appreciate the opportunity to collaborate with Barbara Blodi and all of the contributing authors during the preparation of *Clinical Retina*.

I would like to thank my wife, Betsy, for everything she has done for me over the past 20 years since we met in WAWA. She has been my teacher in so many ways and I am thankful to have her in my life.

I would like to thank my parents, Joan and Bob Quillen, and my brothers, Greg and Bobby Q, for their enthusiasm and support.

Throughout my life I have been blessed with special teachers. Mrs Schracht, Mrs Marrone, Mr Lange, Mr Mazziota, Mr Harris, Fr Burch, Cheston Berlin, George Blankenship, Tom Gardner, Ali Aminlari, Bill Cantore, Joe Sassani, James McManaway, George Rosenwasser, Don Gass, and numerous others have had a lasting impact on my life. They continue to inspire me to this day.

A special thank you to Tim Bennett, CRA, for his assistance in preparing this book. Photographs taken from Tim's collection are scattered throughout this book and CD-ROM package. I appreciate the opportunity to share his gift with you.

Both Barb and I as well as many of the contributing authors have had the good fortune to work with Dr Gass as fellows. Dr Gass is an inspiration to us all. For me, the opportunity to work with Dr Gass in Miami was life changing. He is a remarkable man in every way: honest, kind, thoughtful, insightful. His love of ophthalmology and humility regarding his accomplishments are examples for us all.

I would like to thank George Blankenship for his support and guidance. From the first day I decided to pursue a life in ophthalmology, George has been a friend and mentor.

I would like to thank my partners at the Penn State Department of Ophthalmology for their support over the past ten years. I am proud to be a member of the Penn State Ophthalmology family.

A special thank you to Barry Bowlus and Katharine Dvorak, and the rest of the staff at AMA Press who contributed to the development of *Clinical Retina*. To Barry, we appreciate your enthusiasm for this project and your unyielding commitment to excellence. To Katie, thank you for making this project your own. Your participation has greatly enhanced the quality of this book. —DQ

I am indebted to my parents, Frederick and Ottilie, who instilled in me a love of books, language, and learning. I am also grateful for my brother, Christopher, who has been a welcome mentor throughout my education and my professional career. My husband, Justin, has been a steady, calm, and encouraging influence on me; I thank him for his love, friendship, and constant support during this project. —BB

ABOUT THE EDITORS

David A. Quillen, MD is currently Associate Professor of Ophthalmology and Residency Program Director at the Penn State College of Medicine in Hershey, Pennsylvania. He specializes in medical retina diseases.

He performed his ophthalmology residency training at the Penn State Ophthalmology Residency Program. He completed his Medical Retina fellowship at the Bascom Palmer Eye Institute, University of Miami under the direction of J. Donald M. Gass, MD. Dr Quillen has a strong interest in ophthalmology education and participates in a variety of local and national educational programs.

Dr Quillen is married to Betsy and has three children: Erin, Matthew, and Jack. In addition to ophthalmology, Dr Quillen enjoys dinner and a movie with Betsy, book shopping with Erin, playing and watching sports with Matt, and going to Chocolate World with Jack.

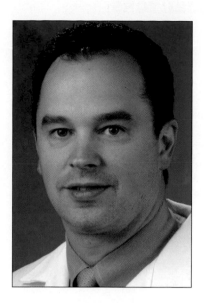

Barbara A. Blodi, MD is Associate Professor at the University of Wisconsin-Madison Medical School in the Department of Ophthalmology and Visual Sciences. She specializes in medical retina diseases.

Dr Blodi graduated from the University of Iowa School of Medicine in 1987 and completed her residency in ophthalmology at Bascom Palmer Eye Institute, University of Miami in 1991. She remained at Bascom Palmer for a fellowship in medical retina with J. Donald M. Gass, MD. This was followed by a year of surgical retina fellowship at the Kellogg Eye Center in Ann Arbor, Michigan, where Dr Blodi continued as a faculty member for two years.

Dr Blodi joined the faculty of the University of Wisconsin in 1997 and became Associate Professor in 2001. She is currently Co-director of the Fundus Photograph Reading Center and collaborates on the design, conduct, and analysis of clinical trials in ophthalmology, specifically in the areas of age-related macular degeneration and diabetic retinopathy.

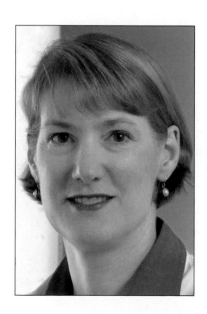

CONTRIBUTORS

G. William Aylward, MD
Moorsfields Eye Hospital
London, England

Alistair J. Barber, PhD
Penn State College of Medicine
Hershey, Pennsylvania

Timothy J. Bennett, CRA
Penn State College of Medicine
Hershey, Pennsylvania

Barbara A. Blodi, MD
University of Wisconsin
Madison

Dean J. Bonsall, MD, FACS
Penn State College of Medicine
Hershey, Pennsylvania

Roy D. Brod, MD
Penn State College of Medicine
Hershey, Pennsylvania

Norman E. Byer, MD
University of California
Los Angeles

David G. Callanan, MD
University of Texas, Southwestern
Arlington

Vanessa Cruz-Villegas, MD
Bascom Palmer Eye Institute
Miami, Florida

Thomas W. Gardner, MD, MS
Penn State College of Medicine
Hershey, Pennsylvania

Justin L. Gottlieb, MD
University of Wisconsin
Madison

J. William Harbour, MD
Washington University
St. Louis, Missouri

Nancy M. Holekamp, MD
Barnes Retina Institute
St. Louis, Missouri

Michael S. Ip, MD
University of Wisconsin Hospital and Clinics
Madison

Mark W. Johnson, MD
Kellogg Eye Center
Ann Arbor, Michigan

T. Mark Johnson, MD
Bert M. Glaser National Retina Institute
Chevy Chase, Maryland

Peter J. Kertes, MD
University of Ottawa Eye Institute
Ontario, Canada

Kimberly A. Neely, MD, PhD
Penn State College of Medicine
Hershey, Pennsylvania

Timothy W. Olsen, MD
University of Minnesota
Minneapolis

Robert E. Parnes, MD
Cumberland Valley Retina Consultants
Hagerstown, Maryland

David A. Quillen, MD
Penn State College of Medicine
Hershey, Pennsylvania

Robert H. Rosa, Jr, MD
Scott and White Clinic
Temple, Texas

Philip J. Rosenfeld, MD, PhD
Bascom Palmer Eye Institute
Miami, Florida

chapter 1

Anatomy and Physiology of the Retina

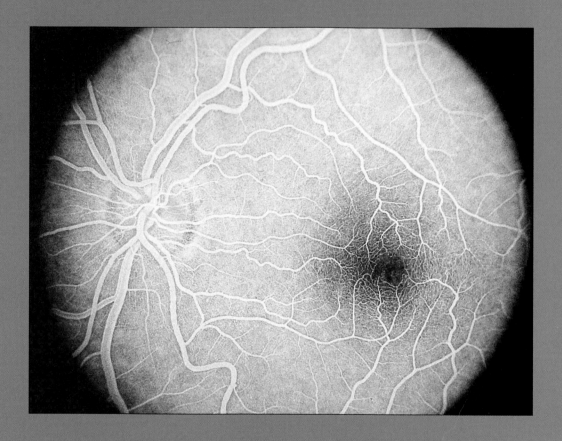

David A. Quillen, MD

Alistair J. Barber, PhD

PARS PLANA

The pars plana is the flat posterior aspect of the ciliary body, extending between the pars plicata of the ciliary body and the ora serrata of the neurosensory retina. The pars plana is located 3.5 mm from the limbus and is 3.5 to 4.5 mm in width. The pars plana consists of a double layer of epithelial cells: the inner, nonpigmented epithelium, which is contiguous with neurosensory retina; and the outer, pigmented epithelium, which is contiguous with the retinal pigment epithelium. The apices of the nonpigmented and pigmented epithelium are fused by tight junctions. The pars plana provides surgical access to the vitreous and retina.

ORA SERRATA

The ora serrata is the anterior border of the neurosensory retina. Topographically, it corresponds to the insertion of the medial and lateral rectus muscles. It has a smooth appearance temporally but is serrated nasally. Ora bays are rounded extensions of the pars plana whereas dentate processes are "teeth-like" extensions of neurosensory retina. There are approximately 20 to 30 dentate processes per eye.

VORTEX VEINS AND CILIARY NERVES

The vortex veins and ciliary nerves are found in the equatorial region of the globe. There is usually one vortex vein per quadrant located between the recti muscles. Vortex veins drain into the superior and inferior ophthalmic veins.

There are two long posterior ciliary nerves and 10 to 20 short posterior ciliary nerves. The ciliary nerves travel in the suprachoroidal space. The two long posterior ciliary nerves are located medially and temporally and carry autonomic fibers to the iris and ciliary body to regulate the pupil size and aqueous humor production, respectively. The short posterior ciliary nerves carry sympathetic nerve fibers that regulate choroidal blood flow.

MACULA

The macula is recognized clinically as the region within the temporal vascular arcades. Histologically, the macula is defined as having the following: two or more layers of ganglion cell nuclei; the presence of xanthophyll pigment; and taller, more pigmented retinal pigment epithelial cells.

FOVEA, FOVEOLA, AND UMBO

The fovea is a 1500-μm area (roughly the size of the optic disc) located slightly inferior and temporal to the optic disc. It has a concave surface due to displacement of the inner retinal layers including the nerve fiber layer, ganglion cell layer, inner plexiform layer, and inner nuclear layer. The central 500 μm of the fovea is devoid of blood vessels (foveal avascular zone [FAZ]). Within the fovea there is a central depression called the *foveola*. The foveola contains only specialized cones and Müller cells. The center of the foveola is known as the *umbo*.

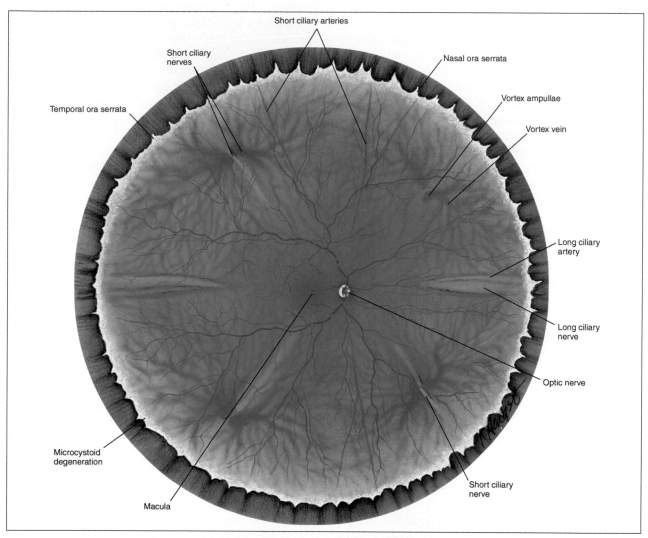

Overview of the anatomy of the pars plana, ora serrata, vortex veins, ciliary nerves, and macula.

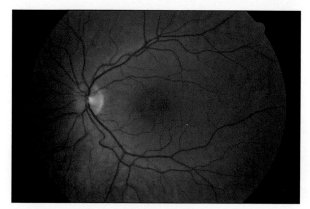

The clinical macula is the region within the temporal vascular arcades. Histologically, the macula is characterized by multiple ganglion cell nuclei, xanthophyll pigment, and taller, more pigmented retinal pigment epithelium.

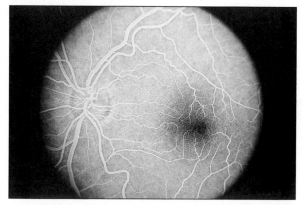

The foveal avascular zone is the central 500-μm area of the fovea devoid of blood vessels. Note the relative hypofluorescence of the central macula.

NEUROSENSORY RETINA

The neurosensory retina is derived from neuroectoderm. The nine layers of the neurosensory retina include the internal limiting membrane (ILM), nerve fiber layer (NFL), ganglion cell layer (GCL), inner plexiform layer (IPL), inner nuclear layer (INL), outer plexiform layer (OPL), outer nuclear layer (ONL), external limiting membrane (OLM), and photoreceptors.

The neurosensory retina includes three types of cells: neurons, glial cells, and vascular cells. The neurons include the photoreceptors, bipolar cells, and ganglion cells for vertical integration of electrical signals from light stimulation. Horizontal and amacrine cells provide horizontal integration and coordination between the other neurons. Glial cells—consisting of Müller cells, astrocytes, and microglia—provide metabolic support for blood vessels and neurons. They play a major role in regulation of the extracellular environment of the retina. Müller cells traverse the entire retinal thickness and contribute to the internal and external limiting membranes. Astrocytes invest blood vessels and neurons in the ganglion cell layer and microglia act as resident macrophages within the retina. The vascular cells include the retinal vascular endothelial cells.

PHOTORECEPTORS

The photoreceptors are specialized neuroepithelial cells derived from neuroectoderm. The two types of photoreceptors are rods and cones. There are approximately 100 million rods and 5 million cones (rod to cone ratio equals 20:1). Rods mediate dim-light vision and have great sensitivity. Cones function in bright light and are responsible for color vision and pattern recognition. Cone *density* is maximal in the fovea and decreases across the macula and peripheral retina. Conversely, rod density is greater in the peripheral retina and decreases in the macula. It is important to note that although the cone *density* is greatest in the fovea, the macula is still rod dominated due to the high ratio of rods to cones.

The inner segments of the photoreceptors contain metabolic machinery whereas the outer segments contain visual pigment. Light energy is converted into electrical signals in the outer segments. In cones, the outer segment discs are attached to the cell membrane. In rods, the outer segment discs are arranged like a "stack of coins" with no attachment to the cell membrane.

RETINAL PIGMENT EPITHELIUM

The retinal pigment epithelium (RPE) consists of a monolayer of cuboidal-shaped cells derived from neuroectoderm. The RPE extends from the margin of the optic disc to the ora serrata where it is contiguous with the pigmented epithelium of pars plana. The RPE has several features: tight junctional complexes including zonula occludens and zonula adherens; apical microvilli; basement membrane infoldings; melanin granules; and phagosomes. The functions of the RPE include the outer blood-retinal barrier; promotion of retinal adhesion; synthesis of extracellular matrix; degradation of photoreceptor outer segments; retinol uptake and transport; absorption of scattered light; supporting the nutritional requirements of outer retina; and response to disease (atrophy, hyperplasia).

RETINAL BLOOD FLOW

Blood travels from the internal carotid artery through the ophthalmic artery before reaching the central retinal artery. Blood traveling through the central retinal artery and its branches supplies oxygen and nutrition to the inner retinal layers from the nerve fiber layer to the inner third of the inner nuclear layer. The retinal vessels lack internal elastic lamina and smooth muscle cells. The retinal vascular endothelial cells are nonfenestrated and contain tight junctions. Pericytes surround the endothelial cells and contribute to the inner blood-retinal barrier. Cilioretinal arteries derived from the ciliary circulation are present in approximately 20% of individuals.

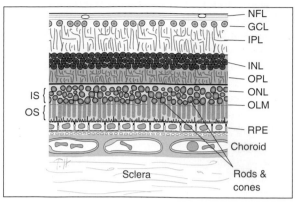

Schematic drawing of the nine layers of the neurosensory retina, retinal pigment epithelium, Bruch's membrane, choroid, and sclera.

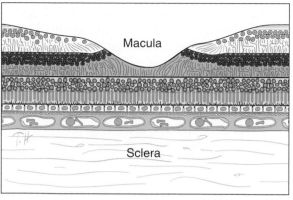

Schematic drawing of the fovea. The normal foveal depression results from displacement of the inner retinal layers including the nerve fiber layer, ganglion cell layer, inner plexiform layer, and inner nuclear layers.

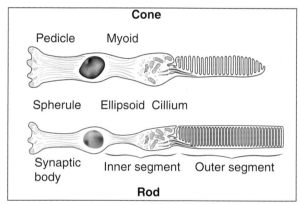

The ratio of rods to cones is 20:1. In cones, the outer segment discs are attached to the cell membrane whereas in rods the discs are arranged like a "stack of coins."

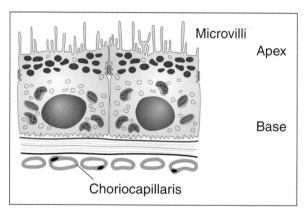

The retinal pigment epithelium is a monolayer of cuboidal-shaped cells derived from neuroectoderm.

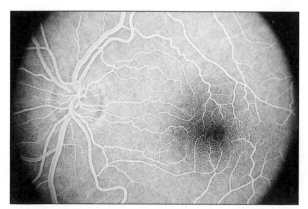

The retinal vascular endothelial cells are nonfenestrated with tight junctions. This forms the inner blood-retinal barrier. Note that fluorescein does not leak from normal retinal vessels.

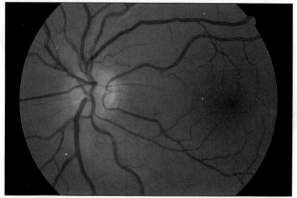

Approximately 20% of individuals have a cilioretinal artery. Cilioretinal arteries arise from the ciliary circulation and supply various portions of the peripapillary retina and macula.

BRUCH'S MEMBRANE

Bruch's membrane is a five-layer structure that consists of the following: the basement membrane of the retinal pigment epithelium, an inner collagenous zone, a middle elastic layer, an outer collagenous zone, and the basement membrane of the choriocapillaris.

CHOROID

The choroid is the posterior portion of the uveal tract; it extends from the ora serrata to the optic disc. The choroid is derived from mesoderm and neuroectoderm. The choroid contains one of the highest rates of blood flow in the body and provides blood supply to the retinal pigment epithelium (RPE) and outer retina (to the outer two thirds of the inner nuclear layer). It also is responsible for the dissipation of heat and is largely responsible for the pigmentation/coloration of the fundus.

Blood reaching the choroid travels through the internal carotid artery to the ophthalmic artery and then flows through branches of the ciliary arteries, which include the medial and lateral posterior ciliary arteries, long and short posterior ciliary arteries, and the recurrent branches of the anterior ciliary arteries. The blood then travels through the large and medium-sized choroidal vessels before reaching the choriocapillaris. Venous drainage from the choriocapillaris is mainly through the vortex veins located in the equatorial region of the globe.

The choriocapillaris is the rich capillary layer of the choroid. In the posterior fundus, the choriocapillaris is arranged in a mosaic of lobules with a central precapillary arteriole and peripheral postcapillary venules. The choriocapillaris contains fenestrated capillary walls.

VITREOUS

The vitreous is a gel-like structure derived from neuroectoderm. It occupies approximately four fifths of the volume of the globe. Although the vitreous is composed of 99% water, it has a viscosity two times that of water due to the presence of hyaluronic acid. In addition, the vitreous contains hyalocytes and type II collagen.

The vitreous base is a 6-mm area that straddles the ora serrata. The vitreous base contains the greatest concentration of collagen. Collagen fibrils attach in a perpendicular fashion to the basement membrane of the nonpigmented epithelium of the pars plana and the internal limiting membrane of the retina. In addition to the vitreous base, the vitreous has attachments at the optic disc, along the retinal vessels, and in the fovea/parafovea area.

NORMAL RETINAL ADHESION

There is a potential space between the neurosensory retina and the RPE. This is the result of the embryologic development of the eye. During the early stages of ocular development, the optic vesicle folds in on itself, becoming the optic cup. The two tissue layers of the optic cup eventually become the outer pigment epithelial layer and the inner neurosensory retinal layer.

The normal retinal adherence is maintained by several factors including the blood retinal barrier, the metabolic activity of RPE and photoreceptors, retinal and choroidal oxygenation, the mechanical interdigitation of RPE microvilli and photoreceptor outer segments, the interphotoreceptor matrix, various hydrostatic and osmotic forces, and possibly retinal tamponade of vitreous.

BLOOD-RETINAL BARRIER

The blood-retinal barrier has two components: the inner and outer blood-retinal barriers. The inner blood-retinal barrier is composed of tight junctions between the retinal vascular endothelial cells. The outer blood-retinal barrier is the result of tight junctions between retinal pigment epithelial cells. Both the inner and outer blood-retinal barriers contribute to the normal retinal homeostasis by restricting various permeabilities from the plasma. The blood-retinal barriers may be disrupted by a variety of conditions including ischemia and inflammation.

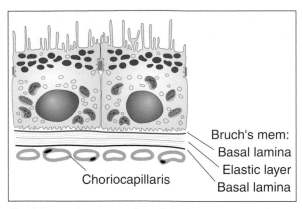

Bruch's membrane consists of the basement membrane of the retinal pigment epithelium, an inner collagenous zone, a middle elastic layer, an outer collagenous zone, and the basement membrane of the choriocapillaris.

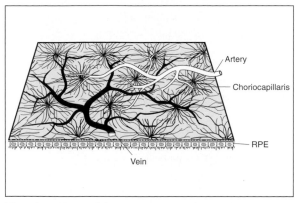

The choroid is a rich vascular network supplying oxygen and nutrition to the retinal pigment epithelium and outer retina. It is arranged in a lobular pattern.

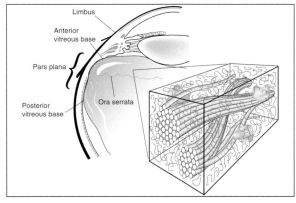

The vitreous is composed of water, hyaluronic acid, hyalocytes, and type II collagen.

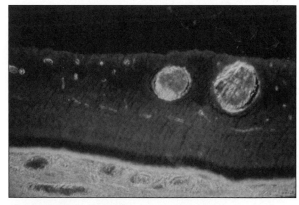

The inner and outer blood retinal barriers are demonstrated in this photomicrograph. The fluorescein is retained within the retinal vessels by the endothelial cell tight junctions and the choriocapillaris by the retinal pigment epithelium. (Reprinted with permission from Elsevier Science. [Eagle RC Jr. Mechanisms of maculopathy. Ophthalmology. 1984;91:613–625].)

PHYSIOLOGY OF THE RETINA

Phototransduction, the conversion of light energy into an electrical signal, occurs as a cascade in three stages: pigment activation, cyclic guanosine monophosphate (cGMP) detection, and hyperpolarization.

The photoreceptor outer segments contain the light-sensitive pigment rhodopsin. Rhodopsin is composed of two parts: a protein called opsin and a molecule of vitamin A aldehyde (retinal). In the dark, the retinal takes the form of 11-cis-retinaldehyde, which is a bent molecule. A photon of light interacts with the 11-cis-retinaldehyde, causing it to rotate about the 11th carbon atom to become all-trans-retinaldehyde. This molecule is straight. This isomeric change in the retinal atom causes a conformational change in the opsin part of the protein, which surrounds the retinal molecule.

Once light causes the change in confirmation of rhodopsin, which is a large membrane-spanning protein, there is a change in the structure and density of the plasma membrane surrounding the protein. This gives rise to stimulation of a g-protein called transducin. Activation of the pigment molecule leads to a reduction in the plasma concentration of the second messenger molecule, cGMP. The g-protein, transducin, stimulates cGMP phopshodiesterase, which in turn converts cGMP to 5'-GMP. Thus the concentration of cGMP in the cytoplasm is dramatically reduced by light.

The outer segment of the photoreceptor has many sodium channels that are gated by cGMP. The Na^+ channels are kept open by high concentrations of cGMP and are therefore open in the dark. When light causes transducin to stimulate conversion of cGMP to 5'-GMP, these Na^+ channels are forced to close.

In the dark Na^+ ions are allowed to move into the outer segment of the photoreceptor through many cGMP-gated sodium channels. This current is balanced by active transport of the Na^+/K^+-ATPase pump in the inner segment of the photoreceptor. Thus, in the dark there is an ion current (called the dark current) of Na^+ ions from the outer to the inner segment of the photoreceptor that is actively driven by the Na^+/K^+-ATPase pump in the inner segment and is passively permitted by cGMP-gated Na^+ channels in the outer segment of the photoreceptor. This current causes a continual depolarization of the plasma membrane at the synaptic terminal part of the photoreceptor, leading to release of neurotransmitters.

In summary, light causes reduction of the concentration of cGMP in the outer segment of the photoreceptor, which in turn closes the sodium channels. Light stops the dark current, which causes the photoreceptor to hyperpolarize (all photoreceptors respond to light with a hyperpolarization). This in turn prevents release of neurotransmitters from the synaptic terminal. It is important to remember that the photoreceptor normally releases neurotransmitter in the dark, when it is not stimulated, and is stopped from releasing neurotransmitter when light stimulates the photoreceptor.

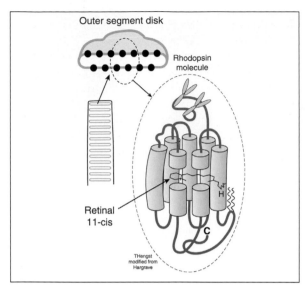

The photoreceptor outer segments contain the light-sensitive pigment rhodopsin. Rhodopsin is composed of two parts: a protein called opsin and a molecule of vitamin A aldehyde (retinal).

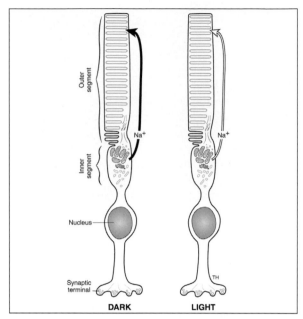

The dark current, mediated by Na⁺ ions, flows from the inner segment to the outer segment of the photoreceptor. In the dark, the current flux is highest. The dark sodium current maintains the receptor in a depolarized state. Under the influence of light, the sodium current decreases and the photoreceptor membrane hyperpolarizes.

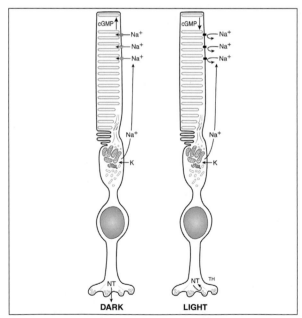

The outer segment of the photoreceptor has many sodium channels that are gated by cGMP. In the dark, the high levels of cGMP keep the sodium channels open. This allows for passive inflow of Na⁺ ions into the outer segment. This current is balanced by active transport of the Na⁺/K⁺-ATPase pump in the inner segment of the photoreceptor. In this depolarized state, neurotransmitter is released from the synaptic terminal. Light causes reduction of the concentration of cGMP, which in turn closes the sodium channels. This causes the photoreceptor to hyperpolarize and decrease neurotransmitter release.

CLINICAL CORRELATION: RETINA

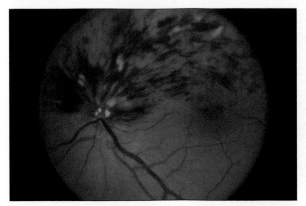

Acute branch retinal vein occlusion with flame-shaped retinal hemorrhages and cotton wool spots involving the nerve fiber layer.

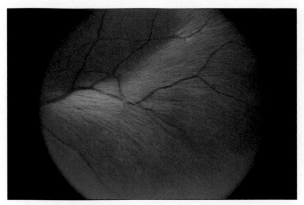

Myelinated nerve fiber layer. Note the arcuate pattern of the nerve fiber layer around the macula. The larger retinal vessels are located within the nerve fiber layer.

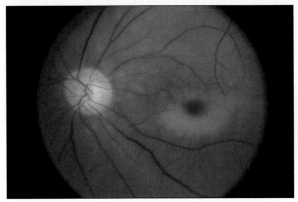

Cherry red spot following a central retinal artery occlusion. The ischemic retinal whitening occurs in the inner retina of the macula where the ganglion cell and nerve fiber layers are thickest. The central red spot is a result of the normal choroidal circulation.

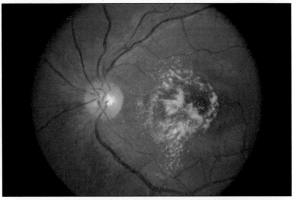

Lipid exudate in the macula following malignant hypertension. The lipid may form a star-pattern within the middle layers of the retina as it radiates from the center of the macula.

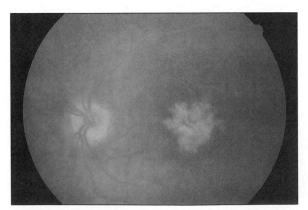

Cystoid macular edema following cataract surgery. The cyst-like spaces form in the outer plexiform layer of the retina (Henle's layer). Fluorescein angiography reveals a classic "petaloid" pattern of hyperfluorescence.

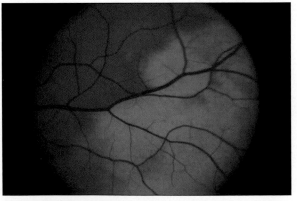

Commotio retinae following a blunt trauma injury. The deep retinal whitening results from shearing of the outer segments of the photoreceptors. Note the normal retinal blood vessels overlying the retinal whitening.

CLINICAL CORRELATION: RETINAL PIGMENT EPITHELIUM

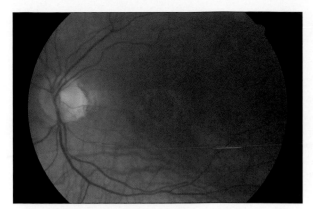

Bull's eye maculopathy in chloroquine toxicity. The hypopigmented region around the center of the fovea results from atrophy of the retinal pigment epithelium.

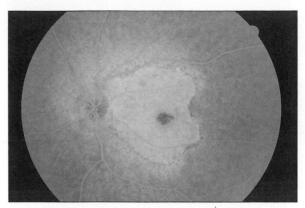

Transmission or "window" defect in age-related macular degeneration with geographic atrophy. Atrophy of the retinal pigment epithelium "unmasks" the underlying choroidal fluorescence.

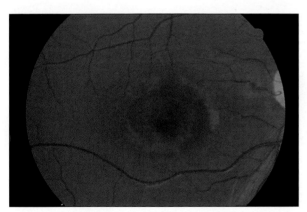

Stargardt disease is characterized by abnormalities of the retinal pigment epithelium (RPE). Lipofuscin accumulation within the RPE results in a vermillion discoloration of the fundus. Atrophy of the RPE may result in a bull's eye maculopathy.

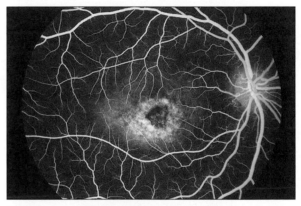

Fluorescein angiography of the same patient demonstrates a "silent choroid" as a result of blockage of the normal choroidal fluorescence. The central hyperfluorescence is a result of atrophy of the retinal pigment epithelium.

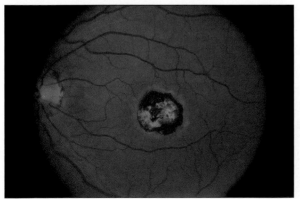

Hyperplastic retinal pigment epithelium (RPE) in a patient with presumed ocular histoplasmosis. In response to disease, the RPE may become atrophic or hyperplastic.

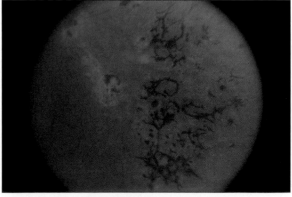

Intraretinal pigment migration in a patient with retinitis pigmentosa. The classic triad of retinitis pigmentosa includes disc pallor, vessel attenuation, and peripheral pigmentary alterations.

CLINICAL CORRELATION: BRUCH'S MEMBRANE AND CHOROID

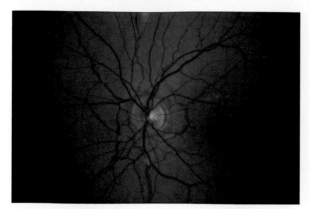

Angioid streaks in a woman with pseudoxanthoma elasticum. Angioid streaks are breaks in the RPE-Bruch's membrane complex. They are often seen radiating from the optic disc.

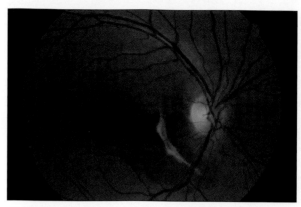

Choroidal ruptures are breaks in the RPE-Bruch's membrane complex following blunt trauma injuries to the eye. They are usually located concentric to the optic disc.

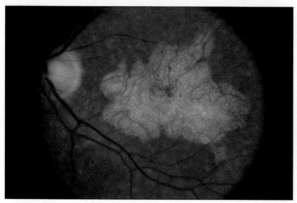

Atrophy of the retinal pigment epithelium in a patient with Stargardt disease reveals the underlying choroidal vessels.

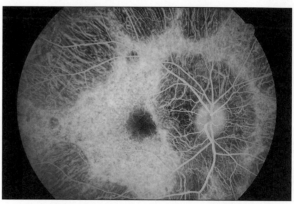

Fluorescein angiogram of a patient with choroideremia demonstrates hyperfluorescence of the choriocapillaris centrally and hypofluorescence in the areas of the retinal pigment epithelial and choriocapillaris atrophy. Note the larger choroidal vessels in the peripapillary and peripheral retina.

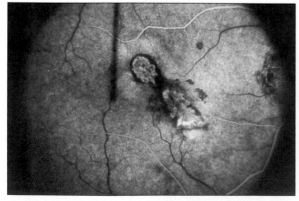

Classic choroidal neovascularization. The new vessel membrane extends from the choroid through Bruch's membrane to the sub-RPE or sub-neurosensory retinal space.

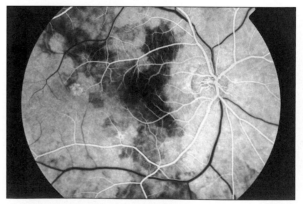

Fluorescein angiogram demonstrating choroidal nonperfusion in a patient with giant cell arteritis. This results from occlusion of the posterior ciliary arteries.

CLINICAL CORRELATION: VITREOUS, RETINAL ADHESION, AND BLOOD-RETINAL BARRIER

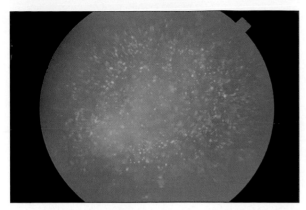

Asteroid hyalosis is characterized by numerous calcium deposits within the vitreous gel. Individuals may be asymptomatic or complain of floaters.

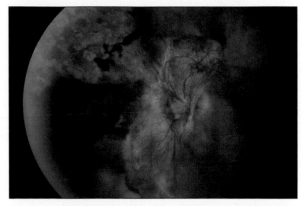

The vitreous provides a scaffold for the growth of new vessels in proliferative diabetic retinopathy. Contraction of the vitreous may cause vitreous hemorrhage or traction retinal detachment.

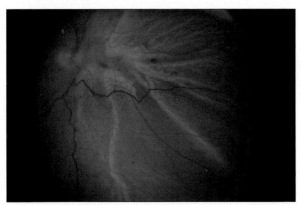

Rhegmatogenous retinal detachment results from a retinal tear or hole. The retinal tear or hole allows fluid to accumulate in the potential space between the neurosensory retina and the retinal pigment epithelium.

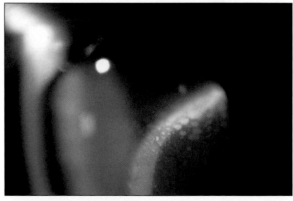

An exudative retinal detachment results from fluid accumulation between the neurosensory retina and the retinal pigment epithelium. This patient had atypical central serous choroidopathy. Note the protein deposits on the posterior surface of the neurosensory retina.

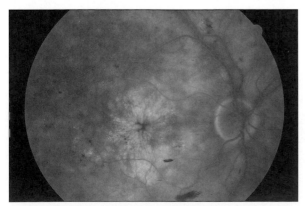

Fluorescein angiography of a patient with diabetic retinopathy demonstrates disruption of the inner blood-retinal barrier. The hyperfluorescence is the result of leakage from the retinal vessels.

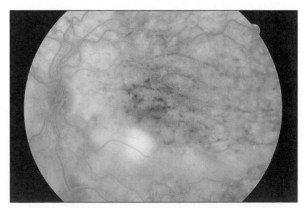

Fluorescein angiography of a patient with toxemia of pregnancy. Leakage of fluid through the retinal pigment epithelium (the outer blood-retinal barrier) results in exudative neurosensory retinal detachments.

SELECTED REFERENCES

1. Bernstein PS. Macular biology. In: Berger JW, Fine SL, Maguire MG, eds. *Age-Related Macular Degeneration.* St. Louis: Mosby, Inc; 1999:1–16.

2. Blanks JC. Morphology and topography of the retina. In: Ogden TE, Hinton DR, eds. *Retina.* 3rd ed. St. Louis: Mosby, Inc; 2001:32–53.

3. Chen J, Flannery J. Structure and function of rod photoreceptors. In: Ogden TE, Hinton DR, eds. *Retina.* 3rd ed. St. Louis: Mosby, Inc; 2001:122–137.

4. Eagle RC Jr. Mechanisms of maculopathy. *Ophthalmology.* 1984;91:613–625.

5. *Fundamentals and Principles of Ophthalmology.* San Francisco: The Foundation of the American Academy of Ophthalmology; 2001:68–95.

6. Gass JD. Muller cell cone, an overlooked part of the anatomy of the fovea centralis: hypotheses concerning its role in the pathogenesis of macular hole and foveomacular retinoschisis. *Arch Ophthalmol.* 1999;117:821–823.

7. Guyer DR, Schachat AP, Green WR. The choroid: structural considerations. In: Ogden TE, Hinton DR, eds. *Retina.* 3rd ed. St. Louis: Mosby, Inc; 2001:21–31.

8. Hargrave PA, McDowell JH. Rhodopsin and phototransduction: a model system for G protein-linked receptors. *FASEB J.* 1992;6:2323–2331.

9. Harris A, Bingaman DP, Ciulla TA, Martin BJ. Retinal and choroidal blood flow in health and disease. In: Ogden TE, Hinton DR, eds. *Retina.* 3rd ed. St. Louis: Mosby, Inc; 2001:68–88.

10. Kandel ER, Schwartz JH, Jessell TM, eds. *Principles of Neural Science.* 4th ed. New York: McGraw-Hill; 2000:507–515.

11. Lagnado L, Baylor D. Signal flow in visual transduction. *Neuron.* 1992;8:995–1002.

12. O'Brien DF. The chemistry of vision. *Science.* 1982;218:961–966.

13. Stryer L. The molecules of visual excitation. *Sci Am.* 1987;257:42–50.

14. Thumann G, Hinton DR. Cell biology of the retinal pigment epithelium. In: Ogden TE, Hinton DR, eds. *Retina.* 3rd ed. St. Louis: Mosby, Inc; 2001:104–121.

chapter 2

Ancillary Testing for Retinal and Choroidal Diseases

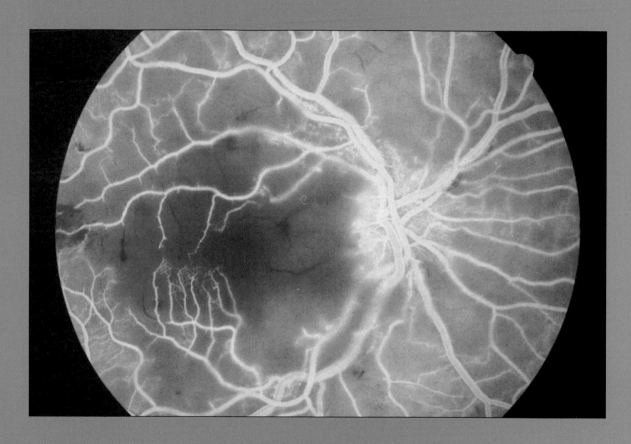

Michael S. Ip, MD

FLUORESCEIN ANGIOGRAPHY

Since fluorescein angiography (FA) was introduced in the early 1960s, it has become one of the most widely used ancillary tests to image the retina. Although direct examination of the retina with slit lamp biomicroscopy and indirect ophthalmoscopy remains indispensable in the diagnosis and management of retinal disease, FA provides additional information concerning the anatomy, physiology, and pathology of the retina and, to a lesser extent, the choroid.

Sodium fluorescein is orange-red in color, with an absorption peak between 465 and 490 nm and an emission peak between 520 and 530 nm. In the intravascular space, sodium fluorescein is 70% to 80% bound to plasma protein.

Clinical Features

Fluorescein angiography provides clinically useful information for nearly the entire spectrum of posterior segment disorders. The diagnosis and treatment of retinal vascular disease, conditions resulting in choroidal neovascularization, inherited retinal disorders, retinal changes as a result of systemic disease processes, inflammatory ocular disease, and some intraocular tumors can often be enhanced with the use of FA. In some instances, FA may be performed to provide baseline images if it is thought that the condition may progress or change over time.

Technique

Fluorescein angiography is performed by injecting sodium fluorescein dye as a bolus into a peripheral vein. Sodium fluorescein dye is available as 5 mL of 10% concentration.

Following injection, the dye enters the choroidal and retinal circulations, and a fundus camera is used to document passage of the fluorescein dye. This process is made possible by illuminating the fundus with a blue light (peak absorption of fluorescein), thereby exciting sodium fluorescein molecules to a higher energy state. The sodium fluorescein molecules then return to their ground state, and in the process release a longer-wavelength yellow-green light. Only the yellow-green light is detected by the photographic film.

Photographic images of both the fellow eye and the eye being evaluated are obtained with the majority of early-phase images taken of the eye under evaluation.

Stereoscopic pairs of photographs are taken to facilitate evaluation of the angiogram. The time elapsed from injection to initial vascular filling, as well as the time elapsed from injection to each photograph taken subsequently, is recorded. The images taken during FA can be either recorded on photographic film or stored electronically.

Side Effects

Adverse effects from FA are generally mild. These include a temporary yellowing of the skin and a yellow-orange color to the urine. Other side effects include nausea, vomiting, pruritus, urticaria, syncope, and local reaction due to extravasation of the dye from the injection site. Reactions that are possibly allergic in nature may be managed with antihistamines, but affected patients should be watched carefully for the development of anaphylaxis. Severe reactions such as bronchospasm, laryngeal edema, and myocardial infarction are infrequent but have been reported. The overall risk of death from FA has been estimated to be 1 in 222 000.

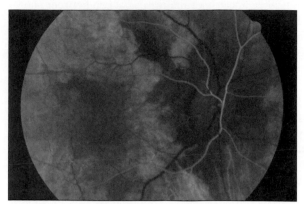

Arterial phase: One to 3 seconds after fluorescein reaches the choroid (the prearterial phase), fluorescein is noted in the retinal arteries. The normal time from injection to arterial filling is approximately 12 seconds. (Note the patchy choroidal filling.)

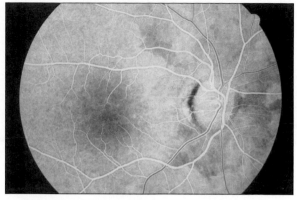

Arteriovenous phase: After filling the retinal arteries, fluorescein dye flows through the precapillary arterioles, capillaries, postcapillary venules, and then to the retinal veins. In the early arteriovenous phase, thin columns of dye are noted along the walls of the larger veins (laminar flow).

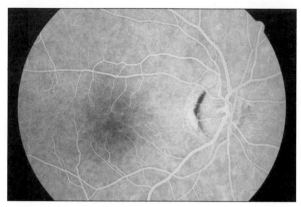

Peak venous phase: Five to 10 seconds after the entire lumen of the veins fill, the peak phase is entered. This typically occurs 20 to 25 seconds after injection, when there is maximal concentration of dye in the retina and choroid.

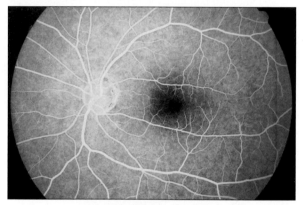

Peak venous phase: The perifoveal capillary network is best visualized in this phase. The foveal avascular zone is the central 400-mm area devoid of blood vessels.

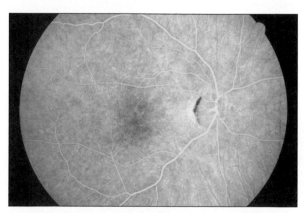

Recirculation phase: Thirty seconds after injection, some of the dye has returned to the heart, and the concentration of dye in the retina begins to fade.

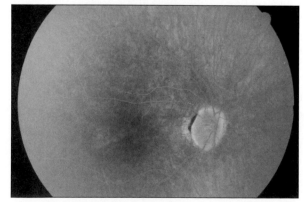

Late phase: Ten minutes after injection, fluorescein dye is generally not present in either the retinal or choroidal circulation, and only faint staining of various structures is noted.

FLUORESCEIN ANGIOGRAPHY: HYPERFLUORESCENCE

Hyperfluorescence may be defined as an increase in normal fluorescence or an abnormal presence of fluorescein at a given time in the fluorescein angiogram.

Pseudofluorescence may be caused by an overlap of the wavelength of light allowed to pass through the exciter and barrier filters. Autofluorescence may be caused by refractile structures in the eye such as optic nerve head drusen, astrocytic hamartomas, large drusen of the retinal pigment epithelium (RPE), and deposits of lipofuscin seen in some macular dystrophies.

Hyperfluorescence in the fluorescein angiogram may be caused by leakage, staining, or pooling of dye and by transmission or "window" defects. Leakage refers to hyperfluorescence in the angiogram due to extravasation of fluorescein dye into the extravascular space resulting from disruption of retinal endothelial tight junctions. Leakage due to loss of retinal endothelial tight junctions may be seen in diabetic macular edema, cystoid macular edema, and venous occlusive diseases. Leakage may appear as areas of hyperfluorescence that increase in size as the angiogram progresses. Retinal neovascularization from proliferative diabetic retinopathy or other causes may result in leakage of fluorescein into the vitreous. This leakage appears as fluffy, hazy hyperfluorescence that is localized over the pathologic area, above the plane of the retina. This type of leakage is typically best viewed in the late phases of the angiogram.

Leakage may also result from the breakdown of the tight junctions between retinal pigment epithelial cells, such as in central serous chorioretinopathy. Subretinal neovascularization, regardless of cause, will also result in leakage, as the new vessels lack tight junctions. Leakage due to subretinal neovascularization is best viewed by assessing both the early and late phases of the fluorescein angiogram. The early phases show irregularly shaped, flat, or sometimes elevated areas of hyperfluorescence that may leak profusely into the subretinal or subpigment epithelial space in the late phases. A lacy pattern to the abnormal subretinal vessels sometimes can be seen on the early-phase angiogram.

Hyperfluorescence due to pooling occurs as a result of dye accumulation within an anatomic or potential space. The increased concentration of fluorescein dye in the area of pooling results in the development of hyperfluorescence. Fluorescein may pool into either the subretinal space or the space created when the RPE separates from Bruch's membrane. When the retina separates from the RPE, a gradual angle is formed where the retina remains attached to the RPE. This feature makes it difficult to determine the extent of retinal detachment both ophthalmoscopically and on the angiogram. Conversely, in the case of a retinal pigment epithelial detachment, the angle between attached and detached RPE is wide because of the firm adhesion between the RPE and Bruch's membrane. This feature allows hyperfluorescent pooling due to retinal pigment epithelial detachments to have clearly discernable borders on the fluorescein angiogram.

Hyperfluorescence due to pooling beneath the RPE may be seen in serous retinal pigment epithelial detachments due to age-related macular degeneration or central serous retinopathy. Hyperfluorescence due to pooling in the subretinal space may be seen in Vogt-Koyanagi-Harada disease, in which pooling of dye occurs as a result of exudative retinal detachment.

Hyperfluorescence may also be due to staining, which represents an accumulation of fluorescein into tissues. Disciform scars from age-related macular degeneration, some large drusen, and damaged RPE may stain. Scleral staining may occur when loss of the RPE and choroid is total, such as in a chorioretinal scar. In this situation, dye leakage from the choroid surrounding the scar stains the sclera in the late phases of the angiogram; typically, no staining is seen in the early phases.

A focal loss of the RPE or decrease in pigment in the RPE can result in a window defect, another type of hyperfluorescence commonly seen on fluorescein angiography. The hyperfluorescence typically appears early in the fluorescein angiogram, at the time of choroidal filling. The brightness of the window defect varies with the brightness of the underlying choroid: window defects are brightest during the early phases of the angiogram and gradually fade. As leakage is not present with window defects, the configuration and area of hyperfluorescence does not change throughout the angiogram. Window defects may be seen in atrophic age-related macular degeneration, in certain toxicities, and occasionally with full-thickness macular holes.

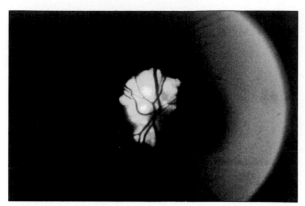

Autofluorescence in a patient with prominent optic disc drusen. Autofluorescence also has been described with astrocytic hamartomas and in some types of macular drusen.

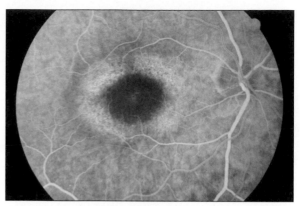

Transmission or "window" defect seen in a fluorescein angiogram of a patient with a bull's eye pattern of macular atrophy resulting from chloroquine toxicity. Loss of the retinal pigment epithelium allows transmission of the underlying choroidal fluorescence.

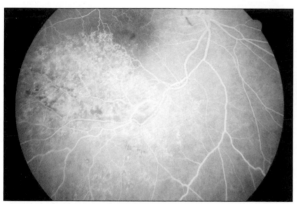

An early-phase angiogram of a patient with a branch retinal vein occlusion. There are irregularities of the retinal vessels in the inferotemporal region of the macula.

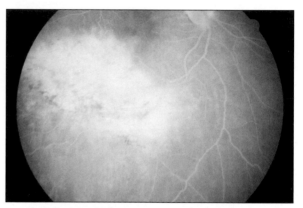

This later-phase angiogram of the same patient demonstrates leakage of dye from the irregular retinal vessels.

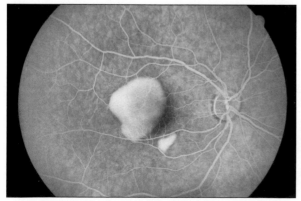

Hyperfluorescence of a serous pigment epithelial detachment. Fluorescein dye accumulates, or pools, in the sub-retinal pigment epithelial space. The presence of a focal hot spot, notch, or irregular filling pattern suggests associated choroidal neovascularization.

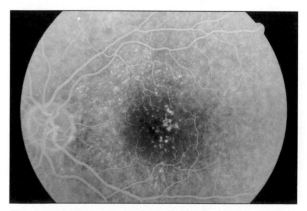

This late-phase angiogram demonstrates staining of drusen. Hyperfluorescence is observed as fluorescein accumulates within the drusen material. Atrophy of the overlying retinal pigment epithelium may contribute as well to the hyperfluorescence seen with drusen.

FLUORESCEIN ANGIOGRAPHY: HYPERFLUORESCENCE (CONT'D)

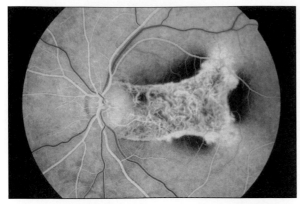

An unusual pattern of atrophy in a young man with a family history of neurofibromatosis. Atrophy of the retinal pigment epithelium allows transmission of hyperfluorescence from the underlying choroidal vessels.

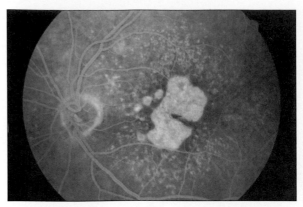

Transmission or "window" defect is seen in age-related macular degeneration with geographic atrophy of the retinal pigment epithelium.

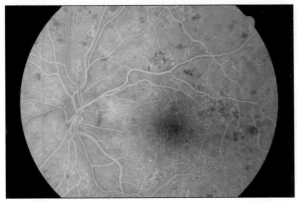

This is an early arteriovenous phase angiogram of a patient with diabetic retinopathy. The small hyperfluorescent spots throughout the macula are microaneurysms.

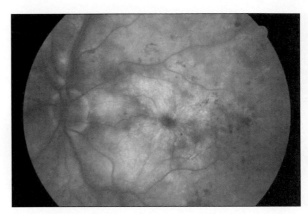

Late-phase angiogram of the same patient demonstrates diffuse leakage of fluorescein dye.

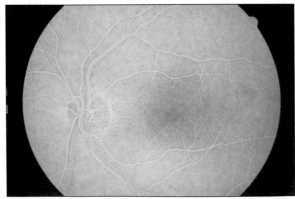

This is an early arteriovenous phase angiogram of a patient with visual loss 6 weeks after uncomplicated cataract surgery. The parafoveal capillaries demonstrate mild irregularities.

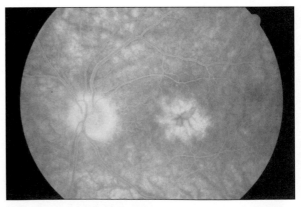

Late-phase angiogram of the same patient reveals the characteristic "petaloid" pattern of hyperfluorescence that occurs with cystoid macular edema.

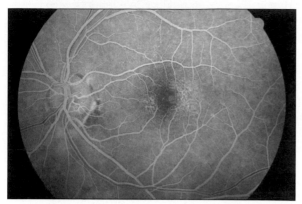

This is an early arteriovenous phase angiogram in a patient with idiopathic juxtafoveal retinal telangiectasis. The nasal and temporal parafoveal capillary networks are telangiectatic.

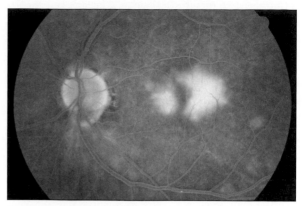

Late-phase angiogram of the same patient demonstrates hyperfluorescence produced by leakage from the irregular retinal capillary beds.

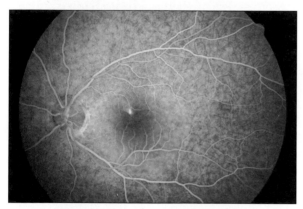

Central serous chorioretinopathy is characterized by a hyperfluorescent spot located superonasal to the center of the fovea.

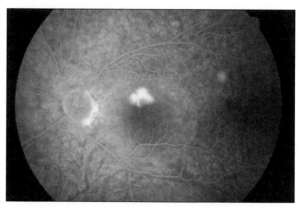

Late-phase angiogram of the same patient demonstrates the classic "smokestack" appearance of hyperfluorescence as a result of fluorescein leakage from the choroid through the RPE subretinal space.

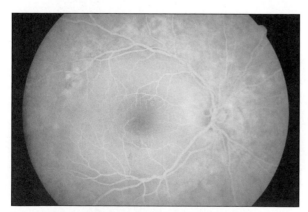

Toxemia of pregnancy is characterized by serous exudative retinal detachments resulting from hypertensive choroidopathy.

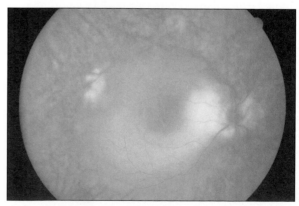

Late-phase fluorescein angiogram of the same patient reveals leakage of fluorescein dye into the subretinal space.

FLUORESCEIN ANGIOGRAPHY: HYPOFLUORESCENCE

Hypofluorescence may be defined as a lack of fluorescence at any given time in the fluorescein angiogram. Hypofluorescence may be the result of either blocked fluorescence or reduced perfusion. Correlation with the clinical examination can often help differentiate the cause. If the area of hypofluorescence seen on the fluorescein angiogram is similar in shape and size to an ophthalmoscopically visible abnormality, such as hemorrhage or pigment, then blocked fluorescence is likely present. Alternatively, if no such material is present ophthalmoscopically, the hypofluorescence is likely due to hypoperfusion.

Hypofluorescence produced by blocked fluorescence results from a condition that reduces the normal retinal and/or choroidal fluorescence. An example of blocked fluorescence is the dark macular region in the normal angiogram that anatomically represents the higher density of melanin in the retinal pigment epithelium of the macula. Blocked fluorescence may also be caused by opacities in the vitreous cavity, preretinal hemorrhage, intraretinal hemorrhage, subretinal hemorrhage, cotton wool spots, dense hard exudates, choroidal nevi or melanoma, retinal pigment epithelial hypertrophy, and a variety of other retinal disorders.

Angiographic characteristics of blocked fluorescence may help localize the pathologic condition to a particular anatomic level. Large retinal vessels and precapillary arterioles are located in the inner retina, at the level of the nerve fiber layer. Capillaries and postcapillary venules are located in the vicinity of the inner nuclear layer, deeper in the retina. Therefore, a blocking abnormality located anterior to the nerve fiber layer will preclude fluorescence from both the inner and outer layers of the retina as well as from the choroidal circulation. Preretinal hemorrhage is an example of this type of blocked fluorescence. A blocking abnormality such as an intraretinal hemorrhage that occurs deep to the nerve fiber layer but anterior to the inner nuclear layer, where the smaller retinal vessels are located, will block fluorescence from the smaller retinal vessels and choroid but not from the larger retinal vessels. Flame-shaped hemorrhages in the nerve fiber layer block underlying fluorescence from the small retinal vessels and choroid but are often not dense enough to completely block fluorescence from the larger retinal vessels. An abnormality in the outer retina or subretinal space can eliminate or reduce choroidal fluorescence, but allow retinal fluorescence to be fully visible. Hemorrhage, pigment, turbid fluid, or dense hard exudate that is located in the deep retina or subretinal space may result in blocked choroidal fluorescence.

Hypoperfusion can produce hypofluorescence as a result of a decrease or absence of retinal and/or choroidal blood flow. Hypofluorescence produced by the absence or decrease of retinal vessels may be readily identified by fluorescein angiography, as these vessels are normally prominent and easily visible. Hypofluorescence may be identified as choroidal in origin when it occurs in the presence of a normal retinal filling pattern. Stereoscopic fluorescein angiography is useful in spatially separating the plane of the retina from the choroid to determine the anatomic location of the hypofluorescence.

Common causes of retinal hypoperfusion include central and branch retinal arterial occlusions and ischemic disease due to diabetes and other causes. Choroidal hypoperfusion may be produced by ophthalmic artery occlusion, giant cell arteritis, hypertensive choroidopathy, lupus choroidopathy, and a variety of other disorders. Patchy choroidal fluorescence is a form of choroidal hypoperfusion that occurs as a normal physiologic condition in some individuals. This phenomenon is the result of the lobular nature of the choriocapillaris. The prechoriocapillaris arterioles are end-arterioles that terminate in a choriocapillaris lobule without anastomoses to adjacent arterioles or lobules. Each lobule fluoresces in an irregular, sometimes hexagonal patch. Some patches fill later than others, resulting in focal areas of patchy choroidal hypofluorescence. These hypofluorescent patches fill normally 2 to 5 seconds later. Defects due to hypoperfusion are best noted in the early phases of the angiogram, as adjacent perfused choroidal vessels leak dye into the area of hypoperfusion in the late phases.

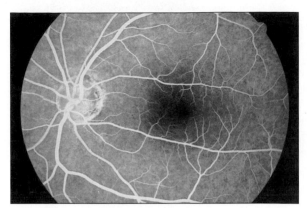

Normal hypofluorescence of the macula results from several factors including the presence of xanthophyll pigment, the foveal avascular zone, and taller, more pigmented retinal pigment epithelial cells.

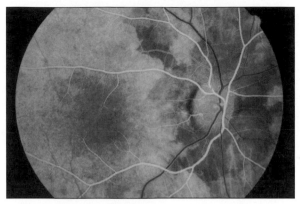

Normal hypofluorescence may occur as patchy filling of the choroid. This early hypofluorescence is observed commonly in the early phase of fluorescein angiography, and normalizes in the later phases of the angiogram.

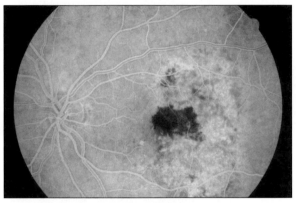

Blocked fluorescence may result from hemorrhage or melanin pigment. This angiogram of a patient with exudative age-related macular degeneration demonstrates hypofluorescence corresponding to subretinal blood.

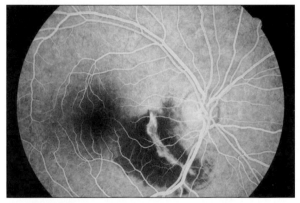

Traumatic choroidal rupture may be associated with subretinal hemorrhage. The normal retinal vessels overlying the blocked, hypofluorescent area confirm the subretinal location of the hemorrhage. The choroidal rupture is the hyperfluorescent lesion concentric to the optic disc.

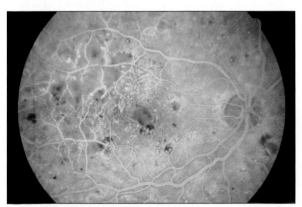

Diabetic retinopathy may be associated with capillary nonperfusion in the macula and peripheral retina. In this angiogram, the foveal avascular zone is enlarged, and the temporal macula has significant capillary dropout.

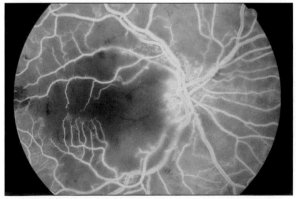

This patient with a Purtscher's-like retinopathy has marked hypofluorescence due to nonperfusion throughout the posterior fundus resulting from occlusion of the retinal capillaries.

FLUORESCEIN ANGIOGRAPHY: HYPOFLUORESCENCE (CONT'D)

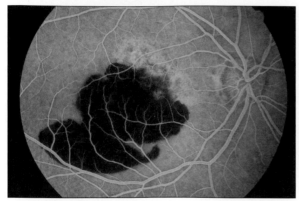

Fluorescein angiogram of a patient with age-related macular degeneration demonstrates a large blocked area of hypofluorescence corresponding to a subretinal hemorrhage. Note the retinal vessels over the area of hypofluorescence fill normally, confirming the subretinal location of the blood.

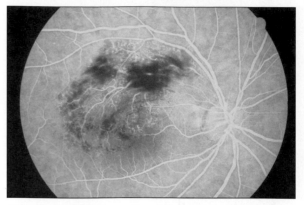

Fluorescein angiogram of a patient with a macular branch retinal vein occlusion. The superficial flame-shaped hemorrhages within the nerve fiber layer block both retinal and choroidal fluorescence.

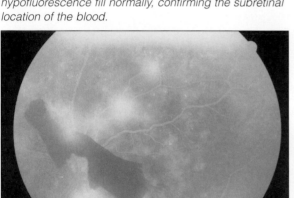

Vitreous and preretinal hemorrhage in a patient with proliferative diabetic retinopathy. Note how the preretinal hemorrhage blocks the underlying optic disc and retinal vessels.

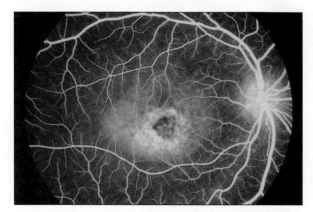

Stargardt disease is characterized by a "silent" choroid on fluorescein angiography. The lipofuscin-packed retinal pigment epithelial cells block the underlying choroidal fluorescence. The central bull's-eye pattern of hyperfluorescence results from retinal pigment epithelial atrophy.

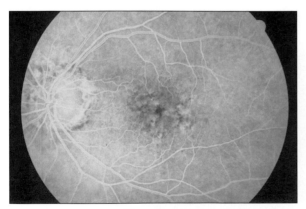

The stippled pattern of hypofluorescence in this patient with age-related macular degeneration results from blocking by focal areas of retinal pigment epithelial hyperpigmentation.

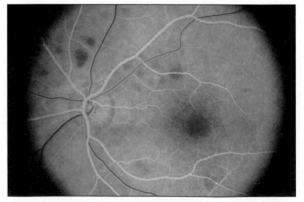

This patient has numerous hypofluorescent spots corresponding to the location of multifocal vitelliform lesions that block fluorescence in the early phases of the angiogram.

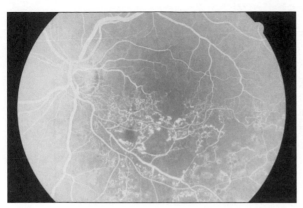

Branch retinal vein occlusions may be associated with capillary nonperfusion. Note the hypofluorescence in the fovea and inferior macula.

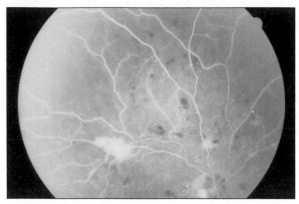

This patient with an ischemic central retinal vein occlusion demonstrates hypofluorescence resulting from intraretinal hemorrhages and profound capillary nonperfusion.

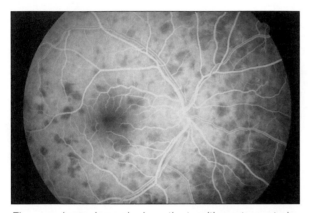

Fluorescein angiography in patients with acute posterior multifocal placoid pigment epitheliopathy is characterized by a "block early, stain late" pattern. The hypofluorescent areas seen in the early phase of the angiogram may result from choroidal nonperfusion.

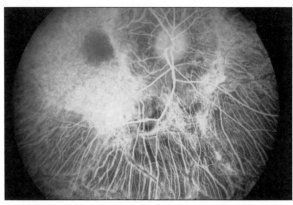

Choroideremia is characterized by loss of the retinal pigment epithelium and choriocapillaris. Loss of the choriocapillaris results in hypofluorescence due to nonperfusion. The larger choroidal vessels are visible in the areas of atrophy.

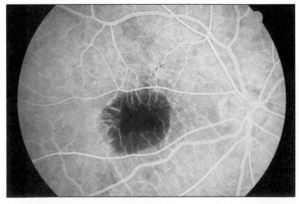

This patient has a well-defined hypofluorescent spot due to nonperfusion following laser photocoagulation for exudative age-related macular degeneration. Intense laser photocoagulation obliterates the choroidal circulation.

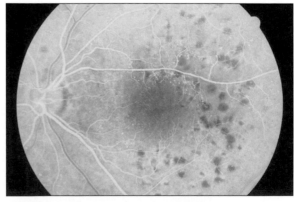

This fluorescein angiogram demonstrates hypofluorescence as a result of retinal capillary nonperfusion and laser photocoagulation. Laser burns may become hyperpigmented over time, resulting in blockage of the normal choroidal fluorescence.

INDOCYANINE GREEN ANGIOGRAPHY

Indocyanine green (ICG) is a water-soluble dye that was developed in 1955. In the 1970s ICG dye was first used to image the posterior segment of the eye. As ICG dye fluoresces too weakly to be used with conventional photographic techniques, initial results were disappointing due to poor image quality. The advent of digital video-angiography systems has improved the quality of ICG angiography, making it now a more widely employed diagnostic test.

Clinical Features

Several properties of ICG dye render it useful as an adjunct to fluorescein angiography (FA). Indocyanine green dye has a peak absorption and emission in the near infrared. These characteristics allow greater transmission of both exciting and emitting energy through hemorrhage, abnormal pigment, turbid subretinal fluid, and the retinal pigment epithelium than the visible light spectrum employed in FA. In addition, ICG dye is 98% bound to serum protein, and thus leaks slowly or not at all from the choroidal circulation, allowing choroidal vascular detail to remain clear.

These properties allow ICG dye to be potentially useful in the diagnosis and management of choroidal neovascularization due to age-related macular degeneration. Indocyanine green angiography may be useful in delineating choroidal neovascularization beneath hemorrhage, serous exudate, and abnormal pigment, allowing ICG-guided treatment of choroidal neovascular lesions that are poorly defined and thus untreatable with FA alone. However, a well-designed, randomized, controlled clinical trial to demonstrate the role of ICG angiography in the management of age-related macular degeneration has yet to be performed.

Indocyanine green angiography has also been used to study other disorders such as central serous retinopathy, inflammatory choroidal disorders, multiple evanescent white dot syndrome, Stargardt disease, and Vogt-Koyanagi-Harada syndrome. For example, in Vogt-Koyanagi-Harada syndrome and in central serous retinopathy, ICG angiography may demonstrate choroidal abnormalities not seen on FA. Indocyanine green angiography may also be useful in distinguishing between choroidal mass lesions such as choroidal melanoma and circumscribed choroidal hemangioma.

Technique

Indocyanine green angiography can be performed alone or in conjunction with FA. To perform ICG angiography, 25 to 50 mg of ICG dye is injected intravenously. The higher doses are used in cases of media opacity, small pupil, or extensive hemorrhage and/or pigment. Fundus images are then taken on a digital videoangiography system. Images are typically obtained at least 20 minutes and sometimes up to 60 minutes after intravenous administration.

Side Effects

Adverse reactions to ICG dye are less frequent than with fluorescein dye. In one large series, the rate of mild adverse reactions to ICG dye was 0.15%. The most common mild adverse reactions included nausea, vomiting, sneezing, and pruritus. Moderate adverse reactions such as syncope, pyrexia, and local tissue necrosis occur in 0.2% of patients. The overall risk of death from ICG angiography has been estimated to be 1 in 333 333.

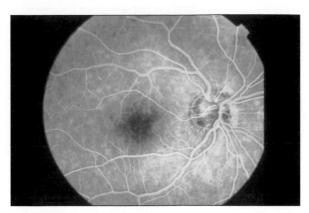

A fluorescein angiogram demonstrates areas of hyperfluorescence in this patient with multiple evanescent white dot syndrome.

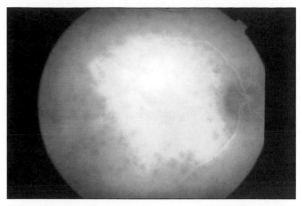

The indocyanine green angiogram may be helpful in the diagnosis of multiple evanescent white dot syndrome, as small areas of hypercyanescence are noted scattered throughout the posterior pole. These areas roughly correspond to those of hyperfluorescence noted on the fluorescein angiogram.

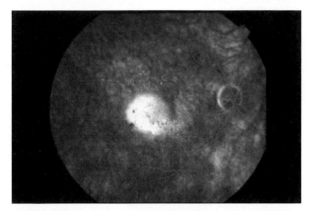

A fluorescein angiogram demonstrating a serous pigment epithelial detachment in a patient with age-related macular degeneration.

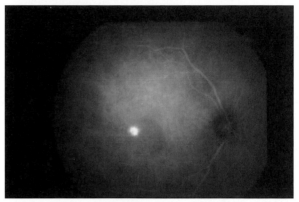

The late-phase indocyanine green angiogram of the same patient demonstrates a hot spot of hypercyanescence. Laser photocoagulation directed at the hot spot may, in some cases, hasten resolution of the serous pigment epithelial detachment.

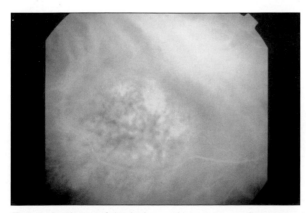

The early phase of the indocyanine green angiogram demonstrates intrinsic vascularity within a circumscribed choroidal hemangioma.

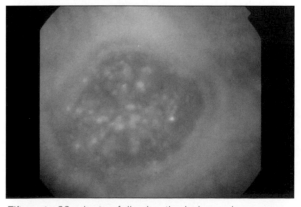

Fifteen to 30 minutes following the indocyanine green angiogram, choroidal hemangiomas may demonstrate a characteristic "wash out" appearance.

ELECTRORETINOGRAPHY

The full-field light-evoked electroretinogram (ERG), which is obtained by a brief flash of light, is the record of a diffuse electrical response generated by the retina. The full-field ERG is characterized by a negative wave-form (termed the a-wave), which represents the photo-receptor response, followed by a positive waveform (termed the b-wave), which represents the Müller and bipolar cell response. Oscillatory potentials are small wavelets on the ascending b-wave. The origin of the oscillatory potentials is unclear; loss of the oscillatory potentials is seen in diabetic retinopathy and in some individuals with congenital stationary night blindness. It is important to note that the full-field ERG is a mass response of the entire retina. The values of the amplitude of each of these main components of the ERG and how quickly they reach their peak (termed implicit time) may help in the evaluation of certain retinal disorders. Furthermore, responses from the cones and rods can be separated as a result of their differential threshold to light, as rods are 10 000 times more sensitive to light than cones.

The photopic ERG tests cone function by keeping the patient in a light-adapted state, thereby bleaching or suppressing the rod response. The ERG response is then evoked with a bright white flash. Cone activity can also be evaluated using the flicker study (cones respond to flicker stimuli greater than 30 cycles per second, while rods do not). The scotopic ERG tests rod function by keeping the patient in a dark-adapted state for 45 minutes or longer and using a dim white or blue flash, below cone threshold, to evoke the ERG response from the rods.

Clinical Features

The ERG is clinically useful in a number of hereditary and degenerative retinal diseases. An extinguished ERG may be seen with retinitis pigmentosa, ophthalmic artery occlusion, diffuse unilateral subacute neuroretinitis, other causes of chorioretinitis (birdshot chorioretinopathy), carcinoma-associated retinopathy, toxic retinopathy, and nutritional deficiencies. In addition, the ERG may help identify eyes with progressive visual loss due to a retained intraocular foreign body. Certain metals such as copper, iron, and magnesium may cause severe and progressive retinal degeneration.

Reduction of the b-wave amplitude is associated with retinal ischemia, and may be helpful in distinguishing ischemic vs nonischemic central retinal vein occlusions. A b-wave to a-wave ratio of less than 1 is associated with an increased risk of neovascular glaucoma. A normal a-wave associated with a reduced b-wave also may be observed in congenital stationary night blindness and X-linked juvenile retinoschisis.

An abnormal photopic ERG in the setting of a normal scotopic ERG is consistent with the diagnosis of cone dystrophy or achromatopsia. A normal ERG can be seen in some optic neuropathies, thus distinguishing optic nerve disease from retinal disease.

Technique

To record the ERG, the eyes are dilated and dark adapted for 45 minutes. Following that, topical anesthesia is administered and a corneal contact lens electrode is applied. The full-field ERG is elicited within a ganzfeld dome, which provides a homogeneous distribution of light over the central 120° of the retina. As the patient fixates on a light-emitting diode, a dim white or blue flash is used to evoke the scotopic or rod-mediated ERG. Next, the photopic- or cone-mediated ERG is evoked.

Side Effects

Side effects of ERG testing are limited to surface irritation and potential corneal abrasion as a result of the corneal electrode. These complications can be minimized with the use of careful technique and proper lens sizing. For example, the common Burian-Allen electrode is available in a variety of sizes to fit premature infants to adults.

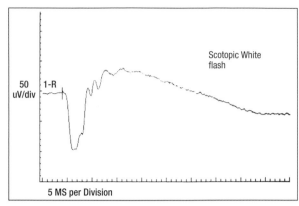

A normal scotopic white electroretinogram is demonstrated. Note the presence of the early a-wave (downward deflection) generated by the photoreceptors, followed by the b-wave (upward deflection), a function of the inner retinal layers (bipolar and Müller cells).

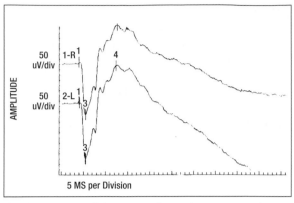

Oscillatory potentials are small wavelets seen on the ascending b-wave. The origin of oscillatory potentials is unclear; they are reduced in ischemic states (eg, diabetic retinopathy).

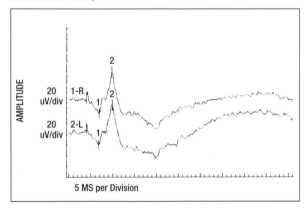

The photopic electroretinogram tests cone function by keeping the patient in a light-adapted state, thereby suppressing the rod response.

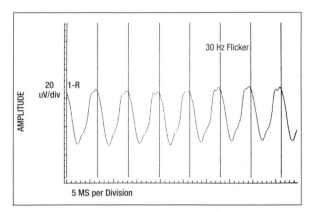

A normal, 30-Hz photopic flicker electroretinogram is demonstrated. This waveform is predominantly cone generated.

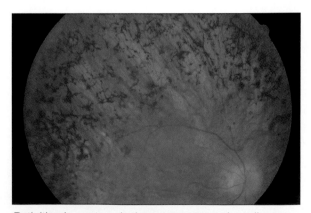

Retinitis pigmentosa is the most common hereditary retinopathy characterized by the degeneration of rods and cones. Clinical features include optic disc pallor, vessel attenuation, and peripheral pigmentary alterations.

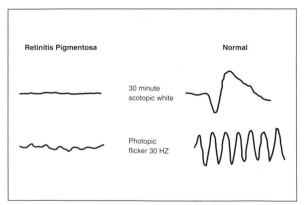

An attenuated scotopic white electroretinogram in a patient with retinitis pigmentosa is consistent with diffuse rod dysfunction. The photopic flicker is also markedly reduced, indicating diffuse cone dysfunction.

ELECTRORETINOGRAPHY (CONT'D)

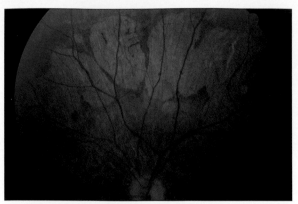

Choroideremia is an X-linked inherited retinal degeneration characterized by diffuse atrophy of the retinal pigment epithelium and choriocapillaris. Visual symptoms include poor night vision and visual field loss.

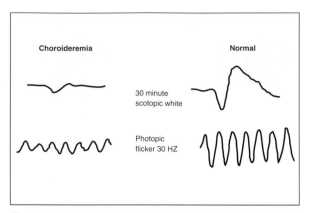

The scotopic electroretinogram in patients with choroideremia is markedly attenuated or extinguished.

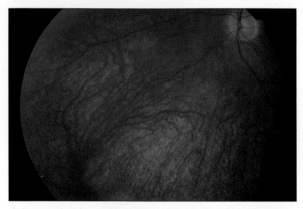

Advanced chloroquine toxicity is manifest by extensive peripheral pigmentary alterations in addition to the characteristic bull's eye maculopathy.

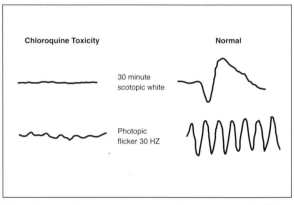

The electroretinogram in advanced chloroquine toxicity maybe severely reduced or nondetectable as a result of diffuse rod and cone dysfunction.

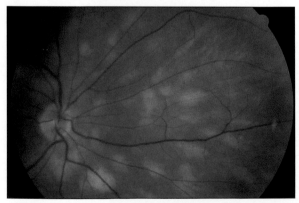

Birdshot chorioretinopathy is a member of the inflammatory white dot syndromes. The cause is unclear, but a strong association has been noted with HLA-A29.

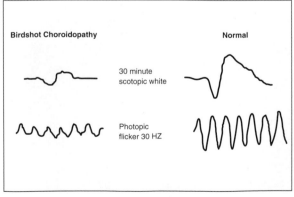

Birdshot chorioretinopathy may be associated with an extinguished electroretinogram (ERG). Other inflammatory conditions associated with abnormal ERGs include diffuse unilateral subacute neuroretinitis and acute zonal occult outer retinopathy.

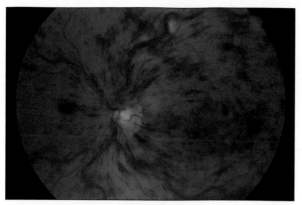

Reduction of the b-wave amplitude is associated with retinal ischemia and may be helpful in distinguishing ischemic vs nonischemic central retinal vein occlusions.

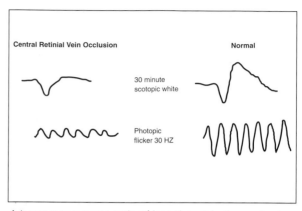

A b-wave to a-wave ratio of less than 1 in the scotopic electroretinogram is associated with an increased risk of neovascular glaucoma.

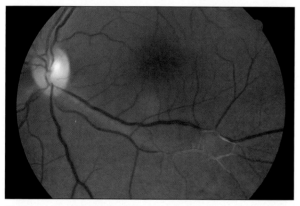

X-linked juvenile retinoschisis is characterized by cyst-like alterations in the fovea. Approximately 50% of patients have peripheral retinoschisis. The histological defect is a splitting of the retina at the nerve fiber layer.

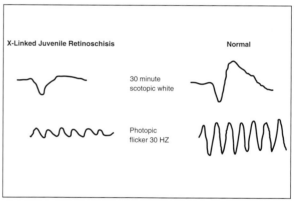

The characteristic electroretinographic abnormality in X-linked juvenile retinoschisis is a normal a-wave but an abnormal b-wave.

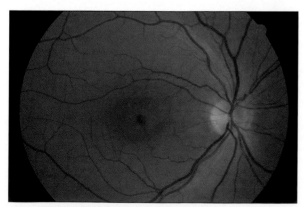

Cone dystrophy is a retinal degeneration affecting primarily cones. Ophthalmoscopic findings may be very subtle clinically (mild temporal disc pallor with or without bull's eye maculopathy).

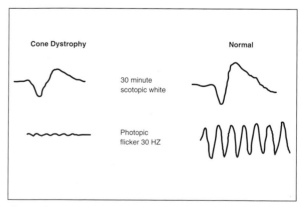

Cone dystrophy is characterized by an extinguished photopic and 30-Hz flicker electroretinogram (ERG). The scotopic ERG may be normal.

ELECTRO-OCULOGRAPHY

The electro-oculogram (EOG) is an electrophysiologic test that measures the function of the retinal pigment epithelium (RPE). The EOG measures the resting potential of the RPE, which depends on metabolic activity of the RPE. Clinically, information is gained from the EOG by comparing the amplitude of the resting potential in the light-adapted vs dark-adapted state. As a result, the EOG is a change in the amplitude of the resting potential under light- and dark-adapted states and is expressed as a ratio of the maximum light-adapted to minimum dark-adapted potentials (the Arden ratio). The normal range for this ratio is between 1.9 and 2.8. A ratio of 1.7 to 1.8 is marginally subnormal, while a ratio of less than 1.7 is considered subnormal. The EOG, like the electroretinogram (ERG), is a mass response. The EOG findings are usually consistent with the ERG with a few notable exceptions. An abnormal EOG associated with a normal ERG is demonstrated in Best's disease and possibly dominant drusen and pattern dystrophy. A normal EOG associated with an abnormal ERG may be seen in patients with X-linked juvenile retinoschisis.

Clinical Features

The most important clinical use of the EOG is to help diagnose patients with Best's disease. The Arden ratio is appreciably reduced in this disease, while the ERG is typically normal to even supranormal. The reduced Arden ratio not only may be reduced in patients with obvious disease, but may also be reduced in patients with the gene for the disease but no clinically evident fundus findings. In cases of Best's disease, in which only one eye manifests fundus changes at an early stage, both eyes will typically show reduced EOG ratios. The EOG may also be used to monitor patients taking chloroquine or hydroxychloroquine, as these drugs are potentially toxic to the RPE.

Technique

The EOG, unlike the ERG, does not use a corneal contact electrode. To perform the procedure, the patient is exposed to ambient room illumination and the eyes are dilated. Electrodes are attached just lateral to the inner and outer canthi of each eye. The subject then alternately fixates between two blinking lights 30° apart in a ganzfeld dome. This procedure is first done in the dark for 12 minutes and then in an illuminated ganzfeld dome for another 12 minutes. Care should be taken to increase the illumination slowly to prevent tearing, which can alter electrode resistance.

Side Effects

As the EOG does not use a corneal contact lens, the possibilities of surface irritation and corneal abrasion are minimized. The EOG may be useful in pediatric patients and in some adult patients unable to tolerate the ERG.

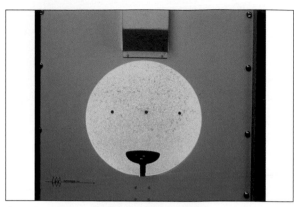

A patient's view of the ganzfeld dome during electro-oculography. Note the two dark fixation lights 30° apart.

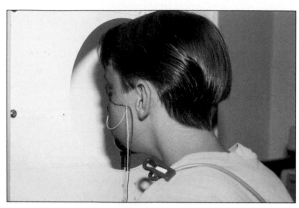

Demonstration of a young child with Best's disease participating in an electro-oculographic study.

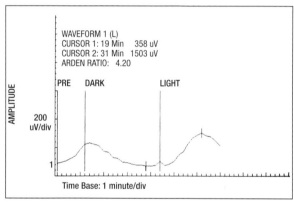

A normal electro-oculogram is demonstrated in this patient with Stargardt disease. The Arden ratio (light peak to dark trough) is 4.2.

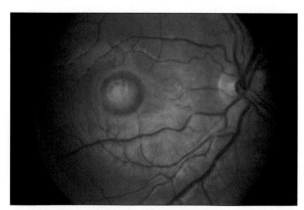

The most common indication for an electro-oculogram (EOG) is Best's disease. The EOG findings may be abnormal in individuals with pattern dystrophy and macular drusen.

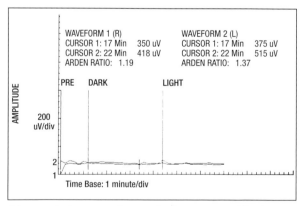

Abnormal electro-oculogram is demonstrated in this patient with Best's disease. The Arden ratio for each eye is less than 1.7.

ECHOGRAPHY

Ultrasound was developed in the early 1900s as a method to detect underwater objects. It was not until the 1960s that ultrasound was developed for ophthalmic applications. Today, ultrasound is a common and often indispensable diagnostic test.

The principle of ultrasonography is based on the piezoelectric effect of certain crystals and ceramic materials. The piezoelectric effect is characterized by the ability of the crystal or ceramic material to convert an electrical pulse, generated by a transmitter, into sound waves and then to receive echoes of the same wavelength and convert them back into electricity. The electrical potentials are then presented on an oscilloscope screen.

Diagnostic ultrasonography projects high frequency sound through soft tissues. The sound waves are partially reflected at various tissue interfaces. The reflections are recorded as either echo spikes (A-scan) or brightness dots (B-scan). Both of these interpretations allow for evaluation of posterior segment structures such as vitreous, choroid, and retina through opaque media.

Clinical Features

Ophthalmic ultrasonography is used for a variety of purposes including measurement of axial length (A-scan), corneal pachymetry (A-scan), diagnostic B-scan, and standardized echography. Only diagnostic B-scan ultrasonography is discussed here. B-scan ultrasonography is useful when opaque media are present, precluding a direct examination of posterior segment structures. In the presence of corneal scars, dense cataracts, and vitreous opacities, B-scan ultrasonography is helpful in identifying and characterizing retinal detachment, choroidal detachment, vitreous detachment, intraocular foreign bodies, and intraocular tumors.

On B-scan ultrasonography, retinal detachment appears as a smooth, mobile, highly reflective membrane. When fully detached, the retina can usually be noted to remain attached at the optic disc and ora serrata. Chronic retinal detachments become less mobile and may often appear thickened.

Choroidal detachment appears as a smooth, convex, and immobile reflective membrane. In contrast to retinal detachment, choroidal detachment can be noted to extend beyond the ora serrata. Choroidal detachment does not extend to the optic disc.

Almost all intraocular foreign bodies are detectable with B-scan ultrasonography. Metallic, stone, glass, and plastic objects are highly reflective and produce high-amplitude echoes. These echoes may be accompanied by acoustic shadowing.

Technique

Ophthalmic ultrasound is a diagnostic technique providing real-time images of tissues. Analysis is facilitated when the clinician partakes in the actual examination itself. Both A-scan ultrasonography and B-scan ultrasonography are performed by a contact or water immersion technique in which fluid coupling is present between the globe and the ultrasound probe. The examination should be performed in a systematic manner obtaining transverse, oblique, longitudinal, and axial scans.

Side Effects

Diagnostic ultrasonography, as described here, uses frequencies in the megahertz range. Significant heat levels are therefore not generated, making this a safe and effective imaging modality.

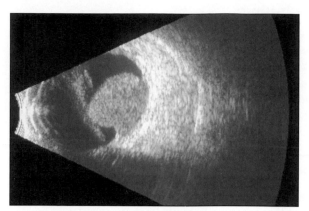

A B-scan image of a patient with a choroidal melanoma. Note the mushroom-shaped outline of the lesion, which results from growth of the lesion through Bruch's membrane.

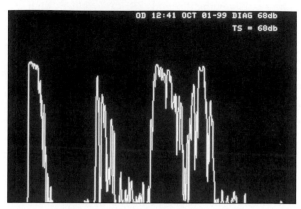

A standardized A-scan of the same lesion demonstrates low to medium internal reflectivity, suggestive of a choroidal melanoma.

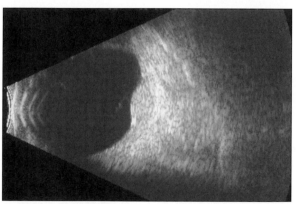

A B-scan image of a patient with a circumscribed choroidal hemangioma. Note the solid convex appearance to this lesion. Often, this is difficult to distinguish from a choroidal melanoma on B-scan ultrasonography alone.

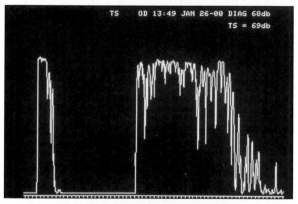

Standardized A-scan of the same patient with choroidal hemangioma, demonstrating medium to high internal reflectivity. This pattern is suggestive of a choroidal hemangioma.

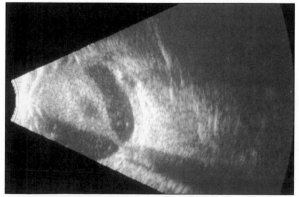

A longitudinal B-scan image of a patient with a funnel retinal detachment. Note the attachment to the optic disc.

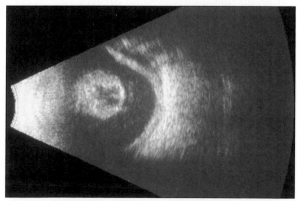

Transverse B-scan image of the same patient with a funnel retinal detachment. As a result of the position from which the scan was obtained, the retinal detachment appears as a circle.

SCANNING LASER OPHTHALMOSCOPY

Scanning laser ophthalmoscopy (SLO) produces high-resolution images of the fundus using less than 1/1000 the illumination required for conventional indirect ophthalmoscopy. In SLO imaging, a laser beam illuminates an area of the ocular fundus, forming a rectangular pattern (raster) on the retina. The light reflected from each retinal point is captured by a photomultiplier. The output of the photomultiplier then determines the brilliance of the spot displayed on a television monitor. The laser beam and electron beam on the monitor are synchronized, forming a picture on the monitor.

Scanning laser ophthalmoscopy is extremely light efficient, with excellent depth of field. This feature is due to the fact that illumination is provided solely from the laser beam and the remainder of the patient's pupil is available for light collection. Scanning laser ophthalmoscopic images have excellent contrast, as compared to those obtained with slit lamp biomicroscopy and standard fundus photography, because of its monochromatic wavelength emission, which minimizes scattering and chromatic aberration.

Clinical Features

The high-quality images and superior depth of field make SLO useful for the diagnosis and management of macular surface disorders such as vitreomacular traction syndrome, macular holes, and macular pucker. Some studies have suggested that SLO is more sensitive than clinical examination alone in detecting early stages of these disorders.

Scanning laser ophthalmoscopy can also be used to perform high-resolution fluorescein or indocyanine green (ICG) videoangiography. Using SLO to perform fluorescein angiography allows for the measurement of capillary flow velocity. Flow velocity is determined by measuring the transit time of blood between two points on the video monitor that are separated by a known distance.

Scanning laser ophthalmoscopy can also be used to perform retinal microperimetry. Arbitrary graphic patterns can be placed in the raster and viewed simultaneously by the patient and observer. Subjective responses to this stimulation are obtained from the patient, and retinal perimetry can be performed to help identify macular scotomata. Determining the location of scotomata in low-vision patients can assist with visual rehabilitation plans.

Technique

Commercial applications for the indications discussed here are available. Scanning laser fluorescein and ICG angiography are obtained just as they would be with a fundus camera. The microperimetry application requires interaction between the patient and observer as the graphic patterns placed in the raster are simultaneously viewed on the video monitor.

Side Effects

Scanning laser ophthalmoscopy uses light levels much lower than most other ophthalmic imaging devices and even conventional ophthalmoscopy. It has been reported that SLO can safely be used for up to 1 hour of continuous viewing, well below that used in clinical practice.

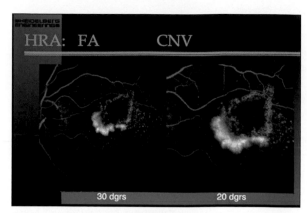

Fluorescein videoangiography using scanning laser ophthalmoscopy. A choroidal neovascular membrane is demonstrated.

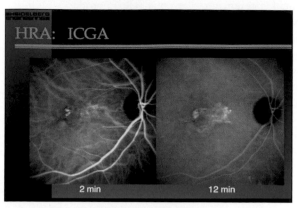

Indocyanine green (ICG) videoangiography using scanning laser ophthalmoscopy. The ICG and fluorescein angiography can be performed simultaneously.

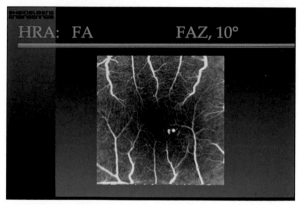

A high-resolution fluorescein angiographic image can be obtained of the central 10°. Note the detail of the perifoveal capillary network.

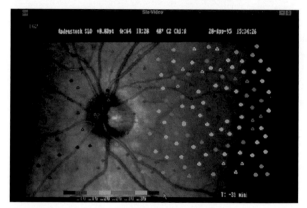

Retinal microperimetry with scanning laser ophthalmoscopy. Projection of such graphic patterns on the retina allows for localization of scotomata as well as fixation training for low-vision patients.

OPTICAL COHERENCE TOMOGRAPHY

Optical coherence tomography (OCT) produces high-resolution, cross-sectional images of posterior pole structures. Unlike other imaging techniques such as computed tomography, magnetic resonance imaging, and ultrasound, OCT uses light waves (810 nm) and is therefore capable of higher-resolution images.

Optical coherence tomography is based on the principle of low coherence interferometry. A diode light source is directed at both the eye and a reference mirror at a known spatial location. The time delay of each optical echo is compared, and thickness data are obtained. Image quality is enhanced by computer processing techniques that eliminate image degradation by microsaccades. A false color display is added to tissues with differing optical scattering properties to further enhance image quality.

Clinical Features

The high-resolution images obtained with OCT have made this technique particularly useful in the evaluation of macular pathology. The differences in optical reflectivity at the anterior and posterior borders of the neurosensory retina allow OCT to provide retinal thickness data. Retinal thickness determination may be helpful in the diagnosis and management of macular edema from a variety of causes.

Optical coherence tomography is also useful in the assessment of macular surface disorders. Stage 1 macular holes are sometimes difficult to detect clinically but OCT images of stage 1 macular holes are quite distinctive. Optical coherence tomography may also help differentiate true, full-thickness macular holes from other entities such as lamellar holes and pseudoholes due to epiretinal membranes.

Optical coherence tomography can also be an effective tool in monitoring the surgical success or failure of vitreoretinal surgery. Following successful macular hole repair, full-thickness retina, often with a normal foveal contour, can be demonstrated with OCT images.

Other diseases for which OCT may have clinical utility include central serous retinopathy and age-related macular degeneration. In central serous retinopathy, OCT is sensitive to even small neurosensory detachments and may be able to detect subclinical elevations of the neurosensory retina. In age-related macular degeneration, OCT can identify intraretinal fluid, subretinal fluid, retinal pigment epithelial detachments, and sometimes choroidal neovascularization.

Technique

Optical coherence tomography is a noncontact technique that requires the subject to be seated at an apparatus resembling a conventional slit lamp and fixate for 2.5 seconds. In this time, 100 retinal points are measured per axial scan.

Side Effects

The power of the diode laser used is well within safety levels set by the American National Standards Institute (ANSI).

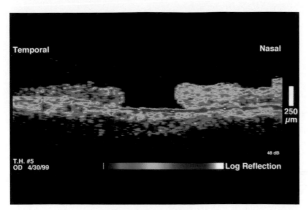

Optical coherence tomogram through a full-thickness macular hole.

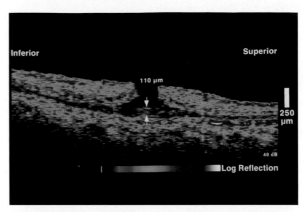

Optical coherence tomogram through a pseudohole. Note the presence of full-thickness retina measuring 110 mm at the base of the pseudohole.

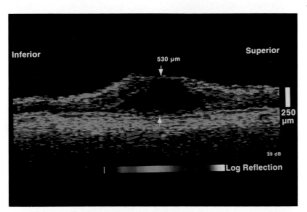

Optical coherence tomogram demonstrating marked intraretinal edema due to diabetic macular edema.

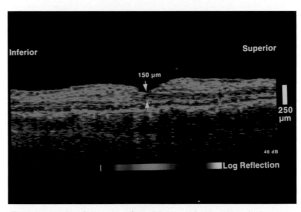

Three months following focal laser photocoagulation, normal foveal thickness and normal foveal contour are restored.

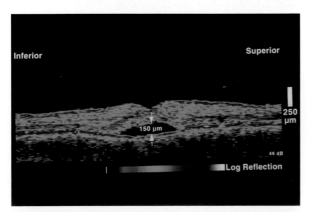

Optical coherence tomogram demonstrating subretinal fluid under the fovea in a patient with central serous retinopathy.

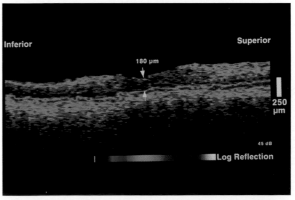

Following 6 months of observation, the subretinal fluid has spontaneously reabsorbed and normal foveal thickness and architecture are demonstrated.

SELECTED REFERENCES

Fluorescein Angiography

1. Berkow JW, Orth DH, Kelley JS. *Fluorescein Angiography: Technique and Interpretation.* San Francisco: American Academy of Ophthalmology; 1991. Monograph 5.
2. Saine PJ. Landmarks in the historical development of fluorescein angiography. *J Ophthalmic Photogr.* 1993;15:17–23.
3. Yannuzzi LA, Rohrer KT, Tindel LJ, Sobel RS, Costanza MA, Shields W, et.al. Fluorescein angiography complication survey. *Ophthalmology.* 1986;93:611–617.

Fluorescein Angiography: Hyperfluorescence

1. Berkow JW, Orth DH, Kelley JS. *Fluorescein Angiography: Technique and Interpretation.* San Francisco: American Academy of Ophthalmology; 1991. Monograph 5.
2. Johnson R, Schatz H, McDonald HR, Ai E. Fluorescein angiography: basic principles and interpretation. In: Ryan SJ, ed. *Retina,* Vol 2. 3rd ed. St. Louis: Mosby, Inc; 2001:875–942.
3. Rabb MF, Burton TC, Schatz H, Yannuzzi LA. Fluorescein angiography of the fundus: A schematic approach to interpretation. *Surv Ophthalmol.* 1978;22(6):387–403.

Fluorescein Angiography: Hypofluorescence

1. Anagnoste SR, Mandava N, Guyer DR, Yannuzzi LA. Fundus angiography. In: Regillo CD, Brown GC, Flynn HW, eds. *Vitreoretinal Disease, The Essentials.* New York: Thieme; 1999:51–64.
2. Berkow JW, Orth DH, Kelley JS. *Fluorescein Angiography: Technique and Interpretation.* San Francisco: American Academy of Ophthalmology; 1991. Monograph 5.
3. Johnson R, Schatz H, McDonald HR, Ai E. Fluorescein angiography: basic principles and interpretation. In: Ryan SJ, ed. *Retina.* Vol 2. 3rd ed. St. Louis: Mosby, Inc; 2001:875–942.

Indocyanine Green Angiography

1. American Academy of Ophthalmology. Indocyanine green angiography (ophthalmic procedures assessment). *Ophthalmology.* 1998;105:1564–1569.
2. Guyer DR, Puliafito CA, Mones JM, Friedman E, Chang W, Verdooner SR. Digital indocyanine green angiography in chorioretinal disorders. *Ophthalmology.* 1992;99:287–291.

Electroretinography

1. Fishman FA, Sokol S. *Electrophysiologic Testing.* San Francisco: American Academy of Ophthalmology; 1990. Monograph 2.
2. Sabates R, Hirose T, McNeel JW. Electroretinography in the prognosis and classification of central retinal vein occlusion. *Arch Ophthalmol.* 1983;101:232–235.
3. Sandberg MA. Objective assessment of retinal function. In: Albert DM, Jakobiec FA, eds. *Principles and Practice of Ophthalmology.* Philadelphia: WB Saunders; 1994:1193–1213.

Electro-oculography

1. Fishman FA, Sokol S. *Electrophysiologic Testing.* San Francisco: American Academy of Ophthalmology; 1990. Monograph 2.
2. Sandberg MA. Objective assessment of retinal function. In: Albert DM, Jakobiec FA, eds. *Principles and Practice of Ophthalmology.* Philadelphia: WB Saunders; 1994:1193–1213.

Echography

1. Guthoff R. *Ultrasound in Ophthalmologic Diagnosis.* New York: Thieme Medical Publishers; 1991.
2. Kendall CJ. *Ophthalmic Echography.* Thorofare, NJ: Slack Inc; 1990.

Scanning Laser Ophthalmoscopy

1. Mainster MA, Timberlake GT, Webb RM, Hughes GW. Scanning laser ophthalmoscopy: clinical applications. *Ophthalmology.* 1982;89:852–857.
2. Sharp PF, Manivannan A. The scanning laser ophthalmoscope. *Phys Med Biol.* 1997;42:951–966.

Optical Coherence Tomography

1. Hee MR, Puliafito CA, Wong C, Duker JS, Reichel E, Rutledge B, et al. Quantitative assessment of macular edema with optical coherence tomography. *Arch Ophthalmol.* 1995; 113:1019–1029.
2. Puliafito CA, Hee MR, Lin CP, Reichel E, Schuman JS, Duker JS, et al. Imaging of macular diseases with optical coherence tomography. *Ophthalmology.* 1995; 102:217–229.

chapter 3

Clinical Features of Retinal Disease

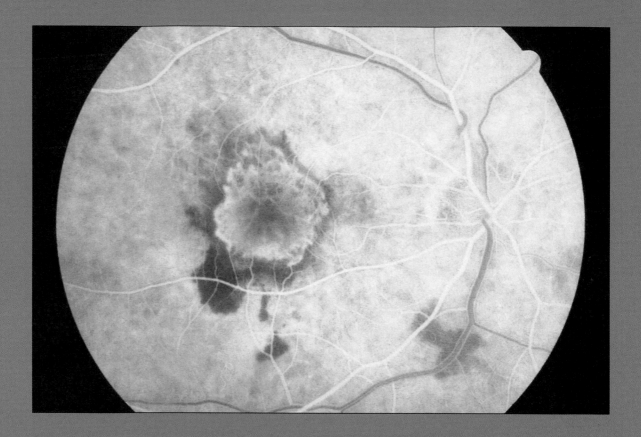

David A. Quillen, MD

Barbara A. Blodi, MD

Timothy J. Bennett, CRA

BULL'S EYE MACULOPATHY

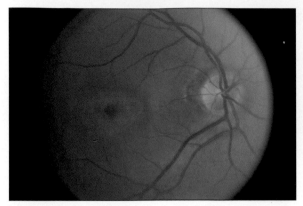

Chloroquine toxicity

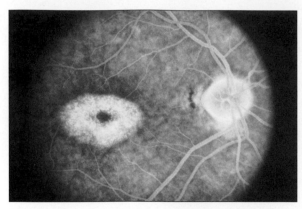

Chloroquine toxicity (fluorescein angiography)

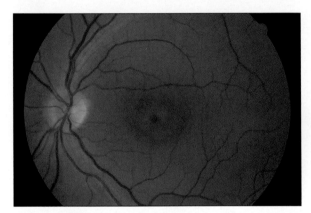

Cone dystrophy

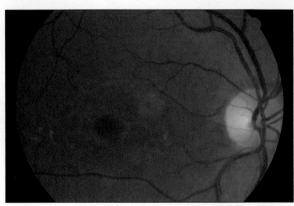

Stargardt disease

Clinical Features

Bull's eye maculopathy refers to a pattern of retinal pigment epithelial alterations in the macula characterized by a central region of hyperpigmentation surrounded by a zone of hypopigmentation reminiscent of an aiming target. These alterations may be subtle clinically but are more prominent with fluorescein angiography. Bull's eye maculopathy is usually bilateral but may be asymmetric. Patients may complain of reduced central acuity (particularly with reading), dyschromatopsia, and paracentral scotomas.

Differential Diagnosis

Conditions associated with bull's eye maculopathy include cone dystrophy, rod-cone dystrophy, chloroquine/hydroxychloroquine toxicity, Stargardt disease, age-related macular degeneration, fenestrated sheen macular dystrophy, concentric annular macular dystrophy, and following intravitreal injection of fomivirsen sodium for cytomegalovirus retinitis. A "pseudo" bull's eye maculopathy may be seen with pattern dystrophies, acute macular neuroretinopathy, chronic macular holes, and resolved unilateral acute idiopathic maculopathy.

CHERRY RED SPOT

Clinical Features

A cherry red spot refers to the macular appearance of a central red spot surrounded by superficial retinal whitening. It is seen most commonly after a central retinal artery occlusion. Occlusion of the central retinal artery results in ischemia and infarction of the inner retina including the nerve fiber and ganglion cell layers. This is manifest by whitening and edema of the inner retina in the macular area where the nerve fiber and ganglion cell layers are thickest. The foveola retains its reddish color because the inner retinal layers are displaced laterally and the underlying choroidal circulation remains intact. Retinal ischemia and infarction account for the cherry red spot observed in cases of intraocular gentamicin toxicity.

A cherry red spot may be observed in a group of neurometabolic storage disorders characterized by the accumulation of glycolipids and phospholipids in the ganglion cell layer of the retina. These disorders include Tay-Sachs disease (GM2 gangliosidosis type 1), Niemann-Pick disease, and cherry red spot myoclonus syndrome (sialidosis type 1). The accumulation of material is most evident in the macula, which contains multiple layers of ganglion cell nuclei. The lack of ganglion cells in the foveola accounts for the central red spot.

Differential Diagnosis

The most common conditions associated with a cherry red spot are central retinal artery occlusion, intraocular gentamicin toxicity, and metabolic storage diseases.

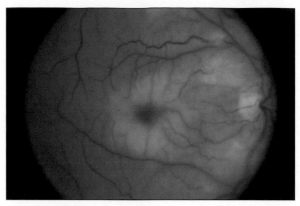

Central retinal artery occlusion

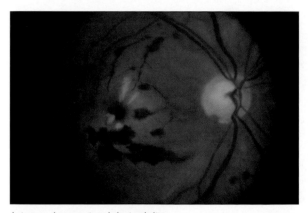

Intraocular gentamicin toxicity

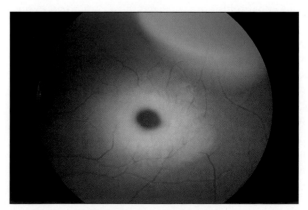

Tay-Sachs disease

CHORIORETINAL FOLDS

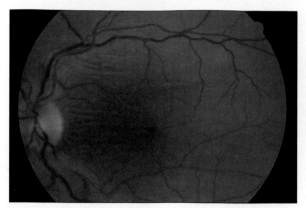

Idiopathic chorioretinal folds

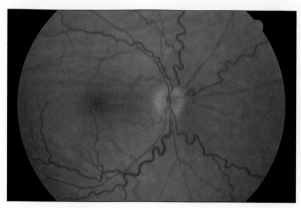

High hyperopia

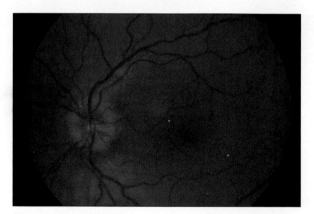

Hypotony maculopathy

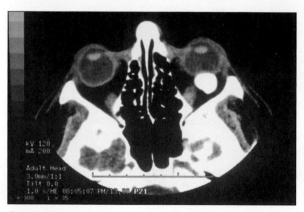

Retrobulbar orbital tumor (computed tomographic scan of osteoma)

Clinical Features

Chorioretinal folds are visualized most commonly in the posterior fundus. They may be unilateral or bilateral, depending on the etiology. Individuals may be asymptomatic or complain of blurred or distorted vision. Idiopathic chorioretinal folds are believed to be caused by scleral shrinkage. Scleral shrinkage decreases the surface area available to the overlying choroid and retina, resulting in chorioretinal folds. Individuals with idiopathic chorioretinal folds usually are asymptomatic, although some degree of hyperopia is common. Imaging studies reveal flattening of the posterior aspect of the globes.

Differential Diagnosis

In addition to idiopathic occurrences, chorioretinal folds may be associated with abnormalities of the optic disc including papilledema and optic disc drusen.

Chorioretinal folds are observed frequently with intraocular hypotony (usually in the setting of glaucoma surgery). When intraocular hypotony is prolonged, the folds may become permanent. Chorioretinal folds in the macula may be associated with posterior microphthalmos and high hyperopia. Radial chorioretinal folds may be observed in exudative age-related macular degeneration (AMD) or other causes of choroidal neovascularization (CNV). Unilateral chorioretinal folds may be associated with a retrobulbar tumor or inflammatory conditions such as posterior scleritis.

CHOROIDAL NEOVASCULARIZATION

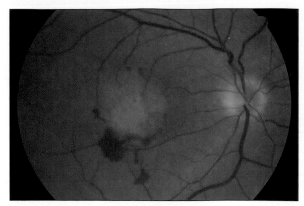

Age-related macular degeneration

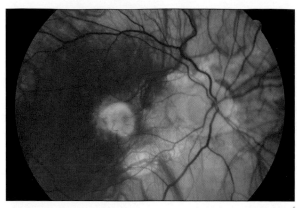

Degenerative myopia

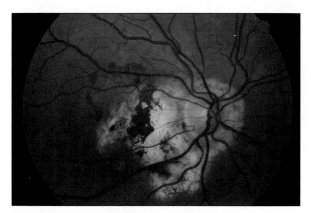

Presumed ocular histoplasmosis

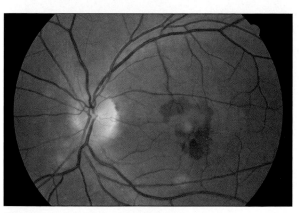

Multifocal choroiditis with panuveitis

Clinical Features

Choroidal neovascularization (CNV) may be observed in a variety of common and unusual conditions. The unifying feature is a disruption of the Bruch's membrane/retinal pigment epithelial complex, which allows vessels from the choriocapillaris to grow into the subretinal pigment epithelial and/or subneurosensory retinal space. CNV is observed clinically as a grayish green subretinal lesion. The lesion is usually associated with subretinal fluid, hemorrhage, and lipid exudation.

Fluorescein angiography is used to distinguish between classic and occult CNV. Classic CNV consists of a lacy vascular network with well-defined borders during the early transit phase of the angiogram. In contrast, occult CNV is characterized by ill-defined hyperfluorescence with poorly demarcated borders. Symptoms associated with CNV include blurred vision, distortion, and central scotoma.

Differential Diagnosis

Age-related macular degeneration (AMD) is the most common condition associated with CNV. The development of CNV is responsible for the vast majority of cases of significant visual loss in individuals with AMD. Other conditions include degenerative myopia; angioid streaks; pattern dystrophies; polypoidal choroidal vasculopathy; presumed ocular histoplasmosis syndrome; multifocal choroiditis; serpiginous choroiditis; Best's disease; Stargardt disease; gyrate atrophy; retinitis pigmentosa; choroidal nevus; choroidal osteoma; choroidal rupture/trauma; status post laser photocoagulation; optic disc drusen; and idiopathic choroidal neovascularization.

COTTON WOOL SPOT

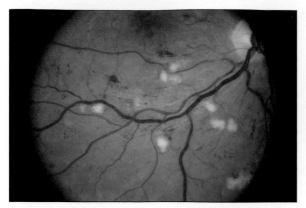

Diabetic retinopathy

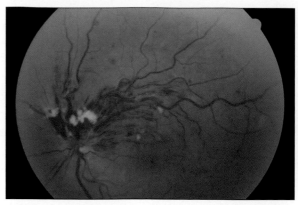

Branch retinal vein occlusion

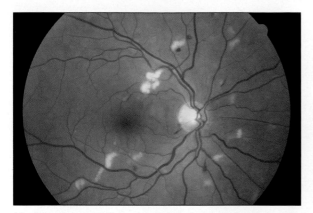

Human immunodeficiency virus retinopathy

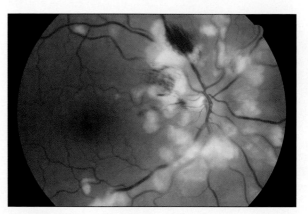

Purtscher's-like retinopathy

Clinical Features

A cotton wool spot is a small area of superficial retinal whitening located in the posterior fundus (often in the macula, with a perivascular and peripapillary distribution). It results from an ischemic insult to the nerve fiber layer and represents interruption of axoplasmic flow. Histologically, cotton wool spots are characterized by thickening of the ganglion cell and nerve fiber layers and the presence of cystoid bodies, which are globular structures within the nerve fiber layer.

Differential Diagnosis

Cotton wool spots are observed most commonly in retinal vascular diseases such as diabetic retinopathy, hypertensive retinopathy, and vascular occlusions. They have been seen in association with anemia, leukemia, and multiple myeloma, and following bone marrow transplantation and radiation therapy of the head and orbits.

Cotton wool spots may be observed in individuals with human immunodeficiency virus. They may be seen in various inflammatory disorders including systemic lupus erythematosus, polyarteritis nodosa, giant cell arteritis, scleroderma, dermatomyositis, cat scratch neuroretinitis, cytomegalovirus retinitis, and Behçet's disease. They have been described in association with interferon therapy.

A variant of the cotton wool spot is seen in Purtscher's-like retinopathy. Purtscher's-like retinopathy is characterized by prominent peripapillary superficial white patches and retinal hemorrhages surrounding a normal optic disc. It was originally described after head trauma but since has been observed in childbirth, pancreatitis, chest compression injuries, renal failure, and connective tissue disorders (dermatomyositis, scleroderma). The pathogenesis remains unclear; however, complement activation with occlusion of the superficial retinal capillaries has been proposed.

CYSTOID MACULAR EDEMA

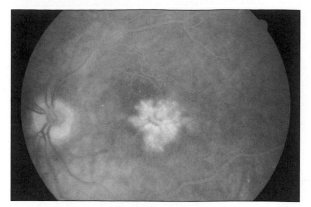

Post-cataract surgery cystoid macular edema
(fluorescein angiogram)

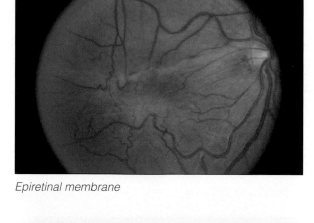

Epiretinal membrane

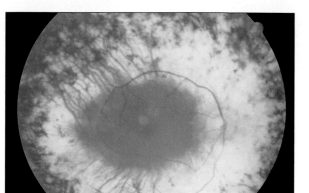

Retinitis pigmentosa

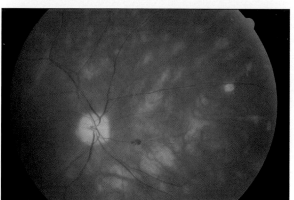

Birdshot chorioretinopathy

Clinical Features

Cystoid macular edema (CME) is characterized by a stellate or honeycomb pattern of retinal thickening in the fovea and parafoveal region. It is visualized most efficiently with the use of a fundus contact lens; often, the cyst-like lesions are seen best with retroillumination. Fluorescein angiography reveals a classic "petaloid" pattern of hyperfluorescence as the dye accumulates in the cystoid spaces. A central yellow spot may be observed in some cases of CME. This feature likely results from the loss of the normal foveal depression and the anterior displacement of xanthophyll pigment.

Histologically, CME is characterized by large cystic spaces containing serous exudate in the outer plexiform layer and small spaces with exudate in the inner nuclear layer. Although the pathogenesis is not completely understood, inflammation likely plays a significant role in the development of CME.

Differential Diagnosis

Cystoid macular edema may develop after any intraocular surgery—particularly cataract surgery. Clinically

significant post-cataract surgery CME occurs in approximately 1% of patients; it is more common in cases of vitreous loss and vitreous incarceration.

CME may be observed in a variety of other conditions including exudative age-related macular degeneration (AMD), epiretinal membrane contraction, and chronic vitreoretinal traction syndromes. CME may be associated with retinal vascular disorders such as diabetic retinopathy and retinal vein occlusions. The condition may result in central visual loss in patients with retinitis pigmentosa as well as inflammatory diseases including birdshot chorioretinopathy, pars planitis, and idiopathic vitritis. CME also has been described in patients with choroidal tumors including choroidal melanomas. CME may develop in individuals with rhegmatogenous retinal detachment. Nicotinic acid toxicity may be associated with a CME-like condition distinguished by the absence of leakage on fluorescein angiography. Latanoprost has been implicated as a cause of CME in pseudophakic and aphakic individuals. X-linked juvenile retinoschisis is characterized by a stellate foveal appearance similar to that of CME. In contrast to CME, the schisis occurs in the nerve fiber layer.

DRUSEN

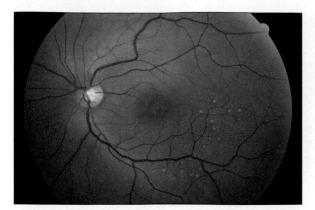

Hard drusen

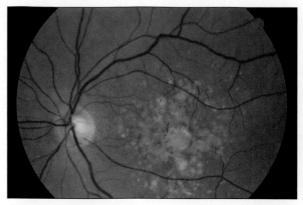

Soft, confluent drusen

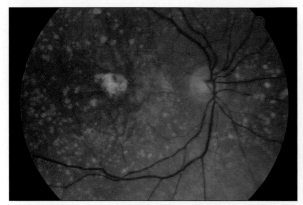

Calcific drusen

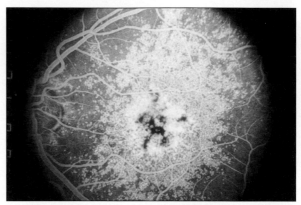

Basal laminar drusen

Clinical Features

Drusen are small, yellowish white, round or oval deposits located between the basement membrane of the retinal pigment epithelium (RPE) and the remainder of Bruch's membrane. They are found most commonly in the macula but may be present in any area of the fundus including the periphery. Drusen are usually bilateral and symmetric. Most individuals with drusen are asymptomatic, although some may complain of blurred vision or distortion. Significant visual loss is associated with the development of choroidal neovascularization (CNV) or atrophy.

Several types of drusen have been described: hard, soft, calcified, and basal laminar/cuticular. Hard drusen are small, yellowish white, discrete deposits. Hard drusen are not associated with the development of advanced age-related macular degeneration (AMD) and are considered by many to be a "normal" aging phenomenon. Soft drusen are larger yellowish deposits with less distinct borders. They may coalesce and become confluent in the foveal/parafoveal region. Soft drusen may be associated with alterations of the RPE, including atrophy and focal hyperpigmentation. Soft drusen and focal hyperpigmentation are associated with an increased risk for the development of CNV. Calcified drusen are small,

refractile deposits associated with AMD and geographic atrophy. They represent dystrophic calcification of drusen. Basal laminar or cuticular drusen are innumerable small, round, discrete nodular deposits that are more apparent on fluorescein angiography. Fluorescein angiography reveals numerous hyperfluorescent pinpoint spots described as having a "stars-in-the-sky" or "Milky Way" appearance. Basal laminar drusen may be associated with vitelliform-like detachments of the RPE and geographic atrophy in the end stage of the disease.

Differential Diagnosis

Drusen are usually observed in the setting of AMD. Occasionally, drusen may be observed in younger individuals (familial or dominant drusen). Basal laminar drusen have been described in patients with type II glomerulonephritis and as a dominantly inherited disorder characterized by a radial pattern of drusen deposition (Malattia levantinese). Unilateral drusen may be associated with an underlying choroidal nevus.

Drusen must be distinguished from Stargardt disease and other fleck dystrophies, the inflammatory white dot syndromes, and fundus albipunctatus.

FLECKED RETINA SYNDROMES

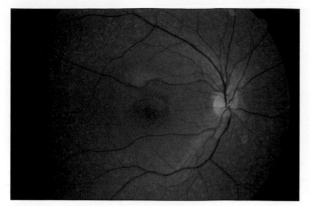

Stargardt disease

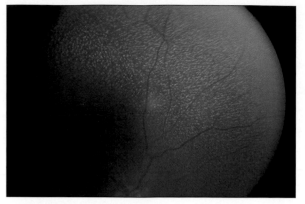

Fundus albipunctatus

Clinical Features

The flecked retina syndromes consist of a diverse group of disorders characterized by the presence of fleck-like lesions at the level of the retinal pigment epithelium (RPE) or retina. True flecks have a triradiate, fish tail, or "pisciform" configuration. The flecks are located at the level of the RPE and may be found in the macula and/or midperipheral retina. They tend to be bilateral and symmetric, although the size and shape of individual flecks may vary. The flecks tend to fade over time. Flecks must be differentiated from round or oval lesions consistent with drusen, several of the congenital stationary night blindness conditions, or the inflammatory white dot syndromes.

Differential Diagnosis

Identifying the location of the fleck-like lesions is important to determine the etiology of a given condition. Stargardt disease/fundus flavimaculatus is the most common flecked retinal syndrome involving the RPE. Other conditions include drusen, fundus albipunctatus, the flecked retina of Kandori, retinitis punctata albescens, Alport's syndrome, and vitamin A deficiency.

Several retinal toxicities may mimic the flecked retina syndromes; these abnormalities are usually found within the retina. They include canthaxanthin, talc, and tamoxifen retinopathies. Other conditions associated with retinal crystals include sickle cell retinopathy, idiopathic juxtafoveal retinal telangiectasis, Bietti's crystalline retinal dystrophy, cystinosis, and oxalosis.

FOVEAL YELLOW SPOT

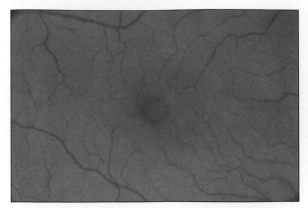

Stage I macular hole

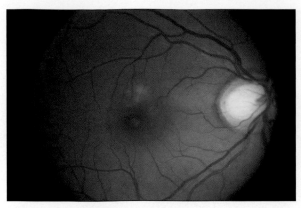

Central serous chorioretinopathy

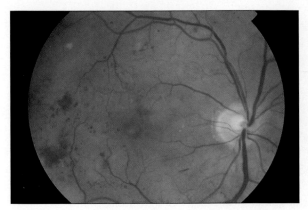

Diabetic retinopathy with macular edema

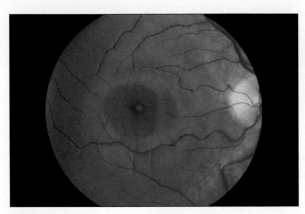

Solar retinopathy

Clinical Features

The macula is recognized clinically as the region within the temporal vascular arcades. Histologically, the macula is defined as having the following: two or more layers of ganglion cell nuclei; taller and more pigmented retinal pigment epithelial cells; and xanthophyll pigment. Under normal circumstances, the foveal depression limits the visibility of the yellow xanthophyll pigment. Loss of the foveal depression is accompanied by anterior displacement of the xanthophyll pigment. This condition is manifest clinically as a yellow spot or ring in the fovea.

Differential Diagnosis

A stage 1 macular hole is the most notable condition characterized by the presence of a yellow spot (or yellow ring) in the fovea. A prominent xanthophyll reflex also may be detected in association with subretinal or intraretinal fluid in the fovea. Conditions include central serous chorioretinopathy, choroidal neovascularization, toxemia of pregnancy, uveal effusion syndrome, optic disc edema, diabetic retinopathy, and cystoid macular edema. Other conditions simulating a prominent xanthophyll reflex include solar retinopathy and pattern dystrophy.

INTRARETINAL HEMORRHAGES

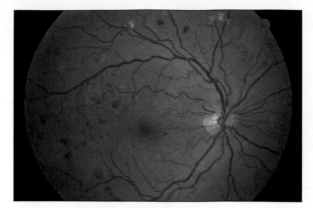

Diabetic retinopathy

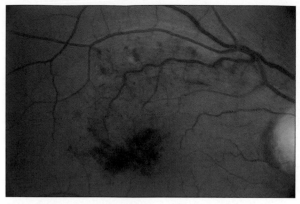

Branch retinal vein occlusion

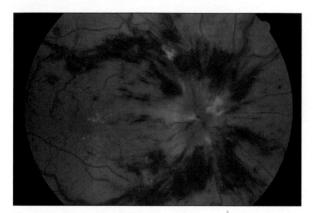

Central retinal vein occlusion

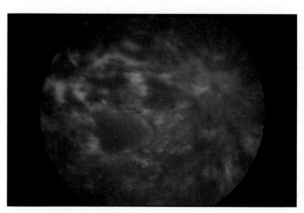

Shaken baby syndrome

Clinical Features

Intraretinal hemorrhages vary in appearance based on their location within the retina. Flame-shaped hemorrhages are superficial, bright red, fan-shaped hemorrhages located in the nerve fiber layer. Dot/blot hemorrhages are small, round, dark red hemorrhages located in the deeper, more vertically oriented layers of the retina. Both flame-shaped and dot/blot intraretinal hemorrhages result from disruption of the retinal capillaries and breakdown of the blood-retinal barrier. Individuals with intraretinal hemorrhages may be asymptomatic or have significant visual loss depending on the etiology.

Differential Diagnosis

Intraretinal hemorrhages are associated with a variety of retinal vascular diseases including diabetes mellitus, hypertension, branch and central retinal vein occlusions, leukemia, anemia, radiation retinopathy, ocular ischemia, retinal macroaneurysms, and sickle cell disease. Intraretinal hemorrhages may be seen with epiretinal membrane contraction. Intraretinal hemorrhages may be observed in inflammatory diseases including human immunodeficiency virus, cytomegalovirus retinitis, sarcoidosis, and Behçet's disease and other conditions associated with vasculitis. They may result from direct or indirect ocular trauma (contusion injury, shaken baby syndrome, childbirth, Valsalva retinopathy, Terson's syndrome, Purtscher's retinopathy). They may occur following acute posterior vitreous separation, in areas of persistent vitreoretinal traction, and with acute retinal tears. Intraretinal hemorrhages have been described following bone marrow transplantation and in association with high-altitude sickness.

LIPID EXUDATES

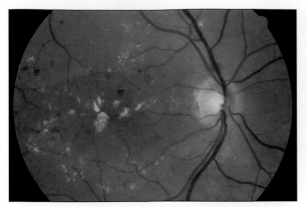

Diabetic retinopathy

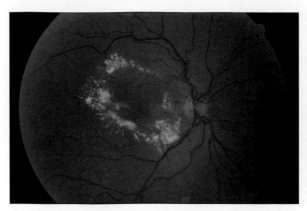

Branch retinal vein occlusion

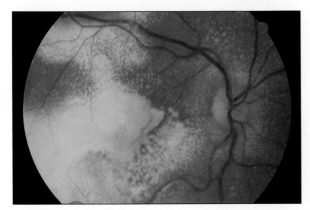

Coat's disease

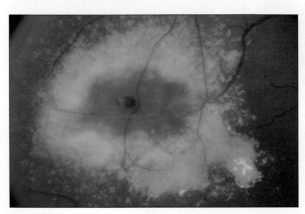

Retinal arterial macroaneurysm

Clinical Features

Lipid exudates have been referred to as "hard exudates." This description reflects the relatively discrete, yellow, refractile nature of the deposits. The lipid deposits are either intraretinal or subretinal, depending on the etiology. Lipid exudates tend to be localized around a given area of pathology forming a round or "circinate" pattern. However, large amounts of lipid exudation may accumulate at sites distant from the abnormality. For example, individuals with Coat's disease or a peripheral retinal capillary hemangioma may present with visual loss as a result of subretinal fluid and lipid exudation in the macula.

Lipid exudates must be distinguished from intra-arterial emboli, retinal crystals, drusen, and the flecked retina syndromes.

Differential Diagnosis

Lipid exudation is usually associated with retinal vascular leakage or abnormal vascular proliferation from either the choroidal or retinal circulation. Retinal vascular leakage may result from congenital vascular abnormalities (Coat's disease, idiopathic juxtafoveal retinal telangiectasis type 1) or acquired retinal vascular disorders (diabetic retinopathy, hypertensive retinopathy, venous occlusive disease, macroaneurysms, radiation retinopathy). In the case of diabetic retinopathy, retinal lipid exudate may be associated with systemic hyperlipidemia. Lipid exudation may occur as an unusual complication of retinitis pigmentosa and chronic retinal detachment.

Lipid exudation from vascular proliferation may be seen in patients with age-related macular degeneration and other causes of choroidal neovascularization. Lipid exudation is associated with choroidal melanoma and retinal capillary hemangiomas.

MACULAR ATROPHY

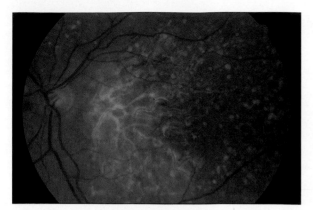

Age-related macular degeneration

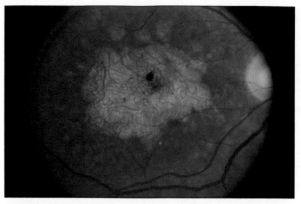

Stargardt disease

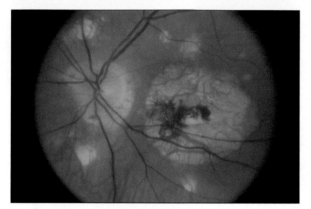

Presumed ocular histoplasmosis

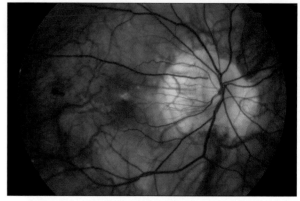

Degenerative myopia

Clinical Features

Macular atrophy is a nonspecific finding observed in a variety of macular, vascular, hereditary, toxic, inflammatory, and traumatic retinal disorders. Macular atrophy may be observed in the young and old, depending on the etiology. Individuals may be asymptomatic or complain of visual loss, distortion, or scotoma.

Macular atrophy is often bilateral but may be asymmetric or unilateral. Areas of macular atrophy may be confined to the macula or be associated with more widespread alterations. In many cases, the region of atrophy assumes a well-defined, geographic, "map-like" pattern. In areas of significant atrophy, the larger choroidal vessels are visible resulting from the loss of retinal pigment epithelium (RPE) and choriocapillaris. Macular atrophy may be associated with RPE alterations or fibrosis.

Differential Diagnosis

Macular atrophy is most commonly observed in age-related macular degeneration (AMD). Geographic atrophy is a significant cause of vision loss in individuals

with nonexudative AMD. The areas of geographic atrophy are well circumscribed, and often develop in a paracentral location before involving the fovea. Calcific drusen are often present. The etiology of geographic atrophy remains unclear but may involve abnormalities in the choroidal circulation.

Other conditions associated with macular atrophy include angioid streaks; central serous chorioretinopathy; myopic degeneration; long-standing cystoid macular edema from any cause; macular phototoxicity; pattern dystrophies; Best's disease and other familial macular dystrophies (North Carolina macular dystrophy; Sorsby's macular dystrophy); choroideremia; cone dystrophy and other causes of bull's eye maculopathy; gyrate atrophy; and Stargardt disease. Macular atrophy may be observed in a variety of inflammatory (histoplasmosis, toxoplasmosis, multifocal choroiditis, serpiginous choroiditis) and traumatic (commotio retinae, choroidal rupture) disorders.

OPTIC DISC EDEMA WITH MACULAR STAR

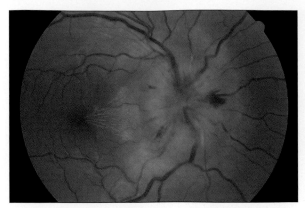

Cat scratch neuroretinitis

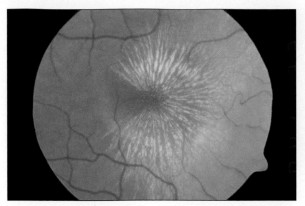

Cat scratch neuroretinitis. (Photograph courtesy Gary Miller, CRA.)

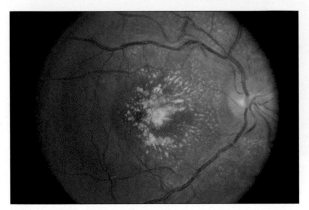

Hypertensive retinopathy

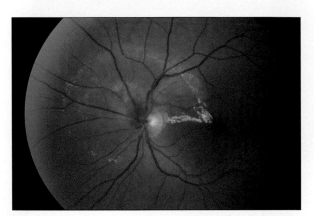

Optic disc capillary hemangioma

Clinical Features

The association of optic disc edema and macular star has been classified as neuroretinitis or Leber's idiopathic stellate neuroretinitis. Patients present with varying degrees of unilateral visual loss; often the visual loss is preceded by a flu-like illness characterized by fevers and lymphadenopathy. Examination reveals an afferent pupillary defect and mild vitritis. Most patients demonstrate optic disc edema associated with fluid exudation from the optic disc through the foveal region. The macular star is formed by a radiating pattern of lipid and protein exudate extending from the optic disc. The star may be more prominent on the nasal aspect of the fovea (half star), and becomes more apparent as the fluid resorbs. The etiology of the star is unclear but most likely represents protein and lipid deposition in Henle's layer. It is important to recognize that the fluid in the macula is from the optic disc and not the result of primary retinal vascular abnormalities in the macula.

Differential Diagnosis

Most cases of unilateral optic disc edema and macular star are related to cat scratch disease. Other conditions include hypertension, Lyme disease, syphilis, tuberculosis, toxoplasmosis, polyarteritis nodosa, capillary angiomas of the optic disc, and other causes of disc edema (pseudotumor cerebri, intracranial arteriovenous malformation). It is important to assess blood pressure before proceeding with laboratory investigation.

PERIPHERAL PIGMENTATION

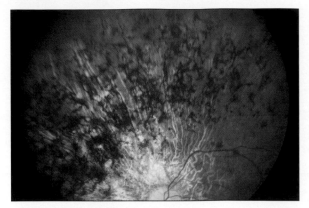

Retinitis pigmentosa

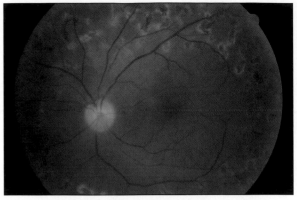

Diabetic retinopathy following laser photocoagulation

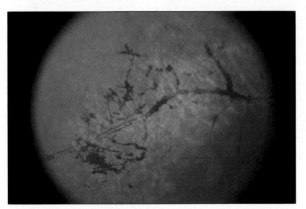

Lattice degeneration

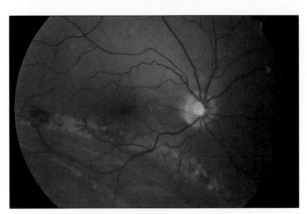

Chronic retinal detachment demarcation line

Clinical Features

Peripheral pigmentation of the fundus may take on a variety of appearances. The most common pigmentary patterns are linear, granular, reticular, clumps, or bone spicule formation.

Differential Diagnosis

Pigmentary clumps and lines are commonly seen within areas of lattice degeneration. In retinitis pigmentosa, a branching or "bone spicule" pattern of peripheral pigmentation develops due to the migration of retinal pigment epithelial pigment along the retinal blood vessels. The pattern of pigment deposition in retinitis pigmentosa typically begins in the midperipheral retina and may be quite subtle on presentation. Midperipheral retinal pigment is also seen in senile reticular pigmentary degeneration, a benign condition that is associated with

peripheral drusen and age-related macular degeneration. Most prominent in the nasal periphery, senile reticular pigmentary degeneration appears as a pigmentary pattern of clumps or branches.

Long-standing subretinal fluid from a chronic rhegmatogenous retinal detachment can cause peripheral pigment to accumulate along the line of detached and attached retina (a demarcation line). Chronic subretinal fluid from an exudative process such as idiopathic central serous chorioretinopathy can, because of gravity, cause a flask-shaped pattern of intraretinal pigment migration in the inferior macula.

Other less common causes of peripheral pigmentation include chloroquine toxicity, Stargardt disease, and pigmented paravenous retinochoroidal atrophy.

PIGMENT EPITHELIAL DETACHMENT

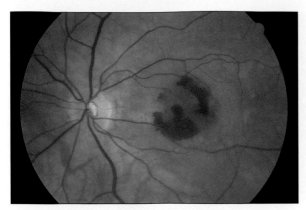

Age-related macular degeneration

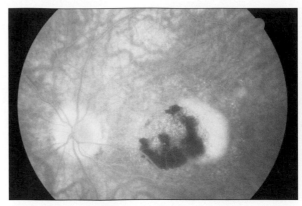

Age-related macular degeneration (fluorescein angiogram)

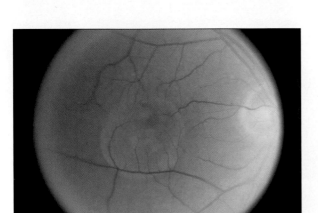

Central serous chorioretinopathy

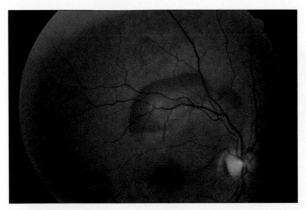

Polypoidal choroidal vasculopathy

Clinical Features

The fundamental clinical feature of a pigment epithelial detachment (PED) is an oval or round elevation of the retinal pigment epithelium (RPE). The elevation is often quite subtle and may be seen only with stereoscopic examination of the macula. The three major types of PEDs—fibrovascular, hemorrhagic, and serous—are named according to the material that is primarily elevating the RPE.

Differential Diagnosis

A fibrovascular PED, a form of occult choroidal neovascularization (CNV), is an area of irregular elevation of the RPE. The fluorescein angiographic features of a fibrovascular PED include stippled hyperfluorescence in the midphase of the angiogram with late leakage or staining. A fibrovascular PED commonly occurs due to choroidal bleeding from occult CNV. A hemorrhagic PED is dark red or gray and, in patients with age-related macular degeneration (AMD), may have drusen on its surface. The differential diagnosis includes idiopathic

polypoidal choroidal vasculopathy or posterior uveal bleeding syndrome. On the fluorescein angiogram, complete hypofluorescence corresponds to the area of hemorrhagic RPE detachment.

Serous PEDs may be seen in AMD and are frequently associated with CNV. On examination, the serous PED appears as a translucent elevation of the RPE with a smooth or dome-shaped surface. In a serous PED, the choroidal pattern is no longer visible and the fluorescein angiographic features consist of uniform filling of dye and persistent pooling of fluorescein throughout the angiogram. Serous pigment epithelial detachments are seen in other conditions, most notably idiopathic central serous chorioretinopathy (ICSC). In ICSC, the serous PED is small and may be masked by the overlying subretinal fluid.

The differential diagnosis of pigment epithelial detachments includes choroidal hemangioma, choroidal melanoma, and subretinal fluid.

PIGMENTED LESIONS

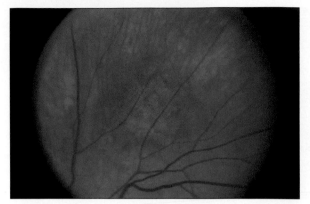

Choroidal nevus

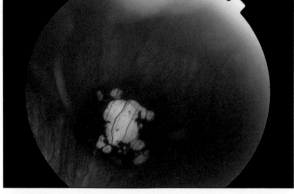

Congenital hypertrophy of the retinal pigment epithelium

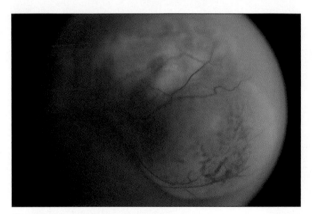

Choroidal melanoma

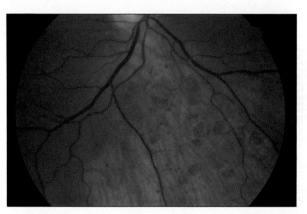

Bear tracks

Clinical Features

Pigmented lesions originating in the retina are typically black with distinct borders. Pigmented lesions originating in the choroid or retinal pigment epithelium (RPE) tend to be gray with less distinct borders.

Differential Diagnosis

The most common pigmented lesion of the choroid, the choroidal nevus, has certain characteristics: it is flat, round or oval, and dark gray. A nevus may vary from a few hundred micrometers to several disc diameters in size. Older nevi often have drusen on the surface and are surrounded by a halo of atrophy. Malignant melanomas are elevated, pigmented lesions of the choroid. Experts in the field of ocular oncology consider certain clinical features highly suggestive of a melanoma, including greater tumor thickness, orange pigment of the surface of the tumor, the absence of drusen, and the presence of subretinal fluid. A rare pigmented tumor of the uveal tract is bilateral diffuse uveal melanocytic proliferation,

a paraneoplastic syndrome consisting of multiple flat pigmented choroidal lesions.

Pigmented lesions may arise from the RPE. Congenital hypertrophy of the RPE (CHRPE), a benign condition typically seen in the mid to far periphery, is characterized by a circular area of heavy pigmentation with a scalloped pattern of atrophy developing in its center. The presence of multiple CHRPE-like lesions has been associated with Gardner's syndrome (familial polyposis). A black sunburst in sickle cell retinopathy represents a solitary lesion of hyperplastic RPE in an area of regressed subretinal hemorrhage. A similar lesion, RPE hyperplasia, can occur after photocoagulation in the macula. A less pigmented tumor, the combined hamartoma of the RPE and retina, typically has a fine, light gray color on its surface and may involve the optic disc.

Pigmentary lesions of the retina may be solitary or appear in clusters. Melanocytomas are solid, benign, dark black tumors often located on or near the optic disc. In grouped pigmentation of the retina, or "bear tracks pigmentation," clusters of circular or oval lesions of varying sizes are found in the retina, in either the macula or the periphery.

PRERETINAL HEMORRHAGE

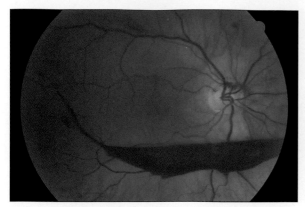

Diabetic retinopathy

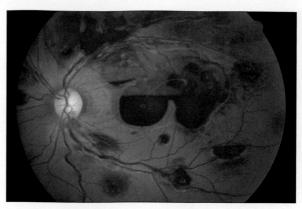

Leukemic retinopathy

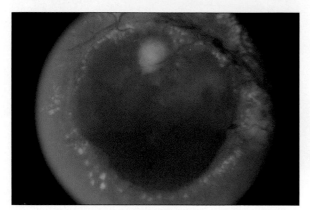

Retinal arterial macroaneurysm

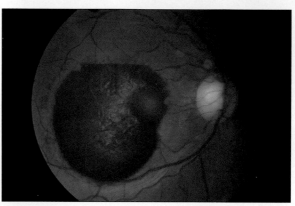

Valsalva retinopathy

Clinical Features

Preretinal hemorrhage is blood anterior to the retina but posterior to the posterior hyaloid of the vitreous. Preretinal hemorrhage typically appears bright red and obscures the retinal blood vessels beneath it. Preretinal hemorrhage often assumes a boat-shaped appearance.

Differential Diagnosis

Proliferative diabetic retinopathy and other proliferative retinopathies are common causes of preretinal hemorrhage. When a partial vitreous detachment in the macula occurs in patients with diabetes, the preretinal or "subhyaloid" hemorrhage takes on a crescent or boat-shaped appearance. In conditions in which the posterior vitreous remains firmly attached throughout the macula, such as in Valsalva retinopathy, the preretinal hemorrhage is often more solid in appearance. In arteriolar macro-aneurysms, the preretinal hemorrhage typically lies in front of intraretinal and subretinal blood.

In Terson's syndrome, blood is trapped between the internal limiting membrane and the neurosensory retina, forming a dome-shaped area of hemorrhage. Over time, the red blood cells may settle to the inferior portion of the dome, creating a red blood cell-serous fluid level. Sub-internal limiting membrane hemorrhage may accompany subhyaloid hemorrhage in Valsalva retinopathy, airbag injuries, trauma, and shaken baby syndrome. Patients with severe leukemia may present with preretinal blood in addition to intraretinal hemorrhage.

Although the exact cause of the hemorrhage is unknown, it is postulated that a certain level of anemia and thrombocytopenia is responsible for the hemorrhages.

RETINAL CRYSTALS

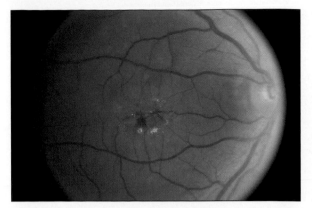

Idiopathic juxtafoval retinal telangiectasis

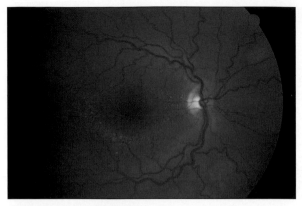

Canthaxanthin retinopathy

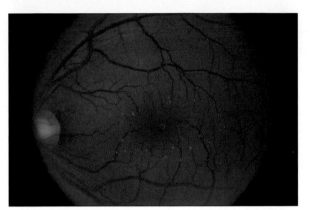

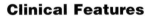
Talc retinopathy

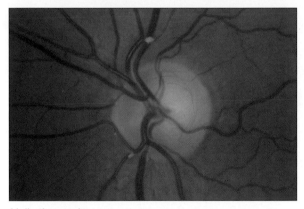

Hollenhorst plaques

Clinical Features

Retinal crystals are small, refractile deposits that are typically found in the inner retina. Because the composition of retinal crystals varies, crystals may appear white, yellow, or gold.

Differential Diagnosis

Retinal crystals can be seen in a number of conditions: degenerative disorders such as idiopathic juxtafoveal retinal telangiectasis; hereditary disorders such as cystinosis, hyperoxaluria, and Bietti's crystalline dystrophy; and toxic retinopathies from such agents as tamoxifen, canthaxanthin, and talc.

In idiopathic juxtafoveolar retinal telangiectasis (IJRT), crystals may be deposited in the inner retina, and are clustered near but not directly under the fovea. In nephropathic cystinosis, an autosomal recessive storage disorder of excess cystine, yellow crystals are deposited in the choroid and retinal pigment epithelium (RPE). In patients with primary and secondary hyperoxaluria,

calcium oxalate crystals are found in the retina and RPE and may form a striking periarterial pattern. The hallmark of Bietti's crystalline tapetoretinal dystrophy is hundreds of retinal crystals scattered throughout the posterior pole.

Breast cancer patients who are treated with high doses of tamoxifen, a nonsteroidal antiestrogen, may have white crystals deposited in the superficial retina. Most commonly found temporal to the fovea, these refractile deposits are thought to represent axonal degeneration. Multiple bright, golden crystals distributed in an oval ring around the fovea are characteristic of canthaxanthin retinopathy. In addition, shiny white deposits within retinal arterioles may be seen in talc retinopathy (talc emboli) and atherosclerotic heart disease (Hollenhorst plaques).

The differential diagnosis of retinal crystals also includes Sjögren-Larsson syndrome, gyrate atrophy, and an idiopathic finding. Refractile deposits can be seen in conditions in which significant retinal atrophy is present, such as chronic retinal detachment, inactive cytomegalovirus infection, or calcified drusen.

RETINAL NEOVASCULARIZATION

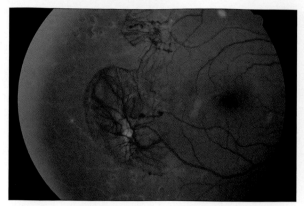

Diabetic retinopathy

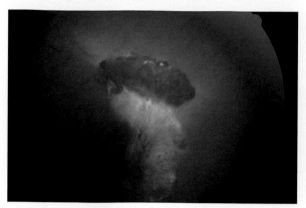

Sickle cell retinopathy

Clinical Features

Neovascularization of the retina begins in the plane between the internal limiting membrane of the retina and the posterior hyaloid of the vitreous. The most common locations for retinal neovascularization are (1) along the vascular arcades and the optic disc (the areas of greatest adherence between the vitreous and the retina) and (2) at the border of perfused and nonperfused retina. The new vessels may form a wheel or frond but may also grow linearly along the retinal surface without forming a network. A hallmark of retinal neovascularization is that the abnormal new vessels can cross both retinal arterioles and veins.

Differential Diagnosis

Retinal neovascularization may be observed in a variety of retinal vascular diseases, inflammatory diseases, and hereditary disorders.

Proliferative diabetic retinopathy is the most common cause of retinal neovascularization. In proliferative diabetic retinopathy, neovascularization of the retina is flat and is usually observed overlying retinal veins. With vitreous contraction, the fronds may become elevated.

Radiation retinopathy can produce retinal neovascularization that is indistinguishable from diabetic new vessels. Vascular occlusive conditions, such as ischemic vein or artery occlusions, may produce retinal neovascularization due to widespread retinal ischemia. The "sea fan" pattern of sickle cell retinopathy forms in the midperipheral retina at the junction of ischemic and nonischemic retina. In retinopathy of prematurity, retinal new vessels form behind the leading edge of the developing retina and may become an elevated ridge of neovascularization. Retinal embolization and leukemia have been associated with neovascularization.

Eales' disease is a chronic inflammatory condition in which anterior or peripheral new vessels may be accompanied by chronic phlebitis and peripheral ischemia. In some conditions, such as sarcoidosis and pars planitis, neovascularization develops as a result of inflammation rather than ischemia.

Retinal neovascularization may be observed in Norrie's disease, incontinentia pigmenti, and familial exudative vitreoretinopathy.

Other conditions simulating retinal neovascularization include shunt vessels on the disc or retina, intraretinal microvascular abnormalities, and retinal angiomas.

RETINITIS

Clinical Features

Necrotizing retinitis typically gives the retina a thickened, opaque appearance, which looks white, yellow, or gray. The area of retinal inflammation may be focal or multifocal, and the borders of the retinitis are generally indistinct. In immunocompetent patients, vitreous cells are found overlying the area of retinitis; in immunocompromised patients, vitreous cells may be absent. Hemorrhage within or at the border of the retinitis is common.

Differential Diagnosis

Retinitis may be focal or multifocal. The differential diagnosis of focal retinitis includes septic embolus, fungal chorioretinitis, toxoplasmosis, and toxocariasis. In a patient with a septic embolus, an area of retinal necrosis may be creamy white, with hemorrhages and cotton wool spots. Candidal chorioretinitis in its early stage appears as a small, white, well-circumscribed lesion in the posterior pole. Toxoplasmosis is a gray-white chorioretinitis adjacent to a pigmented, or partially pigmented, scar that can occur anywhere in the fundus. Toxocariasis, a more difficult diagnosis to make, typically begins in the periphery.

In certain types of multifocal retinitis, such as cat-scratch disease, idiopathic neuroretinitis, multifocal choroiditis, and diffuse unilateral subacute neuroretinitis, the retinitis is characterized by multiple, small intraretinal infiltrates (area less than one-third disc diameter) and may be accompanied by optic disc edema. Other causes of multifocal retinitis include cytomegalovirus retinitis (CMV), acute retinal necrosis, and syphilitic retinitis. Active CMV typically presents with a single area of hemorrhagic full-thickness necrosis in the midperipheral retina, with multiple, small satellite lesions at the border. Acute retinal necrosis, also a viral retinitis from the herpes family, is more likely to present in the peripheral retina, with white plaque-like lesions accompanied by an arteritis (hemorrhage along the arterioles) and vitritis. Less common is the posterior form of acute retinal necrosis, posterior outer retinal necrosis syndrome, which presents with multiple posterior pole lesions and little vitreous inflammation. Syphilitic retinitis may present as patches of gray or white outer retinal infiltrates in the posterior pole or as a multifocal neuroretinitis.

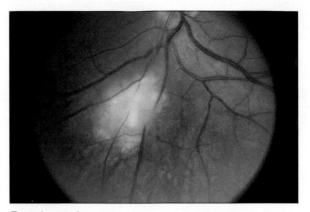

Toxoplasmosis

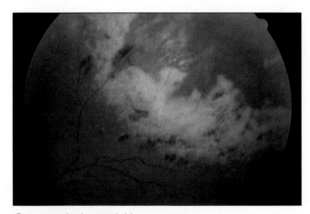

Cytomegalovirus retinitis

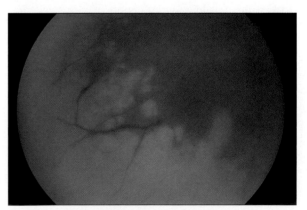

Acute retinal necrosis

RUBEOSIS

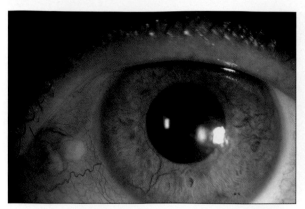

Advanced rubeosis

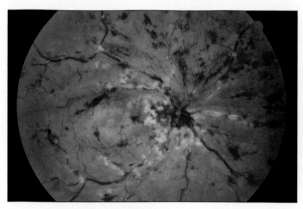

Central retinal vein occlusion

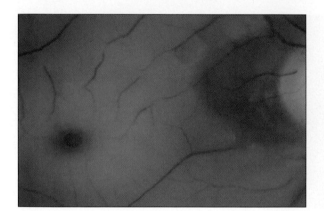

Central retinal artery occlusion

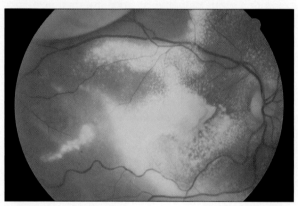

Coat's disease

Clinical Features

Rubeosis is the development of abnormal blood vessels on the surface of the iris as a result of widespread retinal ischemia. The vessels may develop at the pupillary margin where they appear initially as small red buds. As the rubeosis develops, fine blood vessels are seen crossing the iris stroma. Advanced rubeosis consists of larger-caliber vessels and may lead to hyphema. Rubeotic vessels may also form in the angle and are seen as fine red lines crossing the trabecular meshwork. Although rubeosis progresses in the majority of patients, the rubeosis along the pupillary margin may not change over months or years. The main complication of rubeosis is neovascular glaucoma. Frank neovascular glaucoma is characterized by conjunctival injection, corneal edema, anterior chamber cell and flare, iris neovascularization, angle neovascularization with peripheral anterior synechiae, and marked intraocular pressure elevation.

Rubeosis is best visualized during an undilated slit lamp examination of the iris and anterior chamber angle. In a patient in whom rubeosis is suspected, the angle must be examined by gonioscopy as well.

Differential Diagnosis

Patients who develop rubeosis typically have some form of ocular ischemia, such as the ocular ischemic syndrome, retinal vascular disease, chronic retinal detachment, or untreated neoplasm. Ischemic retinal vascular syndromes causing rubeosis include proliferative diabetic retinopathy, radiation retinopathy, ischemic central retinal vein occlusion, central retinal artery occlusion, and end-stage Coat's syndrome. In most retinal vascular causes of ischemia, the development of rubeosis is generally an indication to perform prompt panretinal photocoagulation.

SUBRETINAL FLUID

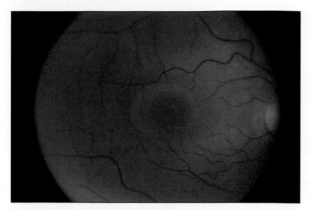

Central serous chorioretinopathy

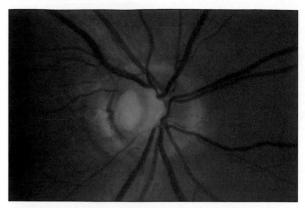

Optic pit

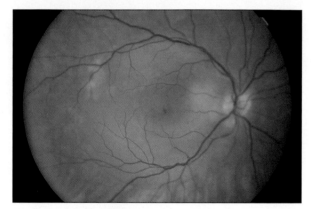

Toxemia of pregnancy

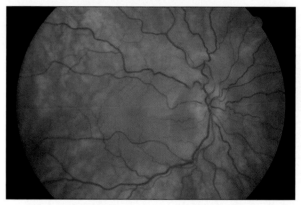

Uveal effusion syndrome

Clinical Features

Subretinal fluid is an accumulation of serous fluid in the subretinal space that forms a separation between the neurosensory retina and the underlying retinal pigment epithelium (RPE). The serous fluid is typically clear, although the choroidal pattern beneath it is somewhat obscured. If fibrin is present, subretinal fluid can be cloudy. The presence of subretinal fluid implies a disruption of the RPE-outer retinal barrier, a physiologic barrier that normally prevents fluid from entering the subretinal space.

Differential Diagnosis

Serous subretinal fluid is an important feature of exudative or neovascular age-related macular degeneration (AMD). In exudative AMD, leaky and abnormal choroidal new vessels grow into the subretinal pigment epithelial space and, as the overlying RPE decompensates, subretinal fluid forms. Subretinal fluid is also seen in idiopathic central serous chorioretinopathy (ICSC). In patients with severe or atypical ICSC, for example, those

patients who have received corticosteroids or who have undergone organ transplant, the subretinal fluid is gray or white. In Harada's disease, a diffuse granulomatous choroiditis, subretinal fluid in the macula is frequently a bilateral finding.

In patients with an optic nerve pit, subretinal fluid may extend in an oval shape from the rim of the optic disc into the macula. This condition is typically unilateral, and the diagnosis must include the identification of the optic pit. Severe hypertension may be a cause of peripapillary and macular subretinal fluid due to occlusion of choroidal arterioles and subsequent ischemic damage to the RPE. In the setting of pregnancy, toxemia may also cause choroidal occlusion and rapid RPE decompensation resulting in subretinal fluid. Both benign choroidal tumors, such as hemangiomas, and malignant tumors such as metastatic carcinoma, can cause breakdown of the RPE-outer retinal barrier leading to an accumulation of fluid in the subretinal space.

Conditions that may be mistaken for subretinal fluid include serous pigment epithelial detachment, intraretinal edema, and cystoid macular edema.

TUMORS

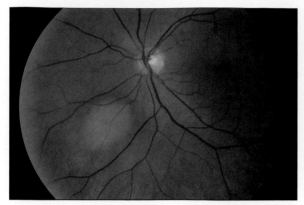

Choroidal metastasis

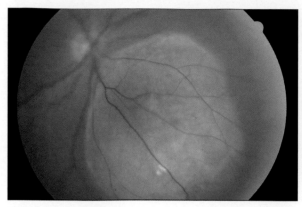

Choroidal melanoma

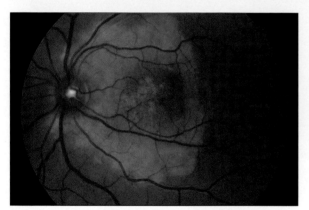

Choroidal osteoma

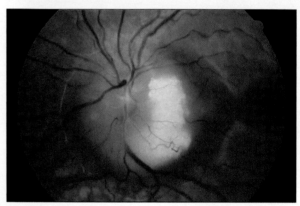

Astrocytic hamartoma (tuberous sclerosis)

Clinical Features

Benign and malignant tumors of the ocular fundus may arise from the uveal tract, retinal pigment epithelium (RPE), and retina. Tumors may present in a spectrum of sizes and colors.

Differential Diagnosis

Nonpigmented tumors of the choroid, such as choroidal hemangioma and metastatic carcinomas, typically appear as solid elevations of the choroid with some overlying subretinal fluid. Choroidal hemangiomas often have an orange-red appearance on presentation and may become yellow or cream colored over time. Metastatic tumors range in color from brown to cream to orange. A distinctive mottled yellow-white infiltration of the RPE is seen in primary ocular-central nervous system lymphomas. Initially, these RPE tumors have an irregular, elevated contour with a characteristic pattern of pigment on the surface. Osteomas are benign choroidal tumors that develop a cream color, most typically found in the peripapillary region. Malignant melanomas are typically elevated, dome-shaped, and pigmented tumors arising from the choroid. However, as many as 25% of melanomas are relatively amelanotic. The presence of lipofuscin (an orange pigment) on the tumor surface and of subretinal fluid often indicates tumor growth.

Although RPE tumors are rare, the combined RPE and retinal hamartoma has a gray, granular appearance that often has an epiretinal membrane on its surface. This benign tumor is difficult to diagnose.

Retinal tumors such as retinoblastoma, retinocytoma, and astrocytic hamartoma may appear white or gray. Vascular tumors such as capillary angiomas in Von Hippel-Lindau disease are red if endophytic or projecting into the retina, and may be associated with large feeding and draining vessels. Typically, cavernous hemangiomas of the retina consist of multiple, deep red clusters of small aneurysmal tumors.

VASCULITIS

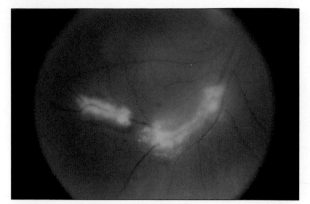

Sarcoidosis

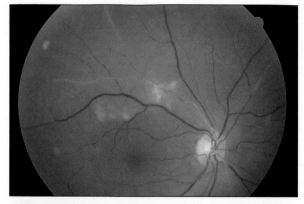

Behçet's disease

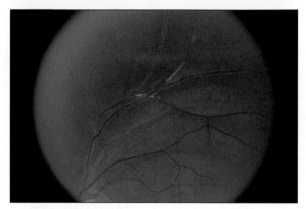

Systemic lupus erythematosus

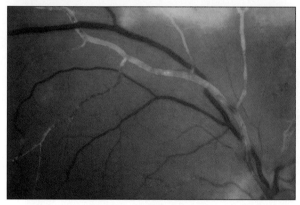

Cytomegalovirus retinitis with frosted branch angiitis

Clinical Features

Vasculitis consists of inflammation of retinal veins (phlebitis) or arterioles (arteritis). The clinical hallmark of retinal phlebitis or arteritis is a sheathing of the involved vessels, which is typically white, gray, or yellow. This vascular sheathing may be quite subtle or absent on biomicroscopy, but is seen as staining or leakage from the retinal vessels on fluorescein angiography. It is not unusual for the angiographic findings of vascular staining and leaking to be more prominent than the biomicroscopic features. Intraretinal hemorrhages may accompany the distribution of the vasculitis.

Retinal vasculitis may be observed as a primary ocular disease or in association with a variety of systemic and infectious conditions. Individuals may be asymptomatic or complain of visual loss, scotoma, and floaters (when the retinal vasculitis is associated with vitritis or vitreous hemorrhage). Pain and redness may be present in those individuals with anterior segment inflammation. Visual loss may be the result of cystoid macular edema, retinal ischemia, and vitreous hemorrhage in eyes with widespread capillary nonperfusion and neovascularization.

Massive perivascular infiltrates can be seen in frosted branch angiitis, a self-limited condition initially described in healthy, young individuals. A similar clinical picture has been reported in immunocompromised patients with cytomegalovirus (CMV) retinitis and

lymphoma. This outpouring of exudate is thought to be secondary to an immune response.

Differential Diagnosis

Vasculitis associated with systemic disease includes sarcoidosis, Behçet's disease, Wegener's granulomatosis, systemic lupus erythematosus, polyarteritis nodosa, inflammatory bowel disease, and multiple sclerosis. Many infectious diseases are associated with retinal vasculitis. These include toxoplasmosis, syphilis, Lyme disease, toxocariasis, tuberculosis, CMV retinitis, and acute retinal necrosis. Primary ocular diseases include birdshot choroidopathy, Eale's disease, and frosted branch angiitis.

Vasculitides that primarily affect retinal veins include sarcoidosis, pars planitis, Eale's disease, and frosted branch angiitis. A number of conditions may affect both arteries and veins such as syphilitic chorioretinitis, Behçet's disease, and primary vasculitis. Behçet's disease may be associated with retinal infiltrates, branch retinal vein occlusions, and vitritis. Those conditions involving primarily the retinal arterioles include toxoplasmosis, acute retinal necrosis, idiopathic branch retinal artery occlusion syndrome, systemic lupus erythematosus, polyarteritis, and Wegener's granulomatosis.

The differential diagnosis of vasculitis includes lipemia retinalis, occluded vessels in retinal vein occlusion, and perivascular sheathing (presumably lipid) in patients with diabetic retinopathy.

VITELLIFORM LESIONS

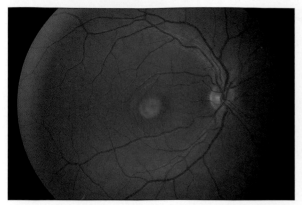

Best's disease

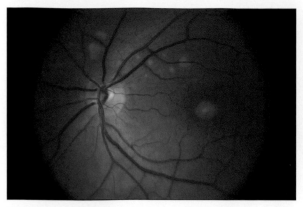

Multifocal Best's disease

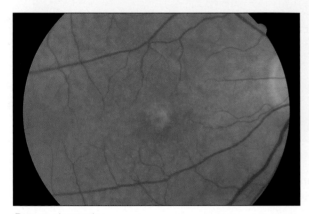

Pattern dystrophy

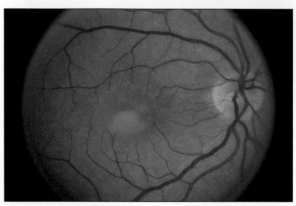

Basal laminar drusen

Clinical Features

Vitelliform, or yellow, lesions in the macula may be single or multiple. Vitelliform lesions refer to deposits of yellow material in the outer retina or retina pigment epithelium (RPE).

Differential Diagnosis

The differential diagnosis of vitelliform lesions includes Best's disease, pattern dystrophy, or basal laminar drusen. In Best's disease, a macular dystrophy, the characteristic round, "sunny side up" egg yolk lesion is a unifocal and bilateral finding. Over several years, the yellow material may settle out of the RPE cells and layer into a "pseudohypopyon" under the retina. The yellow pigment will eventually form a patchy or "scrambled" pattern and eventually leave an area of RPE disruption. The presence of a reduced Arden ratio on the electro-oculogram (EOG) and a positive family history confirm

the diagnosis of Best's disease. Multifocal vitelliform lesions may be seen in Best's disease and in patients with normal EOG findings and no family history.

Multifocal vitelliform macular lesions accompanied by more extensive pigmentary changes on the fluorescein angiogram may signal a pattern dystrophy. These dystrophies appear in adulthood and are often autosomal dominant in inheritance. Pattern dystrophies have a great variety of appearances. The foveomacular dystrophy group, for example, has yellow flecks in the center of the macula and has a vitelliform appearance.

In patients with cuticular or basal laminar drusen, yellow subretinal material may accumulate under the macula in an appearance quite similar to Best's disease. This vitelliform exudation may or may not be associated with underlying choroidal new vessels and can be quite chronic.

Other conditions that may simulate vitelliform lesions include stage 1 macular holes, early cystoid macular edema, hard exudates, and drusen.

VITREOUS HEMORRHAGE

Clinical Features

Vitreous hemorrhage, or red blood cells in the vitreous cavity, may be evenly dispersed or form clumps of cells. Hemorrhage in the formed vitreous initially appears red and, over a period of months, changes in color from red to pink to white. Because of gravity, vitreous hemorrhage tends to be denser inferiorly. The density of blood in the vitreous directly affects visual acuity, which can range from 20/20 to no light perception. A subhyaloid hemorrhage, blood that is trapped between the posterior vitreous surface and inner retina, is more solid and may have a linear or boat-shaped appearance. As the vitreous detaches from the macula, the subhyaloid blood appears more liquid and can move freely under the formed vitreous.

Differential Diagnosis

A common cause of vitreous hemorrhage is posterior vitreous detachment (PVD). At the time of a PVD, the vitreous traction can pull on a retinal blood vessel, creating a vitreous hemorrhage. If the vitreous traction also causes a retinal tear, the torn retinal tissue may bleed into the vitreous cavity. Recurrent vitreous hemorrhage may be due to a bridging vessel between the retinal tear and underlying attached retina. A similar phenomenon may occur in patients with X-linked juvenile retinoschisis. Diabetic retinopathy is a common cause of vitreous hemorrhage. A vitreous hemorrhage in someone with diabetes is presumed to result from neovascularization of the optic disc or retina until proved otherwise. Vitreous hemorrhage following panretinal photocoagulation may be related to persistent neovascularization or vitreous traction on fibrovascular tissue. Other vascular diseases associated with retinal ischemia and neovascularization/vitreous hemorrhage include branch retinal vein occlusion, sickle cell retinopathy, radiation retinopathy, retinal embolization, and leukemia. Inflammatory disorders with vitreous hemorrhage include Eales' disease, pars planitis, sarcoidosis, and systemic lupus erythematosus.

Rarely, exudative age-related macular degeneration may be associated with vitreous hemorrhage. This hemorrhage is the result of "breakthrough bleeding" as subretinal blood moves from the subretinal space into the vitreous.

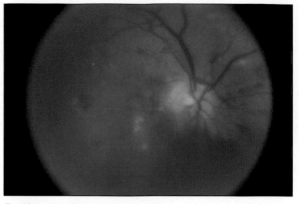
Proliferative diabetic retinopathy

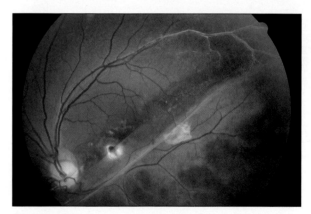
Retinoschisis

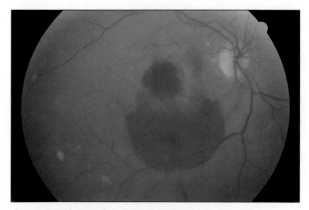
Age-related macular degeneration

VITREOUS OPACITY

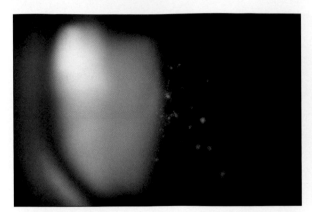

Normal vitreous opacities

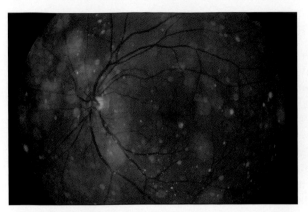

Asteroid hyalosis

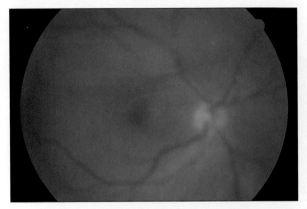

Vitritis (toxoplasmosis)

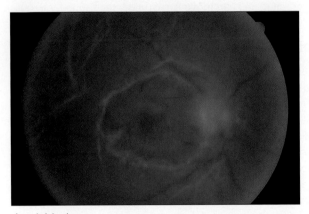

Amyloidosis

Clinical Features

Nonhemorrhagic vitreous opacities may be due to condensed vitreous, white blood cells, tumor cells, or pigment cells. Large strands of vitreous opacities may represent condensation of the vitreous or vitreous degeneration.

Differential Diagnosis

A commonly seen vitreous opacity is a ring of condensed vitreous, a Weiss ring, noted in front of the optic nerve. This Weiss ring is the hallmark of a posterior vitreous detachment (PVD). In addition, a PVD is accompanied by syneresis, or vitreous contraction, which appears as faint vitreous strands or veils.

Vitritis, or white cells in the vitreous, signals inflammation and possibly infection. In intermediate uveitis, such as pars planitis, vitritis is most prominent in the anterior vitreous. In posterior uveitis. such as multifocal choroiditis, cells are initially seen in the posterior vitreous. Chronic inflammation leads to larger clusters of cells. Early bacterial endophthalmitis is characterized by fine cells in the vitreous, while the clinical feature

suggestive of fungal endophthalmitis is white spheres in the vitreous (described as "cotton balls") that may be found overlying a chorioretinal abscess.

Clumps of pigment in the vitreous provide clinical suspicion of a retinal tear or detachment. Red blood cells in the vitreous may be due to a retinal tear, trauma, preretinal neovascularization, or subretinal blood that has diffused into the vitreous cavity. Old blood appears white and may be confused with an inflammatory or neoplastic process. Asteroid hyalosis is a common, benign, degenerative condition in which many yellow-white spheres of calcium soaps are seen in the center of the vitreous. Asteroid hyalosis is unilateral in 90% of cases. In amyloidosis, white amyloid material forms cobweb-like opacities in the vitreous and may, if dense, obscure vision.

Clusters of small, white preretinal nodules can be seen in the inferior vitreous cavity in sarcoidosis. A similar type of vitreous opacity is common in pars planitis, in which preretinal "snowballs" form in front of the peripheral retina or pars plana. White tumor cells in the vitreous (identified by vitreous biopsy) may be a presenting sign of ocular-central nervous system lymphoma, and brown tumor cells can be seen in cases of metastatic cutaneous melanoma.

WHITE DOT SYNDROMES

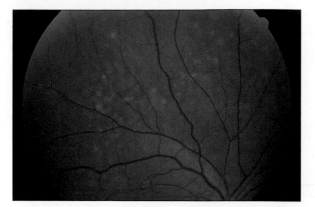

Multiple evanescent white dot syndrome

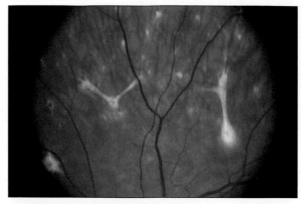

Multifocal choroiditis

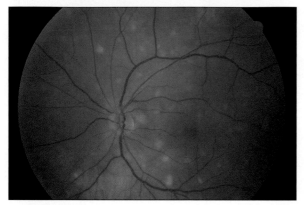

Sarcoidosis

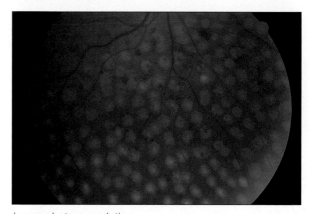

Laser photocoagulation

Clinical Features

The white dot syndromes are a group of disorders characterized by multiple whitish yellow inflammatory lesions located at the level of the retinal pigment epithelium (RPE) and choroid. Symptoms associated with the inflammatory white dot syndromes include blurred vision, visual field loss (blind spot enlargement), photopsias, nyctalopia, and floaters.

The majority of individuals with white dot syndromes are younger than 50 years, with the exception of birdshot chorioretinitis and serpiginous choroiditis, which may affect middle-aged and older adults. Multiple evanescent white dot syndrome (MEWDS), birdshot chorioretinopathy, and multifocal choroiditis with panuveitis are more commonly observed in women. The white dot syndromes may be unilateral or bilateral, depending on the etiology.

Vitritis is usually mild except in cases of birdshot chorioretinopathy and multifocal choroiditis with panuveitis. The white dots may be subtle or prominent, depending on the condition. For example, MEWDS is characterized by faint white dots located in the mid-

peripheral or posterior fundus, whereas multifocal choroiditis with panuveitis is notable for more prominent inflammatory lesions. The white dot lesions may be discrete (MEWDS, multifocal choroiditis, birdshot chorioretinopathy, diffuse unilateral subacute neuroretinitis [DUSN]) or more placoid in appearance (acute posterior multifocal placoid pigment epitheliopathy [APMPPE] and serpiginous choroiditis).

Differential Diagnosis

The classic white dot syndromes include APMPPE, MEWDS, multifocal choroiditis with panuveitis, DUSN, serpiginous choroiditis, and birdshot chorioretinopathy. Other conditions associated with white dot lesions include sarcoidosis, ocular lymphoma, presumed ocular histoplasmosis syndrome, *Pneumocystis* choroidopathy, Behçet's disease, toxoplasmosis, sympathetic ophthalmia, tuberculosis, and syphilis.

Noninflammatory white dot lesions include drusen, Stargardt disease, and other fleck retinal dystrophies, fundus albipunctatus, and early laser photocoagulation burns.

WHITE-CENTERED RETINAL HEMORRHAGES

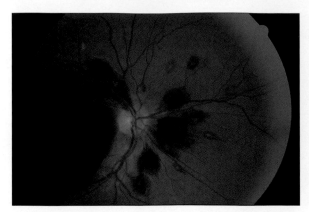

Leukemic retinopathy

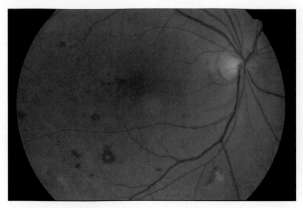

Diabetic retinopathy

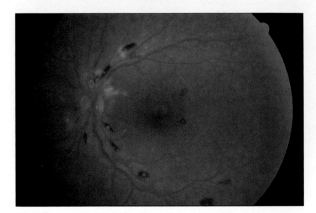

Human immunodeficiency virus retinopathy

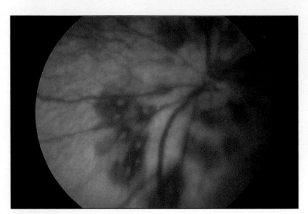

Shaken baby syndrome

Clinical Features

White-centered retinal hemorrhages (Roth spots) were historically described as septic emboli in patients with subacute bacterial endocarditis. However, evidence suggests that they are nonspecific and may be found in a variety of disease states.

Most patients are asymptomatic or have visual loss related to the underlying disease process. White-centered retinal hemorrhages may be isolated or more numerous, depending on the association.

White-centered hemorrhages most likely result from localized capillary rupture from any anoxic insult or sudden elevation in venous pressure. The white center is a fibrin platelet aggregate that results during the physiologic healing process. Previous theories concerning the etiology of the white center have included bacterial infiltrates producing microabscesses (subacute bacterial endocarditis) and collections of abnormal white blood cells (leukemia).

Differential Diagnosis

The differential diagnosis for white-centered retinal hemorrhages is broad. The most common underlying factors are anemia and thrombocytopenia. Conditions in which white-centered hemorrhages have been described include subacute bacterial endocarditis, leukemia, diabetic retinopathy, hypertensive retinopathy, human immunodeficiency virus (HIV) retinopathy, toxoplasmosis, shaken baby syndrome, childbirth, intracranial hemorrhage, anoxia, and carbon monoxide poisoning.

It is important to note that anemia is a common association of subacute bacterial endocarditis, leukemia, and HIV/acquired immunodeficiency syndrome. Anemia may be the underlying factor that links this diverse group of conditions.

TABLE 1

Clinical Features of Retinal Disease

	Bull's Eye Maculopathy	Cherry Red Spot	Choroiretinal Folds
Macular Diseases	Age-Related Macular Degeneration		Age-Related Macular Degeneration
	Macular Hole (chronic)		Hypotony Maculopathy
	Pattern Dystrophy		Idiopathic Chorioretinal Folds
			Posterior Microphthalmos
Retinal Vascular Diseases		Central Retinal Artery Occlusion	
Hereditary Disorders	Stargardt Disease	Tay-Sachs Disease	
	Cone Dystrophy	Niemann-Pick Disease	
	Retinitis Pigmentosa	Cherry Red Spot Myoclonus	
	Fenestrated Sheen Macular Dystrophy		
	Concentric Annular Macular Dystrophy		
Drug Toxicities	Chloroquine/ Hydroxychloroquine	Gentamicin Toxicity	
	Fomivirsen		
Inflammatory Diseases	Acute Macular Neuroretinopathy		Posterior Scleritis
	UAIM		
Tumors			
Trauma	Commotio Retinae		
Peripheral Retinal Diseases			
Vitreous			
Other			Papilledema
			Optic Disc Drusen
			Retrobulbar Tumor

continued

TABLE 1

Clinical Features of Retinal Disease (cont'd)

	Choroidal Neovascularization	Cotton Wool Spot	Cystoid Macular Edema
Macular Diseases	Age-Related Macular Degeneration Myopia Angioid Streaks Pattern Dystrophy Polypoidal Choroidal Vasculopathy Idiopathic		Age-Related Macular Degeneration Post-Intraocular Surgery CME Epiretinal Membrane Vitreoretinal Traction Syndrome Hypotony Maculopathy
Retinal Vascular Diseases		Diabetic Retinopathy Hypertensive Retinopathy Retinal Vascular Occlusions Leukemic Retinopathy Radiation Retinopathy Anemia Bone Marrow Transplantation	Diabetic Retinopathy Branch Retinal Vein Occlusion Central Retinal Vein Occlusion
Hereditary Disorders	Best's Disease Stargardt Disease Gyrate Atrophy Retinitis Pigmentosa		Retinitis Pigmentosa X-Linked Juvenile Retinoschisis
Drug Toxicities		Interferon Toxicity	Latanoprost-related CME Nicotinic Acid Maculopathy Epinephrine Reaction
Inflammatory Diseases	POHS Multifocal Choroiditis Serpiginous Choroiditis	HIV Retinopathy CMV Retinopathy Systemic Lupus Erythematosus Behçet's Disease Giant Cell Arteritis Polyarteritis Nodosa Cat Scratch Disease	Birdshot Chorioretinopathy Intermediate Uveitis Idiopathic Vitritis
Tumors	Choroidal Nevus Choroidal Osteoma		Choroidal Melanoma
Trauma	Choroidal Rupture	Purtscher's Retinopathy Blunt Trauma	
Peripheral Retinal Diseases			Chronic Retinal Detachment
Vitreous			
Other	Laser Photocoagulation Optic Disc Drusen		

TABLE 1

Clinical Features of Retinal Disease (cont'd)

	Drusen	Flecked Retina Syndromes	Foveal Yellow Spot
Macular Diseases	Age-Related Macular Degeneration		Macular Hole, Stage I Central Serous Chorioretinopathy Choroidal Neovascularization Cystoid Macular Edema Pattern Dystrophy Solar Retinopathy Age-Related Macular Degeneration (Drusen)
Retinal Vascular Diseases			Diabetic Retinopathy Toxemia of Pregnancy Branch Retinal Vein Occlusion Central Retinal Vein Occlusion
Hereditary Disorders	North Carolina Macular Dystrophy Dominant Drusen	Stargardt Disease Fundus Albipunctatus Flecked Retina of Kandori Retinitis Punctata Albescens Alport's Syndrome	
Drug Toxicities		Crystalline Retinopathies	
Inflammatory Diseases			
Tumors	Choroidal Nevus		
Trauma			
Peripheral Retinal Diseases			Uveal Effusion Syndrome
Vitreous			
Other	Type II Glomerulonephritis		

continued

TABLE 1

Clinical Features of Retinal Disease (cont'd)

	Intraretinal Hemorrhages	Lipid Exudates	Macular Atrophy
Macular Diseases		Age-Related Macular Degeneration Chronic Central Serous Chorioretinopathy	Age-Related Macular Degeneration Angioid Streaks Central Serous Chorioretinopathy Myopic Degeneration Chronic CME Macular Phototoxicity Pattern Dystrophy
Retinal Vascular Diseases	Diabetic Retinopathy Hypertensive Retinopathy Branch Retinal Vein Occlusion Central Retinal Vein Occlusion Leukemic Retinopathy Radiation Retinopathy Anemia Ocular Ischemic Syndrome Retinal Arterial Macroaneurysm Sickle Cell Retinopathy Bone Marrow Transplantation High-altitude Sickness	Diabetic Retinopathy Hypertensive Retinopathy Branch Retinal Vein Occlusion Central Retinal Vein Occlusion Juxtafoveal Retinal Telangiectasis Radiation Retinopathy Retinal Arterial Macroaneurysm Coat's Disease	

TABLE 1

Clinical Features of Retinal Disease (cont'd)

	Intraretinal Hemorrhages	Lipid Exudates	Macular Atrophy
Hereditary Disorders		Retinitis Pigmentosa	Stargardt Disease
			Best's Disease
			North Carolina Macular Dystrophy
			Sorsby's Macular Dystrophy
			Choroideremia
			Gyrate Atrophy
			Cone Dystrophy
			Rod-Cone Degeneration
Drug Toxicities	Intraocular Gentamicin		Chloroquine/ Hydroxychloroquine
Inflammatory Diseases	HIV Retinopathy		POHS
	CMV Retinitis		Toxoplasmosis
	Sarcoidosis		Multifocal Choroiditis
	Behçet's Disease		Serpiginous Choroiditis
Tumors		Choroidal Melanoma	
		Retinal Capillary Hemangioma	
Trauma	Blunt Trauma	Chronic Retinal Detachment	Commotio Retinae
	Shaken Baby Syndrome		Choroidal Rupture
	Valsalva Retinopathy		
	Terson's Syndrome		
	Purtscher's Retinopathy		
Peripheral Retinal Diseases	Vitreoretinal Traction Syndrome		Retinal Detachment
	Retinal Tear/Detachment		
Vitreous	Posterior Vitreous Detachment		
Other			Laser Photocoagulation

continued

TABLE 1

Clinical Features of Retinal Disease (cont'd)

	Optic Disc Edema with Macular Star	Peripheral Pigmentation	Pigment Epithelial Detachment
Macular Diseases		Central Serous Chorioretinopathy	Age-Related Macular Degeneration Central Serous Chorioretinopathy Polypoidal Choroidal Vasculopathy
Retinal Vascular Diseases	Hypertensive Retinopathy		
Hereditary Disorders		Retinitis Pigmentosa Stargardt Disease Pigmented Paravenous Retinochoroidal	
Drug Toxicities		Chloroquine Toxicity Siderosis	
Inflammatory Diseases	Cat Scratch Disease Toxoplasmosis Lyme Disease Syphilis Tuberculosis Polyarteritis Nodosa	DUSN Viral Retinitis	
Tumors	Optic Disc Capillary Hemangiomas	BDUMP	
Trauma		Commotio Retinae Choroidal Rupture	
Peripheral Retinal Diseases		Choroidal Effusion (late) Chronic Retinal Detachment Reticular Pigmentary Degeneration Lattice Degeneration	
Vitreous			
Other	Papilledema Optic Neuropathy	Scatter Laser Photocoagulation	

TABLE 1
Clinical Features of Retinal Disease (cont'd)

	Pigmented Lesions	Preretinal Hemorrhage	Retinal Crystals
Macular Diseases			
Retinal Vascular Diseases	Juxtafoveal Retinal Telangiectasis Sickle Cell Retinopathy (Black Sunburst)	Diabetic Retinopathy Branch Retinal Vein Occlusion Sickle Cell Retinopathy Leukemic Retinopathy Retinal Arterial Macroaneurysm	Juxtafoveal Retinal Telangiectasis Sickle Cell Retinopathy
Hereditary Disorders		X-Linked Juvenile Retinoschisis	Bietti's Crystalline Retinal Dystrophy Cystinosis Hyperoxaluria
Drug Toxicities			Tamoxifen Toxicity Canthaxanthine Toxicity Talc Retinopathy
Inflammatory Diseases	Toxoplasmosis (inactive scar)		
Tumors	Choroidal Nevus Choroidal Melanoma CHRPE Bear Tracks Melanocytoma		
Trauma		Terson's Syndrome Valsalva Retinopathy Shaken Baby Syndrome	
Peripheral Retinal Diseases		Retinal Tear	
Vitreous		Posterior Vitreous Detachment	
Other			

continued

TABLE 1

Clinical Features of Retinal Disease (cont'd)

	Retinal Neovascularization	Retinitis	Rubeosis
Macular Diseases			
Retinal Vascular Diseases	Diabetic Retinopathy		Diabetic Retinopathy
	Branch Retinal Vein Occlusion		Central Retinal Artery Occlusion
	Radiation Retinopathy		Central Retinal Vein Occlusion
	Sickle Cell Retinopathy		Ocular Ischemic Syndrome
	Retinopathy of Prematurity		Coat's Disease
	Leukemic Retinopathy		Radiation Retinopathy
	FEVR		Retinopathy of Prematurity
			Eale's Disease
Hereditary Disorders	Norrie's Disease		
	Incontinentia Pigmenti		
Drug Toxicities	Talc Retinopathy		
Inflammatory Diseases	Eale's Disease	Toxoplasmosis	
	Pars Planitis	CMV Retinitis	
	Sarcoidosis	HSV Retinitis	
		Acute Retinal Necrosis	
		PORN	
		Cat Scratch Disease	
		Toxocariasis	
		Syphilis	
		Fungal Chorioretinitis	
		Behçet's Disease	
Tumors			Retinoblastoma
			Choroidal Melanoma
Trauma			
Peripheral Retinal Diseases	Chronic Retinal Detachment		Chronic Retinal Detachment
Vitreous		CNS Lymphoma	
Other			

TABLE 1

Clinical Features of Retinal Disease (cont'd)

	Subretinal Fluid	Vasculitis	Vitelliform Lesions
Macular Diseases	Age-Related Macular Degeneration		Age-Related Macular Degeneration
	Central Serous Chorioretinopathy		Pattern Dystrophies
Retinal Vascular Diseases	Coat's Disease	Eale's Disease	
	Toxemia of Pregnancy	Ocular Ischemic Syndrome	
Hereditary Disorders			Best's Disease
Drug Toxicities			
Inflammatory Diseases	Vogt-Koyanagi-Harada Syndrome	Behçet's Disease	
	Posterior Scleritis	Sarcoidosis	
		Systemic Lupus Erythematosus	
		Pars Planitis/ Multiple Sclerosis	
		Toxoplasmosis	
		Syphilis	
		Tuberculosis	
		Viral Retinitis/ARN	
		Toxocariasis	
		Birdshot Chorioretinopathy	
		Lyme Disease	
		Leukemic/Lymphoma	
		Frosted Branch Angiitis	
Tumors	Choroidal Melanoma		
	Choroidal Hemangioma		
	Choroidal Metastasis		
Trauma			
Peripheral Retinal Diseases			
Vitreous		Idiopathic Vitritis	
		CNS Lymphoma	
Other	Optic Pit		

continued

TABLE 1

Clinical Features of Retinal Disease (cont'd)

	Vitreous Hemorrhage	White-Centered Hemorrhages	White Dot Syndromes
Macular Diseases	Age-Related Macular Degeneration		Drusen
Retinal Vascular Diseases	Diabetic Retinopathy	Diabetic Retinopathy	
	Branch Retinal Vein Occlusion		
	Sickle Cell Retinopathy	Leukemic Retinopathy	
	Leukemic Retinopathy	Hypertensive Retinopathy	
	Retinal Arterial Macroaneurysm	Anemia	
	Eale's Disease		
	Coat's Disease		
	Peripapillary Arterial Loops		
	Retinopathy of Prematurity		
Hereditary Disorders	X-Linked Juvenile Retinoschisis		Stargardt Disease
			Fundus Albipunctatus
			Retinitis Punctata Albescens
			Flecked Retina of Kandori
Drug Toxicities			

TABLE 1

Clinical Features of Retinal Disease (cont'd)

	Vitreous Hemorrhage	White-Centered Hemorrhages	White Dot Syndromes
Inflammatory Diseases	Sarcoidosis Pars Planitis	HIV Retinopathy *Candida* Endophthalmitis Toxoplasmosis	APMPPE MEWDS DUSN Multifocal Choroiditis Serpiginous Choroiditis Birdshot Chorioretinitis Sarcoidosis Histoplasmosis Pneumocystis Choroidopathy Behçet's Disease Toxoplasmosis Sympathetic Ophthalmia Syphilis
Tumors			
Trauma	Terson's Syndrome Shaken Baby Syndrome Optic Disc Evulsion	Shaken Baby Syndrome Childbirth	
Peripheral Retinal Diseases	Retinal Tear/Detachment		
Vitreous	Posterior Vitreous Detachment		Lymphoma
Other		Subacute Bacterial Endocarditis Intracranial Hemorrhage Carbon Monoxide Poisoning/Anoxia	Laser Photocoagulation

continued

SELECTED REFERENCES

Bull's Eye Maculopathy

1. Kempen JH. Drug-induced maculopathy. *Int Ophthalmol Clin.* 1999;39:67–82.
2. Stone TW, Jaffe GJ. Reversible bull's-eye maculopathy associated with intravitreal fomivirsen therapy for cytomegalovirus retinitis. *Am J Ophthalmol.* 2000;130:242–243.

Cherry Red Spot

1. Brown GC, Eagle RC, Shakin EP, Gruber M, Arbizio VV. Retinal toxicity of intravitreal gentamicin. *Arch Ophthalmol.* 1990;108:1740–1744.
2. Brady RO. Ophthalmologic aspects of lipid storage diseases. *Ophthalmology.* 1978;85:1007–1013.
3. Federico A, Battistini S, Ciacci G, de Stefano N, Gatti R, Durand P, et al. Cherry-red spot myoclonus syndrome (type I sialidosis). *Dev Neurosci.* 1991;13:320–326.

Chorioretinal Folds

1. Cohen SM, Gass JD. Bilateral radial chorioretinal folds. *Int Ophthalmol.* 1994;18:243–245.
2. Leahey AB, Brucker AJ, Wyszynski RE, Shaman P. Chorioretinal folds. A comparison of unilateral and bilateral cases. *Arch Ophthalmol.* 1993;111:357–359.

Choroidal Neovascularization

1. Campochiaro PA, Soloway P, Ryan SJ, Miller JW. The pathogenesis of choroidal neovascular neovascularization in patients with age related macular degeneration. *Mol Vis.* 1999;5:34.
2. Cohen SY, Laroche A, Leguen Y, Soubrane G, Coscas GJ. Etiology of choroidal neovascularization in young patients. *Ophthalmology.* 1996;103:1241–1244.
3. Marano F, Deutman AF, Leys A, Aandekerk AL. Hereditary retinal dystrophies and choroidal neovascularization. *Graefes Arch Clin Exp Ophthalmol.* 2000;238:760–764.

Cotton Wool Spot

1. Brown GC, Brown MM, Hiller T. Cotton wool spots. *Retina.* 1985;5:206–214.
2. McLeod D, Kohner EM. Cotton wool spots and giant cell arteritis. *Ophthalmology.* 1996;103:701–702.
3. Shami MJ, Uy RN. Isolated cotton wool spots in a 67-year-old woman. *Surv Ophthalmol.* 1996;40(5):413–415.

Cystoid Macular Edema

1. Gass JDM, Norton EWD. Cystoid macular edema and papilledema following cataract extraction: a fluorescein funduscopic and angiographic study. *Arch Ophthalmol.* 1966;76:646–661.
2. Rossetti L, Autelitano A. Cystoid macular edema following cataract surgery. *Curr Opin Ophthalmol.* 2000;11:65–72.
3. Schumer RA, Camras CB, Mandahl AK. Latanoprost and cystoid macular edema: Is there a causal relation? *Curr Opin Ophthalmol.* 2000;11:94–100.

Drusen

1. Abdelsalam A, Del Priore L, Zarbin MA. Drusen in age-related macular degeneration: pathogenesis, natural course, and laser photocoagulation-induced regression. *Surv Ophthalmol.* 1999;44:1–29.
2. Bressler NM. Clinicopathologic correlation of drusen and retinal pigment epithelial abnormalities in age-related macular degeneration. *Retina.* 1994;14:130–142.

Flecked Retina Syndromes

1. Armstrong JD, Meyer D, Xu S, Elfervig JL. Long-term follow-up of Stargardt's disease and fundus flavimaculatus. *Ophthalmology.* 1998;105:448–457.

Foveal Yellow Spot

1. Gass JD. Reappraisal of biomicroscopic classification of stages of development of a macular hole. *Am J Ophthalmol.* 1995;119:752–759.

Intraretinal Hemorrhages

1. Kivlin JD, Simons KB, Lazoritz S, Ruttum MS. Shaken baby syndrome. Ophthalmology. 2000;107:1246–1254.
2. Yu T, Mitchell P, Berry G, Li W, Wang JJ. Retinopathy in older persons without diabetes and its relationship to hypertension. *Arch Ophthalmol.* 1998;116:83–89.

Lipid Exudates

1. Chew EY. Diabetic retinopathy and lipid abnormalities. *Curr Opin Ophthalmol.* 1997;8:59–62.
2. Duker JS, Jalkh AE. Lipid exudates in age-related macular degeneration. *Am J Ophthalmol.* 1993;116:140–147.

Macular Atrophy

1. Marmor MF, McNamara JA. Pattern dystrophy of the retinal pigment epithelium and geographic atrophy of the macula. *Am J Ophthalmol.* 1996;122:382–392.
2. Sunness JS, Gonzalez-Baron J, Applegate CA, Bressler NM, Tian Y, Hawkins B, et al. Enlargement of atrophy and visual acuity loss in the geographic atrophy form of age-related macular degeneration. *Ophthalmology.* 1999;106:1768–1779.

Macular Disc Edema with Macular Star

1. Dreyer, RF, Hopen, G, Gass, JD, Smith, JL. Leber's idiopathic stellate neuroretinitis. *Arch Ophthalmol.* 1984;102:1140–1145.

2. Ormerod, LD, Dailey, JP. Ocular manifestations of cat-scratch disease. *Curr Opin Ophthalmol.* 1999;10:209–216.

3. Solley WA, Martin DF, Newman NJ, King R, Callanan DG, Zacchei T, et al. Cat scratch disease: posterior segment manifestations. *Ophthalmology.* 1999;106:1546–1553.

Peripheral Pigmentation

1. Bastek JV, Siegel EB, Straatsma BR, Foos RY. Chorioretinal juncture. Pigmentary patterns of the peripheral fundus. *Ophthalmology.* 1982;89(12):1455–1463.

2. Gass JDM. *Stereoscopic Atlas of Macular Diseases: Diagnosis and Treatment,* 4th ed. St. Louis: Mosby, Inc; 76–77.

Pigment Epithelial Detachment

1. Macular Photocoagulation Study Group. Subfoveal neovascular lesions in age-related macular degeneration: Guidelines for evaluation and treatment in the Macular Photocoagulation Study. *Arch Ophthalmol.* 1991;109:1242–1257.

2. Tornambe, PE. Treatment of retinal pigment epithelial detachments. *Ann Ophthalmol.* 1984;16:884–886.

Pigmented Lesions

1. Shields GL, Shields JA, Kiratli H, De Potter P, Cater JR. Risk factors for growth and metastasis of small choroidal melanocytic lesions. *Ophthalmology.* 1995;102:1351–1361.

2. Tiret A, Parc, C. Fundus lesions of adenomatous polyposis. *Curr Opin Ophthalmol.* 1999;10:168–172.

Preretinal Hemorrhage

1. Guyer DR, Schachat AP, Vitale S, Markowitz JA, Braine H, Burke PJ, et al. Leukemia retinopathy: relationship between fundus lesions and hematologic parameters at diagnosis. *Ophthalmology.* 1989;96:860–864.

Retinal Crystals

1. Kaiser-Kupfer MI, Kupfer C, Rodrigues MM. Tamoxifen retinopathy: a clinicopathologic report. *Ophthalmology.* 1981;88:89–93.

2. Moisseiev J, Lewis H, Bartov E, Fine SL, Murphy RP. Superficial retinal refractile deposits in juxtafoveal telangiectasis. *Am J Ophthalmol.* 1990;109:604–605.

Retinal Neovascularization

1. Jampol LM, Goldbaum MH. Peripheral proliferative retinopathies. *Surv Ophthalmol.* 1980;25:1–14.

2. Kinyoun JL, Lawrence BS, Barlow WE. Proliferative radiation retinopathy. *Arch Ophthalmol.* 1996;114:1097–1100.

Retinitis

1. Forster DJ, Dugel PU, Frangieh GT. Rapidly progressive outer necrosis in the acquired immune deficiency syndrome. *Am J Ophthalmol.* 1990;110:341–348.

2. Walters G, James TE. Viral causes of the acute retinal necrosis syndrome. *Curr Opin Ophthalmol.* 2001;12:191–195.

Rubeosis

1. Brown GC, Magargal LE. The ocular ischemic syndrome: clinical, fluorescein angiographic and carotid angiographic features. *Int Ophthalmol.* 1988;11:239–251.

2. Sivak-Callcott JA, O'Day DM, Gass JDM, et al. Evidence-based recommendations for the diagnosis and treatment of neovascular glaucoma. *Opthalmology.* 2001;108:1767–1778.

Subretinal Fluid

1. Gass JDM, Little HL. Bullous retinal detachment and multiple retinal pigment epithelial detachments in patients receiving hemodialysis. *Ophthalmology.* 1995;75:810–821.

Tumors

1. Collaborative Ocular Melanoma Study Report No. 5. Factors predictive of growth and treatment of small choroidal melanoma. *Arch Ophthalmol.* 1997;115:1537–1544.

Vasculitis

1. Graham EM, Stanford MR, Whitcup SM. Retinal vasculitis. In: Prepose JS, Holland GN, Wilhemus KR, eds. *Ocular Infection and Immunity.* St. Louis: Mosby-Year Book Inc; 1996:538–551.

2. Stanford MR, Verity DH. Diagnostic and therapeutic approach to patients with retinal vasculitis. *Int Ophthalmol Clin.* 2000;40:69–83.

Vitelliform Lesions

1. Dubovy SR, Hairston RJ, Schatz H, et al. Adult-onset foveomacular pigment epithelial dystrophy: clinicopathologic correlation of three cases. *Retina.* 2000;20:638–649.

2. Gass JDM. Autosomal dominant pattern dystrophies of the pigment epithelium. In: Gass JDM. *Stereoscopic Atlas of Macular Diseases: Diagnosis and Treatment.* St Louis: Mosby-Year Book, Inc; 1997:314–325.

Vitreous Hemorrhage

1. Davis, M. Vitreous contraction in proliferative retinopathy. *Arch Ophthalmol.* 1965;74:741–751.

Vitreous Opacity

1. Akiba J, Ishiko S, Yoshida A. Variations of Weiss's ring. *Retina.* 2001;21:243–246.

2. Gill MK, Jampol LM. Variations in the presentation of primary intraocular lymphoma: case reports and a review. *Surv Ophthalmol.* 2001;45:463–471.

3. Moss SE, Klein R, Klein BE. Asteroid hyalosis in a population: the Beaver Dam eye study. *Am J Ophthalmol.* 2001;132:70–75.

White Dot Syndromes

1. Brown J Jr, Folk JC. Current controversies in the white dot syndromes. Multifocal choroiditis, punctate inner choroidopathy, and the diffuse subretinal fibrosis syndrome. *Ocul Immunol Inflamm.* 1998;6:125–127.

2. Polk TD, Goldman EJ. White dot chorioretinal inflammatory syndromes. *Int Ophthalmol Clin.* 1999;39:33–53.

3. Shah GK, Kleiner RC, Augsburger JJ, Gill MK, Jampol LM. Primary intraocular lymphoma seen with transient white fundus lesions simulating the multiple evanescent white dot syndrome. *Arch Ophthalmol.* 2001;119:617–620.

White-Centered Retinal Hemorrhages

1. Duane TD, Osher RH, Green WR. White-centered hemorrhages: their significance. *Ophthalmology.* 1980;87:66–69.

2. Ling R, James B. White-centered retinal hemorrhages (Roth spots). *Postgrad Med J.* 1998;74:581–582.

chapter 4

Macular Diseases

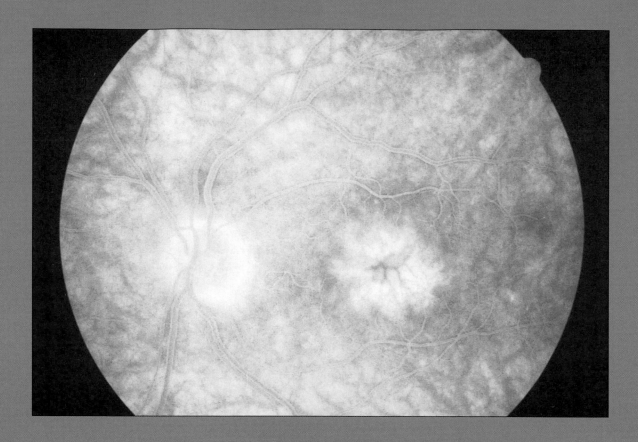

T. Mark Johnson, MD

Mark W. Johnson, MD

AGE-RELATED MACULAR DEGENERATION: NONEXUDATIVE

Age-related macular degeneration (AMD) is the leading cause of legal blindness in people aged 65 years or older in the United States. Approximately 90% of individuals with AMD have the nonexudative or "dry" form of the disease. Types of nonexudative AMD include drusen, retinal pigment epithelial alterations, and geographic atrophy. Risk factors for AMD include age, family history of AMD, and cardiovascular factors including hypertension and a history of cigarette smoking.

Symptoms

The majority of people with nonexudative AMD are asymptomatic. Individuals with drusen may complain of mild distortion or visual loss. Individuals with more extensive retinal pigment epithelial alterations or geographic atrophy complain of difficulty reading or recognizing details, and have paracentral or central scotomas. Visual loss associated with geographic atrophy is slow; abrupt changes in vision suggest the possibility of choroidal neovascularization (CNV).

Clinical Features

The characteristic finding in AMD is drusen. Drusen are small, discrete yellowish white deposits. They are observed most commonly in the macula but may be found in every area of the fundus. Drusen tend to be bilateral and symmetric. Several types of drusen have been observed: hard, soft, calcified, and basal laminar/cuticular (see "Drusen" in Chapter 3). Retinal pigment epithelial (RPE) alterations include atrophy and hyperpigmentation. Geographic atrophy is characterized by well-demarcated round or oval patches of atrophy in the parafoveal/foveal region. The atrophic patches may enlarge or coalesce over years. In general, the center of the fovea is involved late in the disease process.

Ancillary Testing

Fluorescein angiography may be performed to examine for evidence of CNV or progression of geographic atrophy. This evaluation is particularly important for patients with sudden alterations in vision. Drusen appear as focal areas of hyperfluorescence that are not associated with late leakage. Geographic atrophy demonstrates a classic transmission or "window" defect as a result of RPE loss.

Pathology/Pathogenesis

Drusen are localized deposits found between the basement membrane of the RPE and the remainder of Bruch's membrane. Two types of deposits have been identified: basal laminar and basal linear. Basal laminar deposit is composed of wide-spaced collagen located between the plasma membrane and the basement membrane of the RPE. Basal linear deposit consists of granular and vesicular, electron-dense, lipid-rich material located external to the basement membrane of the RPE in the inner collagenous zone of Bruch's membrane. Geographic atrophy is characterized by well-demarcated areas of RPE atrophy with sclerosis of the underlying choriocapillaris.

The pathogenesis of AMD is not completely understood. Twin and family studies suggest genetics may have a significant influence on the development and progression of AMD. Alterations in choroidal blood flow also may play a role.

Treatment/Prognosis

There is no known treatment for nonexudative AMD. The Age-Related Eye Disease Study (AREDS) demonstrated a reduction in the progression of AMD in patients taking zinc, beta-carotene, vitamin C, and vitamin E. Laser-induced drusen reduction is associated with improved visual acuity and contrast sensitivity in eyes at 1 year. The long-term effects of laser-induced drusen reduction on visual function require additional observation, and several studies are investigating the role of grid laser treatment for the prevention of CNV in patients with drusen.

The majority of individuals with nonexudative AMD do very well with excellent visual function. Visual loss is the result of progressive geographic atrophy or CNV. The estimated risk for the development of CNV in patients with bilateral drusen is 10% to 15% over 5 years. Clinical features associated with an increased risk of CNV are soft drusen, areas of focal hyperpigmentation, and CNV in the fellow eye.

Systemic Evaluation

Age-related macular degeneration may be associated with cardiovascular risk factors including hypertension and a history of cigarette smoking. A general physical examination and smoking cessation are strongly recommended.

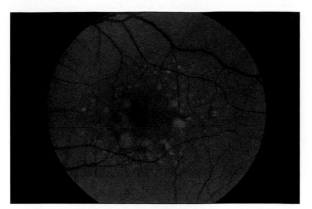

A variety of different types of drusen may be observed in patients with age-related macular degeneration. "Soft" drusen are larger, yellowish deposits with slightly ill-defined borders. "Hard" drusen are small, discrete deposits located at the level of the retinal pigment epithelium.

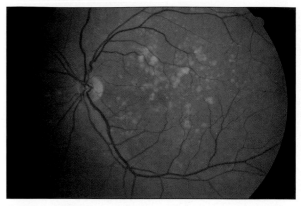

Patients with drusen are usually asymptomatic; rarely, patients may complain of reduced or distorted vision.

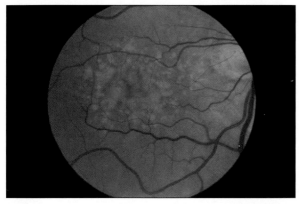

The risk of developing exudative age-related macular degeneration is greater in patients with soft, confluent drusen and focal areas of hyperpigmentation.

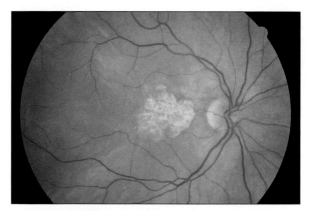

Geographic atrophy is responsible for most cases of visual loss in patients with nonexudative age-related macular degeneration. The atrophic patches may enlarge or coalesce over years. In general, the center of the fovea is involved late in the disease process.

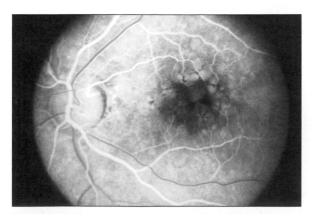

Early-phase fluorescein angiogram of a patient with age-related macular degeneration demonstrates variable hyperfluorescence of the soft drusen.

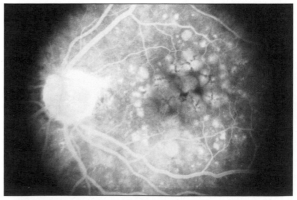

Late-phase fluorescein angiogram of the same patient in the previous figure reveals late staining of the drusen material. Note the linear streaks of hypofluorescence corresponding to areas of focal hyperpigmentation.

AGE-RELATED MACULAR DEGENERATION: NONEXUDATIVE (CONT'D)

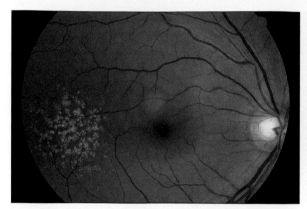

This patient has numerous hard drusen located in the temporal macula of each eye. Hard drusen have not been associated with an increased risk of choroidal neovascularization.

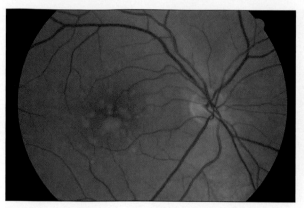

This patient has a few soft, confluent drusen located near the fovea. She was asymptomatic.

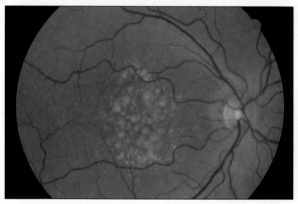

Over time, soft drusen may coalesce to form larger deposits, simulating a pigment epithelial detachment. Patients may experience a hyperopic shift in their refractive error.

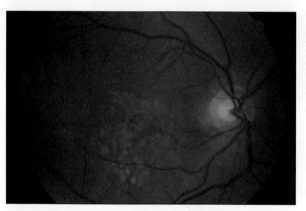

This 64-year-old man had numerous soft drusen with areas of focal hyperpigmentation. He subsequently experienced visual loss related to the development of occult choroidal neovascularization.

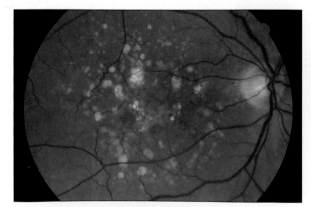

Calcific drusen are usually observed in the setting of geographic atrophy. Calcific drusen are highly refractile and represent dystrophic calcification of the drusen material.

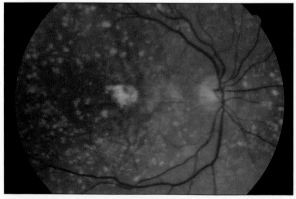

This 90-year-old man had visual loss related to age-related macular degeneration with geographic atrophy. Note the presence of calcific drusen. Also note the absence of drusen in the region of atrophy.

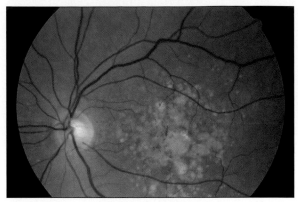

This pair of fundus photographs demonstrates the progression of age-related macular degeneration. Note the soft, coalescent drusen.

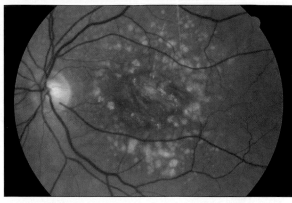

Over a 5-year period, the macular degeneration progresses with the development of geographic atrophy and calcific drusen.

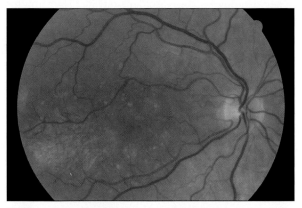

This patient had age-related macular degeneration with geographic atrophy that was most notable in the temporal macula.

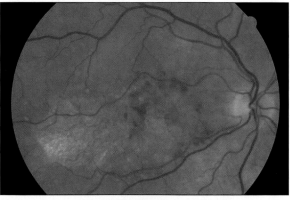

Three years later, the same patient presented with sudden vision loss. The patient had subretinal blood and fluid consistent with choroidal neovascularization. Approximately 20% of patients with geographic atrophy develop choroidal neovascularization.

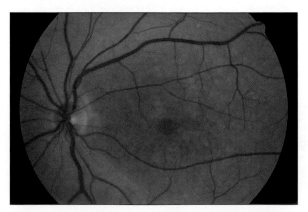

The extent of geographic atrophy is unclear on this fundus photograph of a 68-year-old woman with age-related macular degeneration.

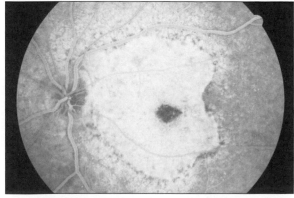

A fluorescein angiogram of the same patient highlights the transmission or "window" defect corresponding to the extensive area of retinal pigment epithelial atrophy.

AGE-RELATED MACULAR DEGENERATION: EXUDATIVE

Age-related macular degeneration (AMD) is the leading cause of legal blindness in people 65 years of age or older in the United States. Approximately 10% of individuals with AMD have the exudative form of the disease. Exudative AMD accounts for the majority of cases of significant visual loss in AMD. Manifestations of exudative AMD may include choroidal neovascularization (CNV), pigment epithelial detachment (PED), retinal pigment epithelial tear, massive subretinal hemorrhage, fibrovascular scar formation, radiating chorioretinal folds, and vitreous hemorrhage.

Symptoms

Individuals with exudative AMD may complain of visual loss, metamorphopsia, scotoma, micropsia, photopsia, and formed hallucinations (Charles Bonnet syndrome). In cases of unilateral exudative AMD, symptoms include poor depth perception and the need to close the "bad" eye to see fine detail.

Clinical Features

Choroidal neovascularization appears as a grayish green lesion associated with subretinal fluid, subretinal hemorrhage, and/or lipid exudation. In many individuals, the most significant findings are subretinal fluid with or without subretinal hemorrhage. Serous PEDs are round or oval, sharply demarcated dome-shaped elevations of the retinal pigment epithelium (RPE). Additional complications of CNV include RPE tear, massive subretinal hemorrhage (usually in patients receiving anticoagulant therapy), radiating chorioretinal folds, and rarely vitreous hemorrhage. Ultimately, most individuals develop a fibrovascular scar in the macula.

Ancillary Testing

Fluorescein angiography is used to determine the type and location of the CNV. The type of CNV is divided into two categories: classic or occult. Classic CNV is characterized by a lacy vascular network with well-demarcated borders during the early phase of the angiogram followed by late leakage. Occult CNV includes fibrovascular PEDs that appear as poorly defined areas of hyperfluorescence early followed by late leakage, and late leakage of undetermined source. Location is defined in terms of the relationship of the CNV to the center of the fovea: extrafoveal (200 μm to 2500 μm), juxtafoveal (1 μm to 199 μm), and subfoveal (under the fovea).

Fluorescein angiography may help to distinguish a nonvascularized, serous PED (commonly seen in central serous chorioretinopathy) from a fibrovascular PED seen in AMD. Fluorescein angiographic features suggesting a fibrovascular PED include hot spots, notched PEDs, and an irregular filling pattern.

Indocyanine green (ICG) angiography may be considered for lesions associated with subretinal hemorrhage or PED in which the borders of CNV are not clearly defined. Patterns of ICG angiography in AMD include focal hot spots, plaques of hyperfluorescence, and combination lesions.

Pathology/Pathogenesis

Abnormalities in the RPE/Bruch's membrane complex allow capillaries from the choroidal circulation to gain access to the sub-RPE and subneurosensory retinal space. Neovascular proliferation is associated with the accumulation of subretinal fluid, blood, and exudate—ultimately leading to fibrovascular scarring. The stimulus for angiogenesis remains unknown.

Treatment/Prognosis

The Macular Photocoagulation Study (MPS) demonstrated the effectiveness of laser photocoagulation in reducing the risk of severe visual loss in eyes with CNV that meet the eligibility criteria. Treatment benefit was significant for extrafoveal, juxtafoveal, and subfoveal classic CNV membranes. Persistence and recurrence of CNV (greater than 50%) limit the long-term efficacy of laser treatment. Photodynamic therapy (PDT) has become the preferred treatment for patients with predominantly classic subfoveal CNV. Photodynamic therapy uses the light-activated dye verteporfin to obtain closure of the CNV without the associated retinal damage of traditional thermal laser. Unfortunately, the effects are temporary, and most patients require 4 to 6 treatments over the course of 2 years. No effective treatment has yet been developed for occult CNV.

Experimental therapies for exudative AMD include submacular surgery, macular translocation, feeder vessel photocoagulation, antiangiogenic drug therapy, and radiation therapy.

Systemic Evaluation

Age-related macular degeneration may be associated with cardiovascular risk factors including hypertension and a history of cigarette smoking. A general physical examination and smoking cessation are strongly recommended.

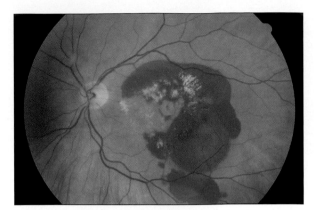

Exudative age-related macular degeneration is characterized by the presence of subretinal fluid, subretinal hemorrhage, and lipid exudate.

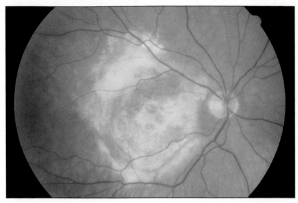

Over time, fibrovascular proliferation results in the development of a disciform scar in the macula.

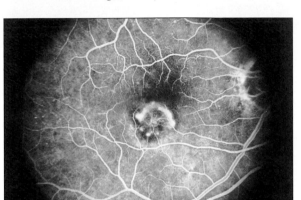

Exudative age-related macular degeneration is caused by the proliferation of new vessels from the choroidal circulation to the subretinal pigment epithelial and/or subneurosensory retinal space. Fluorescein angiogram of "classic" choroidal neovascularization shows a well-defined area of lacy hyperfluorescence in early view.

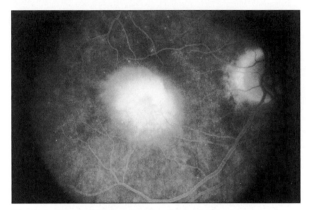

The late-phase angiogram is characterized by prominent hyperfluorescence as a result of leakage.

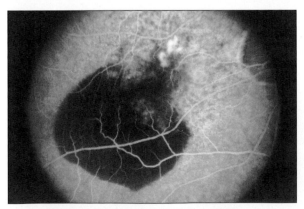

Occult choroidal neovascularization includes fibrovascular pigment epithelial detachments that appear as poorly defined areas of hyperfluorescence early followed by late leakage, and late leakage of undetermined source. The early phase of the fluorescein angiogram demonstrates blocking of fluorescence due to large subretinal hemorrhage.

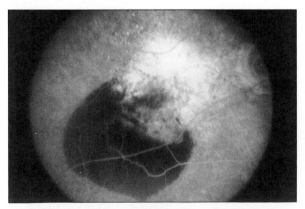

Superonasal to fovea is a small component of classic choroidal neovascularization (CNV). The late-phase angiogram demonstrates a larger area of poorly defined leakage consistent with a larger occult CNV.

AGE-RELATED MACULAR DEGENERATION: EXUDATIVE (CONT'D)

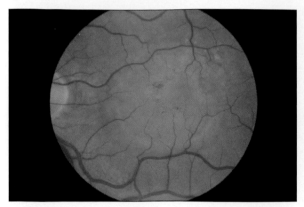

Pigment epithelial detachment is a well-defined, dome-shaped elevation of the retinal pigment epithelium. It results from fluid and blood accumulation between the RPE and Bruch's membrane.

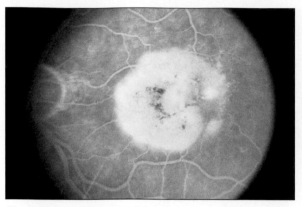

Fluorescein angiogram of the pigment epithelial detachment in the previous figure shows irregular fluorescein filling of the pigment epithelial detachment with an adjacent area of late leakage indicative of occult choroidal neovascularization.

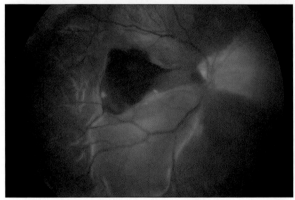

Massive subretinal hemorrhage may be seen in patients with exudative age-related macular degeneration. These patients often have a history of anticoagulation therapy. The prognosis for visual recovery is poor.

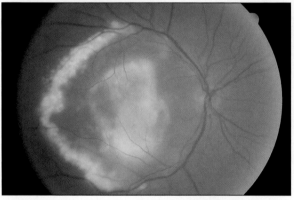

Exudative age-related macular degeneration with chronic choroidal neovascularization leakage may demonstrate a "Coats-like" response with massive lipid exudate surrounding the choroidal neovascularization complex.

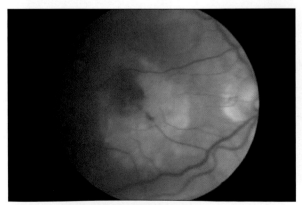

A retinal pigment epithelial tear or rip may occur spontaneously or following laser photocoagulation for choroidal neovascularization. Fundus examination reveals a round or oval region of retinal pigment epithelial atrophy adjacent to a region of "clumped up" retinal pigment epithelium.

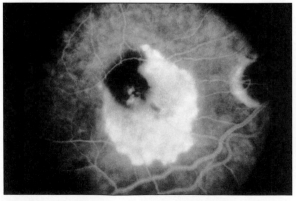

The fluorescein angiogram of the fundus picture in the previous figure demonstrates hyper- and hypofluorescence corresponding to the retinal pigment epithelial alterations.

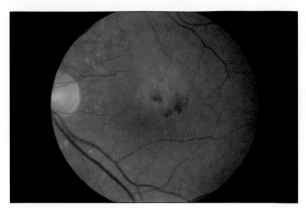

Laser photocoagulation may reduce the risk of visual loss related to exudative age-related macular degeneration. This 68-year-old woman presented with choroidal neovascularization in her left eye.

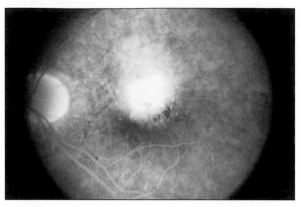

The fluorescein angiogram of the same patient revealed subfoveal classic choroidal neovascularization with late leakage.

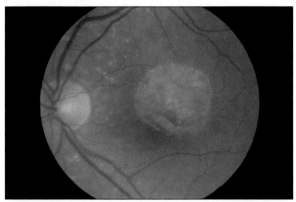

Laser photocoagulation was performed. This fundus photograph taken 6 weeks after laser photocoagulation reveals a well-demarcated area of atrophy in the treated area. The subretinal blood and fluid have resolved.

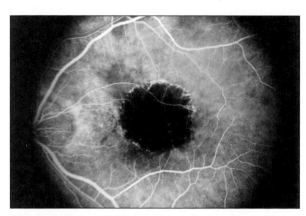

The fluorescein angiogram demonstrates hypofluorescence corresponding to the treated area.

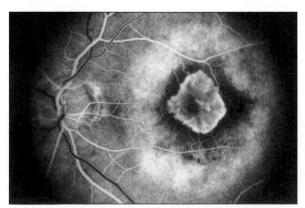

Photodynamic therapy with verteporfin has become the treatment of choice for subfoveal, classic choroidal neovascularization (CNV). This fluorescein angiogram reveals classic CNV before treatment.

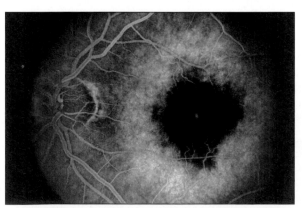

This fluorescein angiogram reveals the early effect of photodynamic therapy. Three weeks following treatment, marked hypofluorescence occurs as a result of closure of the choroidal neovascularization.

ANGIOID STREAKS

Angioid streaks are characteristic linear, narrow subretinal streaks that radiate from a peripapillary area to the macula and midperipheral fundus. Angioid streaks typically appear in the second decade and are usually bilateral. They may be associated with systemic disease in approximately 50% of patients. Visual loss usually results from secondary choroidal neovascularization (CNV).

Symptoms

Patients with angioid streaks are usually asymptomatic. Visual symptoms arise secondary to CNV in about 50% of eyes. The presence of CNV is heralded by decreased vision, central scotoma, and metamorphopsia.

Clinical Features

Angioid streaks are linear, subretinal streaks that radiate from a peripapillary region to the macula and midperipheral fundus. The streaks are usually bilateral and may be variable in appearance. Streaks range in color from reddish brown and gray to yellow. About 10% of patients have diffuse angioid streaks that radiate concentrically as well as radially, producing a "cracked eggshell" appearance. The streaks may widen and lengthen with time. About one third of patients have a diffuse mottling of the fundus, termed a peau d'orange appearance.

Choroidal neovascularization may occur with angioid streaks. Choroidal neovascularization is suggested by the presence of subretinal fluid and subretinal hemorrhage. Subretinal hemorrhage without CNV may also occur along the angioid streaks with minor ocular trauma.

Ancillary Testing

Fluorescein angiography is performed in patients with suspected CNV. Usually, CNV is detected in the macula along the track of an angioid streak. The fluorescein pattern of angioid streaks is variable. The streaks may hyperfluoresce early and stain in the late phase of the study.

Pathology/Pathogenesis

Angioid streaks represent full-thickness breaks in Bruch's membrane with disruption of the underlying choriocapillaris and the overlying retinal pigment epithelium. Bruch's membrane is thickened and basophilic, with evidence of calcium deposition. The pathogenesis of angioid streaks is unknown. Calcification and a loss of elasticity of Bruch's membrane may lead to ruptures of Bruch's membrane with minor trauma or due to the forces exerted by the extraocular muscles on the globe. Disruption in Bruch's membrane may result in the development of choroidal neovascularization.

Treatment/Prognosis

Laser therapy has been used to treat CNV developing in association with angioid streaks. Laser photocoagulation techniques similar to those used for the treatment of CNV associated with age-related macular degeneration have been studied. Visual loss may be stabilized in patients with successfully treated membranes. Most case series demonstrate a high rate of recurrence of CNV. Photodynamic therapy may be effective in reducing the risk of visual loss in patients with subfoveal CNV.

Systemic Evaluation

Angioid streaks may occur in association with several systemic diseases. In one series, 50% of patients with angioid streaks had evidence of systemic disease. Pseudoxanthoma elasticum is an inherited disorder of connective tissue characterized by papular and reticular skin changes, producing a "chicken skin" appearance. Patients may also suffer from occlusive vascular disease, upper gastrointestinal hemorrhage, and hypertension. Paget's disease of bone is characterized by gross deformities of the skull, spine, and pelvis due to coarsely thickened and sclerotic bone. Angioid streaks may also be seen with sickle cell disease, lead poisoning, Ehlers-Danlos syndrome, and abetalipoproteinemia.

Systemic evaluation may include skin biopsy (pseudoxanthoma elasticum), radiographs (Paget's disease of bone), hemoglobin electrophoresis (sickle cell disease), and serum lead levels.

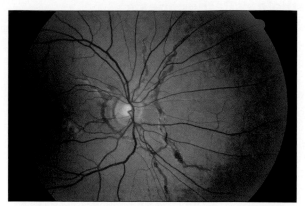

This fundus photograph reveals multiple angioid streaks radiating from the optic disc in a woman with pseudoxanthoma elasticum. Note the subretinal location of the streaks.

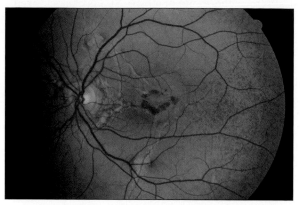

The fellow eye of the same patient reveals multiple angioid streaks and subfoveal hemorrhage suggesting the presence of choroidal neovascularization.

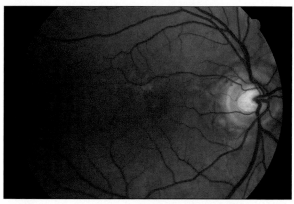

This 42-year-old woman with pseudoxanthoma elasticum was found to have multiple angioid streaks in each eye. Her right eye had prominent peripapillary streaks and one streak extending through the macula with atrophy in the fovea.

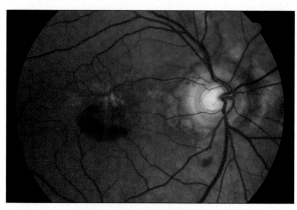

Same patient approximately 3 years later. She presented with sudden visual loss related to choroidal neovascularization with subretinal hemorrhage along the margin of the angioid streak.

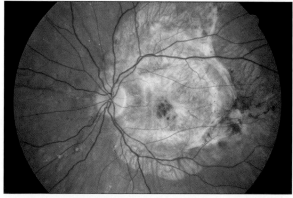

Visual loss in patients with angioid streaks is usually related to the development of choroidal neovascularization. Fibrovascular proliferation commonly results in the formation of a macular scar.

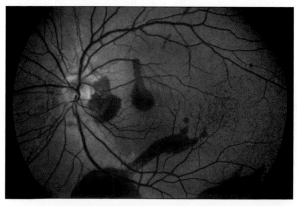

This patient developed subretinal hemorrhage following incidental eye trauma. Also note the "peau d orange" pigment mottling in the temporal macula.

CENTRAL SEROUS CHORIORETINOPATHY

Central serous chorioretinopathy (CSC) is characterized by self-limited localized serous retinal detachments of the macula. Central serous chorioretinopathy usually occurs in young individuals, with a male preponderance of 8:1. Although typically unilateral, CSC may be bilateral. Common associations include stress, type-A personality traits, hypertension, and headache. Central serous chorioretinopathy is most commonly idiopathic but has been described with pregnancy, systemic lupus erythematosus (SLE), hemodialysis/organ transplantation, and other hypercortisolemic states, including exogenous corticosteroid use and Cushing's syndrome.

Symptoms

Patients with CSC present with visual blurring, distortion, micropsia, and an area of visual darkening (positive scotoma).

Clinical Features

Visual acuity may be decreased to a variable degree. Approximately 50% of patients with CSC retain better than 20/30 visual acuity. Subretinal fluid produces a hyperopic shift in the patient's refraction. Amsler grid testing often reveals central or paracentral distortion. Macular examination demonstrates a localized oval or round area of subretinal fluid. Some cases may have an associated retinal pigment epithelial (RPE) detachment. Retinal pigment epithelial alterations are observed commonly in both eyes.

Retroretinal precipitates on the back surface of the retina also may be observed. The presence of subretinal fibrin suggests very active leakage and is more common with pregnancy, SLE, or corticosteroid use. Resolved episodes of CSC may produce mottled changes in the RPE. Atypical findings include inferior, dependent RPE atrophic tracks from prolonged, recurrent serous detachments, multiple bullous serous retinal detachments associated with subretinal fibrin and shifting subretinal fluid, and choroidal neovascularization (CNV).

Ancillary Testing

Fluorescein angiography demonstrates a focal leakage point in the early phase of the angiogram with pooling of fluorescein in the subretinal fluid in the later phases of the angiogram. About 30% of patients have more than one leakage point evident. Recurrent leakage points tend to occur within 1 mm of the previous leakage points. In approximately 10% of cases, a classic "smokestack" pattern of hyperfluorescence is observed. Transmission or "window" defects are common in both eyes. Indocyanine green angiography demonstrates choroidal hyperpermeability.

Pathology/Pathogenesis

The precise pathogenesis of CSC is not completely understood. Central serous chorioretinopathy is most likely the result of increased capillary permeability in the choriocapillaris. Why choriocapillaris hyperpermeability develops is unclear. Central serous chorioretinopathy has been produced in monkeys following daily intravenous injections of epinephrine; the adrenergic effect of epinephrine may cause damage to the choriocapillaris and subsequent choriocapillaris hyperpermeability. The disorder has been observed in various hypercortisolemic states including exogenous corticosteroid use, Cushing's syndrome, pregnancy, SLE, and hemodialysis/organ transplantation. Cortisol may influence the constrictive action of catecholamines on arterioles; cortisol also may contribute to hypertension and increase capillary fragility.

Treatment/Prognosis

The majority of cases of CSC are self-limited with a duration of approximately 6 weeks. The prognosis for visual recovery is excellent, with 90% of patients recovering 20/30 or better visual acuity. Focal laser photocoagulation has been demonstrated to hasten the resolution of subretinal fluid but has no clear effect on long-term visual prognosis. In general, focal laser treatment is reserved for patients with persistent subretinal fluid for more than 4 months, occupational requirements for earlier visual rehabilitation, or development of degenerative changes in the area of detached retina. A well-defined leakage point greater than 500 mm from the center of the foveal avascular zone should be present. A light-intensity burn is placed over the leakage site.

Although some evidence indicates that laser treatment may reduce the recurrence rate of CSC, no randomized trials have confirmed this observation. Due to the potential complications of laser photocoagulation including a paracentral scotoma or secondary CNV, laser therapy continues to be reserved for chronic cases. Recurrent episodes of CSC are observed in 30% to 50% of patients. Most recurrences occur within 1 year of the initial episode.

Systemic Evaluation

Systemic evaluation should focus on possible precipitating factors such as corticosteroid usage, pregnancy, and hypertension.

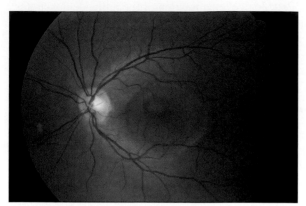

Central serous chorioretinopathy is characterized by the presence of a localized oval or round area of subretinal fluid.

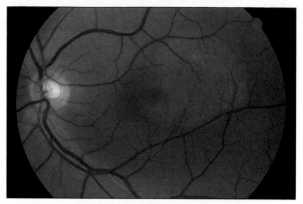

During the early resolution phase of central serous chorioretinopathy, protein deposits may form on the posterior surface of the retina. Other common findings are pigment epithelial detachments and pigmentary alterations.

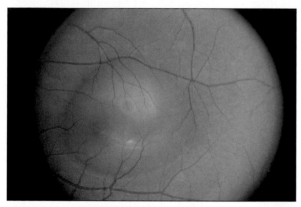

The presence of subretinal fibrin suggests very active leakage and is more common with pregnancy, systemic lupus erythematosus, and corticosteroid use.

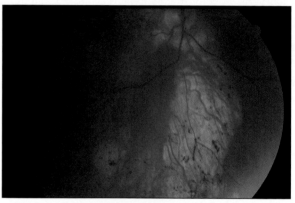

Dependent retinal pigment epithelial atrophic tracks result from prolonged, recurrent central serous chorioretinopathy. The tracts often originate in the peripapillary region and extend inferiorly; macular involvement is associated with visual loss.

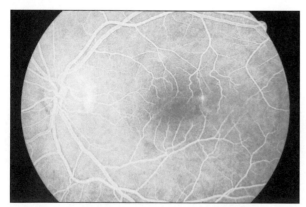

The typical fluorescein angiographic finding of central serous chorioretinopathy is a single hyperfluorescent spot that increases in size and intensity throughout the study.

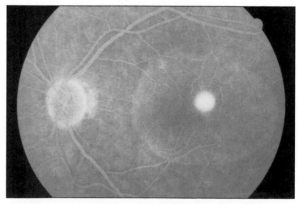

Late-phase fluorescein angiographic image of the same patient reveals increased size and intensity of fluorescein leakage.

CYSTOID MACULAR EDEMA

Cystoid macular edema (CME) is most commonly encountered after cataract surgery but may arise in association with a number of conditions including retinal vascular disease, retinitis pigmentosa, uveitis, and secondary to the use of several drugs such as epinephrine, latanoprost, and nicotinic acid. Postcataract CME is most commonly observed 1 to 3 months postoperatively. Risk factors include vitreous loss/incarceration, intracapsular extraction technique, and use of iris clip intraocular lenses.

Symptoms

Most patients present with decreased vision. Some patients may note metamorphopsia or micropsia due to macular edema.

Clinical Features

Refraction may demonstrate a hyperopic shift. Cystoid macular edema is difficult to detect without the use of a fundus contact lens. The condition is characterized by a stellate or honeycomb pattern of retinal thickening in the fovea and parafoveal region. Macular biomicroscopy shows thickening of the retina with loss of the normal foveal reflex. This feature may manifest as a yellow spot in the fovea.

Ancillary Testing

Fluorescein angiography is the gold standard test for the evaluation of CME. Accumulation of edema fluid in the outer plexiform layer leads to the characteristic petaloid pattern of cystoid spaces observed around the fovea. While angiography is more sensitive than clinical examination for the determination of CME, it correlates poorly with visual acuity. Characteristic features are leakage from perifoveal capillaries leading to the late accumulation of dye within the cystoid spaces. Late staining of the optic disc may also occur. Clinical CME complicating nicotinic acid therapy shows no leakage on fluorescein angiography.

Pathology/Pathogenesis

Cystoid macular edema arises from accumulation of edema fluid within the retina due to disruption of the normal blood-retinal barrier. Inflammatory mediators are hypothesized to trigger the breakdown of the blood-retinal barrier. Vitreous traction may impair the normal pumping action of Müller cells and further contribute to the development of edema.

Pathological examination of the retina demonstrates Müller cell edema and accumulation of edema fluid within the outer plexiform layer. In chronic cases, cysts may coalesce into larger cysts or lamellar/full-thickness macular holes.

Treatment/Prognosis

Preoperative topical nonsteroidal anti-inflammatory drugs (NSAIDs) reduce the incidence of angiographic CME. The clinical benefit of CME prophylaxis is less clear. Many cases of postoperative CME will resolve spontaneously over several weeks to months. Topical NSAIDs and steroids have been demonstrated to be effective in the resolution of postoperative CME; in fact, corticosteroids may have some synergy with NSAIDs in the treatment of this disorder. Patients whose conditions fail topical therapy are considered for periocular steroid therapy. The role of carbonic anhydrase inhibitors and hyperbaric oxygen are controversial. Nd:YAG laser therapy may be used to perform vitreolysis in cases of CME associated with vitreous incarceration in the surgical wound after cataract surgery. In cases of chronic CME, pars plana vitrectomy has been shown to improve the visual outcome in aphakic and pseudophakic patients.

The therapy of CME associated with chronic uveitis is primarily directed at treatment of the underlying inflammation.

Systemic Evaluation

Postoperative CME is not associated with systemic disease. Patients with uveitis and associated CME may have underlying systemic inflammatory diseases that require evaluation.

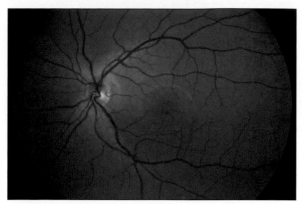

Cystoid macular edema (CME) is difficult to detect without the use of a fundus contact lens. Findings that suggest the presence of CME include loss of the normal foveal reflex and a yellow spot in the center of the fovea.

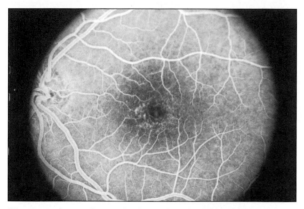

Fluorescein angiography is an invaluable tool in the diagnosis of cystoid macular edema. The early findings include leakage from the perifoveal capillaries.

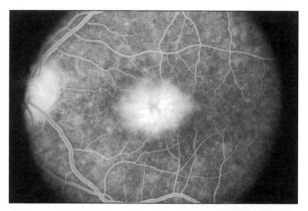

Fluorescein leaks throughout the study, often resulting in a characteristic "petaloid" pattern of dye pooling in the late views.

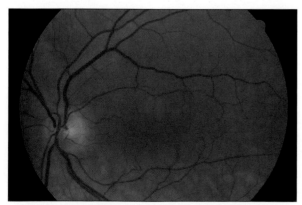

Cystoid macular edema (CME) is observed most commonly following intraocular surgery. Other causes of CME include retinal vascular occlusions, posterior uveitis, retinal degeneration, and drug toxicities. This 68-year-old woman had idiopathic vitritis with bilateral CME.

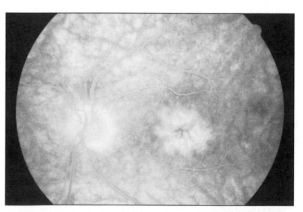

Fluorescein angiogram of the same patient reveals the classic petaloid pattern of late hyperfluorescence.

EPIRETINAL MEMBRANE

Epiretinal membranes are proliferations of glial tissue that produce mechanical distortion of the macula that may or may not be associated with visual symptoms. Numerous terms are used to describe epiretinal membranes, including macular pucker and cellophane maculopathy. While epiretinal membranes may occur secondary to numerous ocular processes, the most common form is idiopathic.

Symptoms

Patients with epiretinal membranes present with a variable reduction in visual acuity. Alterations in the normal anatomy of the macula may lead to significant distortion, binocular diplopia, or even macropsia. Visual loss tends to be stable from the time of diagnosis.

Clinical Features

Macular examination demonstrates the presence of a glistening, crinkled sheen to the retinal surface corresponding to the location of the epiretinal tissue. Contracture of the epiretinal membrane may lead to distortion of the retinal vasculature and retinal folds. Severe cases may be associated with the presence of foveal ectopia. Retinal examination may demonstrate retinal whitening, retinal edema, or occasional retinal or preretinal hemorrhage. Irregularities of the retinal vasculature are common.

Epiretinal membranes may have gaps resulting in the appearance of a macular pseudohole. Differentiating a pseudohole from a full-thickness macular hole is performed clinically using the slit beam or laser aiming beam test.

Ancillary Testing

In general, the diagnosis of epiretinal membrane is established clinically. Ancillary testing is rarely required. Fluorescein angiography may be obtained to examine the extent of macular distortion and to what degree—if any—the epiretinal membrane is associated with vascular leakage. Optical coherence tomography may allow better visualization of the relationship of the epiretinal membrane to the retinal surface and may be helpful in excluding vitreomacular traction and distinguishing pseudoholes from full-thickness macular holes.

Pathology/Pathogenesis

The most common form of epiretinal membrane is the idiopathic variety, which usually forms after posterior vitreous detachment (PVD). In the absence of a PVD, other ocular conditions should be considered. Epiretinal membranes may arise in association with retinal vascular disease including retinal venous occlusions and diabetic retinopathy, uveitis, hereditary retinopathies, trauma, or following retinal detachment.

The precise pathogenesis of epiretinal membranes remains unclear. They appear to arise as glial proliferations on the retinal surface. In some cases, inflammatory mediators may play a role in the stimulation of glial proliferation.

Treatment/Prognosis

Asymptomatic epiretinal membranes are common and require no therapy. Patients with significant visual symptoms secondary to epiretinal membrane proliferation may elect to undergo pars plana vitrectomy with removal of the epiretinal tissue. Approximately 70% to 80% of patients will gain at least two lines of visual acuity with successful removal of the epiretinal tissue. Vitrectomy for epiretinal membrane removal is associated with a significant risk of cataract progression.

Systemic Evaluation

Epiretinal membranes are generally not associated with systemic diseases.

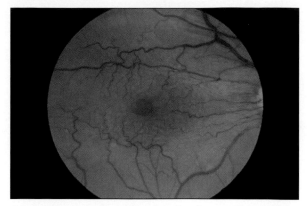

An epiretinal membrane is visualized as a glistening, crinkled sheen on the surface of the retina. A pseudohole is present in this patient.

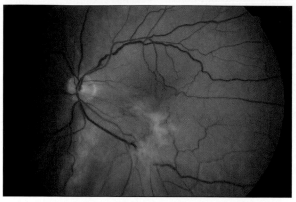

More severe cases of epiretinal membrane are associated with retinal and vascular distortion.

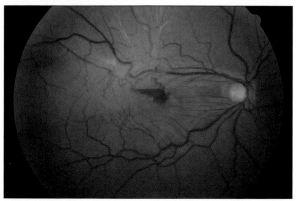

This fundus photograph demonstrates a severe epiretinal membrane with vascular distortion, preretinal hemorrhage, and retinal whitening due to axoplasmic stasis.

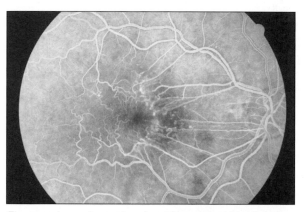

Fluorescein angiography of another patient highlights the retinal vascular distortion caused by contraction of the epiretinal membrane. Leakage of fluorescein may be seen in severe cases.

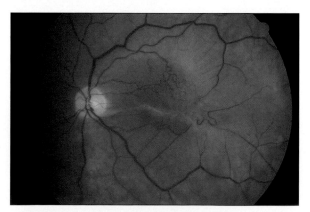

Preoperative fundus photograph of a patient with a prominent epiretinal membrane associated with significant macular distortion and vision loss.

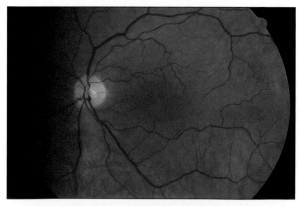

The postoperative photograph of the same patient demonstrates resolution of macular distortion. The patient's vision improved from 20/300 to 20/25.

HYPOTONY MACULOPATHY

Hypotony is low intraocular pressure (usually less than 5 mm Hg) leading to functional and structural changes in the eye. Hypotony occurs in a number of clinical settings and may result from reversible or irreversible causes. The most common setting for hypotony maculopathy is in association with glaucoma filtration surgery, in which 1.3% to 3% of patients may develop maculopathy. Central visual loss may result from irregular folding of the retina and choroid in the macula.

Symptoms

Patients present with central visual loss and metamorphopsia in the setting of hypotony.

Clinical Features

Visual acuity may be significantly impaired with hypotony. Retinal examination demonstrates irregular retinal and choroidal folds radiating temporally from the optic nerve. The peripapillary choroid is frequently engorged and may mimic papilledema. In severe cases, the insertion of the inferior oblique muscle may visibly produce an internal compression of the macula.

Prolonged hypotony leads to the formation of permanent pigment lines in the macular region. Severe chronic cases of hypotony may result in atrophia bulbi.

Ancillary Testing

Diagnostic testing is primarily directed toward the identification of the cause of hypotony. Anterior segment imaging with gonioscopy or ultrasound biomicroscopy may be useful in the diagnosis of cyclodialysis clefts.

Pathology/Pathogenesis

There are a wide variety of causes of hypotony. In general, hypotony can be classified according to mechanisms including external fistula, internal fistula, ciliary body insufficiency, inflammation, and others. External fistulas are the result of accidental or surgical trauma and link the internal ocular compartments with the ocular surface. Internal fistulas connect the suprachoroidal space with the aqueous or vitreous and include problems such as cyclodialysis and retinal detachment. Ciliary body inflammation may result from medications or surgical interventions. Inflammation produces a reduction in aqueous production as well as an increase in uveoscleral outflow. Rare causes of hypotony include ocular ischemia, giant cell arteritis, uremia, and myotonic dystrophy.

Treatment/Prognosis

Hypotony maculopathy requires identification and correction of the etiology of hypotony. A variety of techniques are described for the management of overfiltering blebs. The visual prognosis is variable. While several case series have described good visual recovery with reversal of hypotony, other series have poorer visual outcomes despite normalization of intraocular pressure. In cases of prolonged hypotony, the chorioretinal folds persist even after the intraocular pressure is normalized.

Systemic Evaluation

Hypotony maculopathy usually does not have systemic manifestations. Rare systemic causes of hypotony include myotonic dystrophy and ocular ischemia related to carotid occlusive disease or giant cell arteritis.

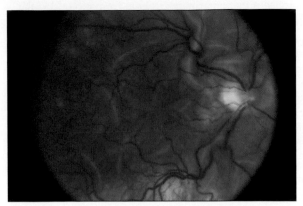

This fundus photograph demonstrates optic disc swelling and macular distortion in a patient with prolonged hypotony after trabeculectomy.

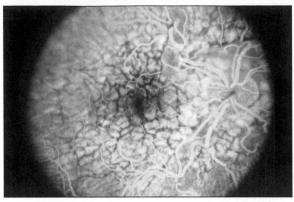

Fluorescein angiography of the same patient reveals prominent, irregular chorioretinal folds.

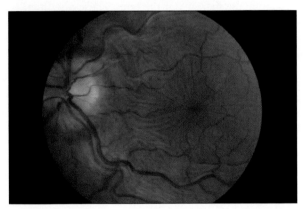

Hypotony maculopathy resulting from a traumatic cyclodialysis cleft. The patient had numerous chorioretinal folds throughout the macula.

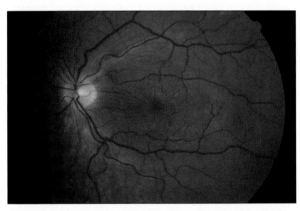

The macular changes in the same patient resolved after laser therapy to close the cyclodialysis cleft and restore normal intraocular pressure. Macular folds may become permanent in long-standing cases.

MACULAR HOLE

Idiopathic macular holes are full-thickness defects that arise in the macula in less than 1% of the population. They are most prevalent in the 50- to 80-year age group, and appear to be more common in women. Approximately 10% of patients develop bilateral macular holes.

Macular holes also may arise in association with trauma, myopia, and chronic cystoid macular edema. Rarely, tangential traction from an epiretinal membrane may cause a full-thickness macular hole. Most apparent macular holes arising within epiretinal membranes are not full thickness and are classified as macular pseudoholes.

Symptoms

Patients present with a variable degree of visual loss depending on the size of the hole, the location of the hole relative to the foveola, and the size of any associated neurosensory retinal detachment. Associated symptoms include central scotoma and metamorphopsia. The visual loss may be noted incidentally on covering the fellow eye.

Clinical Features

The clinical features vary depending on the stage of the macular hole at presentation. The macular findings are appreciated best with the use of a fundus contact lens. In patients with a stage 1 macular hole, a yellow spot (stage 1A) or yellow ring (stage 1B) is visualized in the center of the fovea. Stage 2 macular holes are characterized by a full-thickness macular hole less than 400 µm in diameter. Fine retinal striae radiating from the hole may be visualized. Stage 3 macular holes are larger than 400 µm in diameter and may have an associated cuff of subretinal fluid. Stage 4 macular holes are similar to stage 3 holes except that a total posterior vitreous detachment (PVD) is present. The base of the hole may contain yellow-white deposits on the retinal pigment epithelium (RPE). Eyes with a vitreofoveolar separation often have an operculum overlying the macular hole.

Differentiating a true macular hole from a pseudohole is performed with a slit beam or laser aiming beam test. A slit beam centered over the macular hole is perceived as being bent, pinched, or interrupted in the location of the macular hole. A 50-µm laser aiming beam will "disappear" when projected into the hole.

Ancillary Testing

Macular holes are diagnosed by clinical examination. Ancillary testing may provide insight into pathogenesis but rarely affects management decisions. B-scan ultrasonography may demonstrate the vitreoretinal relationship that contributes to hole formation. Macular holes and the posterior hyaloid membrane also may be imaged with optical coherence tomography (OCT). Fluorescein angiography may reveal a central hyperfluorescent transmission or "window" defect as a result of xanthophyll pigment displacement and retinal pigment epithelial atrophy in long-standing cases.

Pathology/Pathogenesis

The precise pathogenesis of macular holes is becoming better understood. Imaging with OCT and ultrasonography suggests that localized perifoveal vitreous detachment (an early stage of age-related PVD) results in static and dynamic tractional forces that lead to a full-thickness foveolar dehiscence.

In pathologic sections macular holes are full-thickness retinal defects. Glial cells extend across the retinal surface along the margins of the hole. These are often continuous with an adjacent epiretinal membrane. The parafoveal retina demonstrates cystic changes in the outer plexiform layer. The retinal pigment epithelial cells in the area of the hole are distended with lipofuscin and lose their apical microvillous processes.

Treatment/Prognosis

Stage 1 holes are estimated to have a 50% to 60% rate of progression to full-thickness macular hole. Some stage 1 holes are relatively asymptomatic; therefore, the true rate of progression in the general population may be lower. Stage 2, stage 3, and stage 4 holes have been demonstrated to have a better visual outcome with vitrectomy compared to observation. Vitrectomy involves complete removal of the core vitreous and the posterior hyaloid membrane, including all epiretinal tissue. Removal of the internal limiting membrane may be employed in some cases. The use of adjuvant therapies such as autologous serum and growth factors is controversial. Following vitrectomy, a fluid-gas exchange is performed followed by tamponade with the patient in a face-down position.

The rate of hole closure with surgery approaches 80% to 90%. Visual recovery is variable, with holes of shorter duration and holes less than 500 µm in diameter experiencing the greatest benefit. Complications of surgery include retinal detachment, cataract progression, and visual field defects.

Systemic Evaluation

Macular holes are not associated with systemic disease.

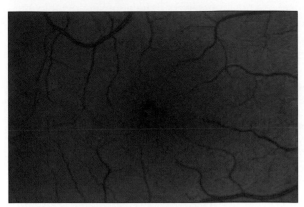

Stage 1A macular hole is characterized by a central yellow spot without retinal dehiscence. The central yellow spot results from the loss of the normal foveal depression.

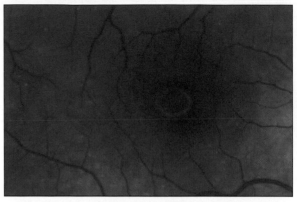

A yellow ring without retinal dehiscence is the characteristic finding in patients with stage 1B macular holes. Approximately 50% of stage 1 macular holes resolve spontaneously.

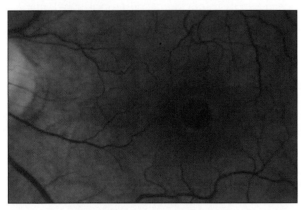

Stage 2 macular hole in this patient with 20/200 visual acuity exhibits eccentric retinal dehiscence. Stage 2 macular holes are small, full-thickness macular holes less than 400 μm in diameter.

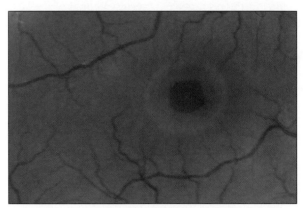

Stage 3 macular holes are full-thickness macular holes greater than 400 μm in diameter without a posterior vitreous detachment (PVD). Stage 4 macular holes are similar to stage 3 macular holes except that a total PVD is present.

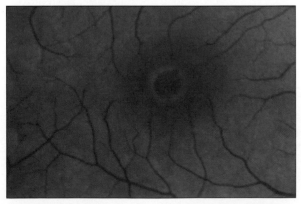

Fundus photograph of woman with a stage 2 macular hole with eccentric retinal dehiscence and 20/200 visual acuity.

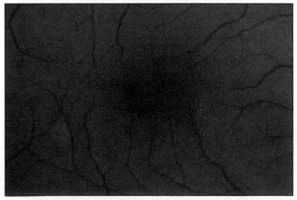

This photograph of the same patient demonstrates resolution of the macular hole after pars plana vitrectomy with membrane peeling and gas tamponade. Her visual acuity improved to 20/30.

MYOPIC DEGENERATION

Simple myopia is one of the most common ocular disorders encountered, with a prevalence estimated at 10% to 30% of the population. Degenerative myopia is a less common condition associated with greater visual disability.

Symptoms

Patients with degenerative myopia may present with progressive visual loss associated with progressive myopic changes. Central visual impairment may result from lacquer cracks, atrophic maculopathy, choroidal neovascularization (CNV), or macular hole formation.

Clinical Features

The clinical features of degenerative myopia are the result of slowly progressive enlargement of the globe. Stretching of the posterior pole results in drag of the choroid and the retinal pigment epithelium (RPE) from the optic nerve, leaving an atrophic temporal crescent. Extensive ectasia of the sclera in the posterior segment leads to formation of a staphyloma with posterior herniation of the retina and choroid. Enlargement of the globe leads to thinning of the RPE and choriocapillaris, resulting in a "tigroid" appearance of the fundus and more pronounced visualization of the larger choroidal vessels.

Macular examination may demonstrate atrophic areas resulting from loss of the RPE and choriocapillaris. Lacquer cracks represent spontaneous ruptures of Bruch's membrane. Lacquer cracks appear as irregular yellow or whitish lines and are typically located in the base of a staphyloma. The acute development of a lacquer crack may be heralded by a subretinal hemorrhage.

The most significant visual complications of degenerative myopia are CNV, macular hole formation, and macular atrophy. Choroidal neovascularization has been estimated to occur in 5% to 10% of patients whose axial length is greater than 26.5 mm. In this setting, CNV is typically small and often has an associated pigmented rim. Subretinal fluid and hemorrhage may be present. The CNV may be associated with a lacquer crack.

Spontaneous involution of a CNV in degenerative myopia may leave a pigment clump referred to as Fuchs' spot. Macular hole in degenerative myopia may be associated with a posterior retinal detachment.

Ancillary Testing

Fluorescein angiography is useful in the evaluation of patients with degenerative myopia. Lacquer cracks appear as early hyperfluorescent lines that remain hyperfluorescent in the late phases of the angiogram without leakage. Lacquer cracks that were not visible with clinical examination may be evident on angiography. Angiography is important in the evaluation of CNV. Typical early hyperfluorescence with late leakage is present. Late leakage tends to be more localized than that observed with CNV associated with age-related macular degeneration.

Pathology/Pathogenesis

The pathogenesis of degenerative myopia remains unclear. The clinical features appear to result from progressive enlargement of the globe with stretching and subsequent damage to the ocular tissues.

Treatment/Prognosis

Macular holes and associated retinal detachments are generally repaired with pars plana vitrectomy and gas tamponade. In cases of extreme posterior staphyloma, an external approach with a scleral buckle applied to the macular region has been used.

The optimal management of CNV associated with myopia remains unclear. Some CNVs may resolve spontaneously without treatment, with relative stabilization of visual acuity. A small, randomized trial of laser photocoagulation of CNV located outside the fovea demonstrated a beneficial effect of laser therapy at 2 years' follow-up in terms of visual acuity. No significant benefit was noted at 5 years, and a significant number of recurrences were noted. Laser treatment of CNV in myopia is further marred by progressive expansion of laser scars with longer follow-up.

Photodynamic therapy is capable of stabilization of visual acuity with a limited number of patients regaining significant amounts of vision. Subretinal surgery for the removal of CNV in degenerative myopia has been limited, but early results show a low rate of visual improvement and a significant recurrence rate. Limited macular translocation has been used successfully in small case series of CNV associated with myopia.

Systemic Evaluation

Degenerative myopia may be observed in systemic conditions including Marfan's syndrome, Ehlers-Danlos syndrome, Stickler's syndrome, and Down's syndrome.

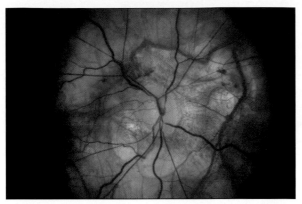

Myopic degeneration is characterized by peripapillary atrophy, straightening of the retinal vessels, and macular abnormalities. This patient had a prominent posterior staphyloma with marked peripapillary atrophy.

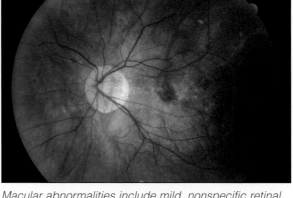

Macular abnormalities include mild, nonspecific retinal pigment epithelial alterations, lacquer cracks, atrophy, choroidal neovascularization (CNV), Fuchs' spots, and macular holes. This patient had a pigmented Fuchs' spot following spontaneous resolution of CNV.

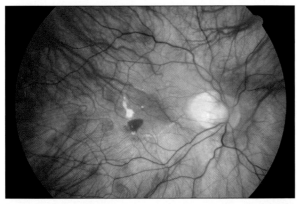

Lacquer cracks represent spontaneous ruptures of Bruch's membrane. The development of a new lacquer crack may be associated with subretinal hemorrhage.

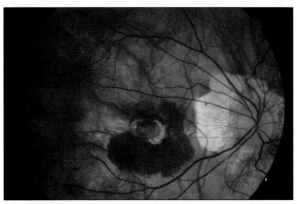

The finding of subretinal hemorrhage usually indicates the presence of choroidal neovascularization (CNV). The CNV associated with myopic degeneration is often small and pigmented. Fluorescein angiography typically reveals a classic pattern of new vessels.

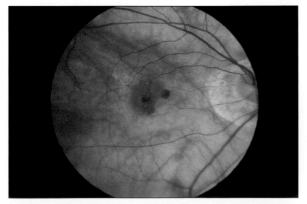

Fundus photograph of a patient with a myopic fundus revealing subretinal hemorrhage and a pigmented choroidal neovascular membrane.

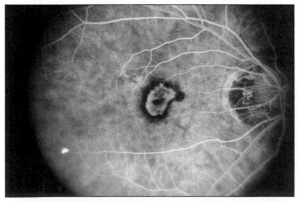

Fluorescein angiogram of the same patient demonstrates classic choroidal neovascularization with a well-defined pattern of hyperfluorescence. The surrounding hypofluorescence results from hemorrhage and retinal pigment epithelial hyperplasia.

PATTERN DYSTROPHY

The pattern dystrophies represent a spectrum of disorders characterized by alterations of the retinal pigment epithelium (RPE) in patients with relatively few visual symptoms. Numerous entities that were described individually are now considered to be variations of pattern dystrophy. These disorders include adult vitelliform dystrophy, butterfly dystrophy, reticular dystrophies, and fundus pulverulentis (coarse mottling).

Symptoms

Patients with pattern dystrophy are often visually asymptomatic. They may be noted to have retinal pigment epithelial changes of the macula on routine examinations. Some patients have mild blurring or visual distortion. A family history of pattern dystrophy may be present.

Clinical Features

Visual acuity is relatively normal, with most patients retaining better than 20/40 acuity. Macular examination demonstrates alterations in the RPE pattern. These alterations generally consist of deposits of yellow, orange, or brown pigment in dots, flecks, branching lines, or other patterns. The pigment deposits typically appear in midlife. Occasionally, different patterns may be seen in the 2 eyes of the same patient or in different members of the same pedigree. The optic nerve and the retinal vasculature remain normal.

Ancillary Testing

Fluorescein angiography demonstrates more extensive RPE changes than are evident on clinical examination. Areas of RPE pigment deposition produce hypofluorescence. The intervening RPE often demonstrates transmission defects that do not leak.

Color vision testing may demonstrate a mild tritan defect. The electroretinographic findings are normal in most cases. The electro-oculographic recordings may be subnormal, indicating a more diffuse dysfunction of the RPE.

Pathology/Pathogenesis

Pattern dystrophies are usually inherited in an autosomal dominant fashion. A variety of genetic mutations have been described in families with pattern dystrophies. The majority of described mutations occur on the peripherin/RDS gene. A variety of mutations on the peripherin/RDS gene appear to be capable of producing a pattern dystrophy. Other genetic loci are capable of producing a phenotype consistent with a pattern dystrophy.

The precise pathogenesis of pattern dystrophies is unknown. Pathological studies on patients with pattern dystrophies are limited.

Treatment/Prognosis

Fortunately, most patients with pattern dystrophy retain good visual acuity and relatively normal visual function with long-term follow-up. Visual loss, when it occurs, is associated with atrophy or the development of choroidal neovascularization (CNV) (infrequent). There are no known treatments for visual loss secondary to nonexudative pattern dystrophy. Laser photocoagulation may be considered for CNV complications.

Systemic Evaluation

In general, pattern dystrophies are not known to have systemic features. However, pattern dystrophy may be seen in patients with pseudoxanthoma elasticum, myotonic dystrophy, and Kjellin's syndrome.

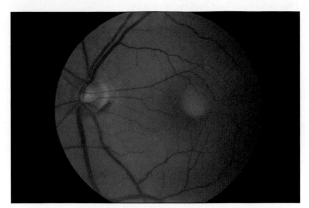

Pattern dystrophies manifest in a variety shapes and figures. The pattern is usually symmetric in both eyes. This patient had bilateral, central yellow deposits of the adult foveomacular vitelliform type.

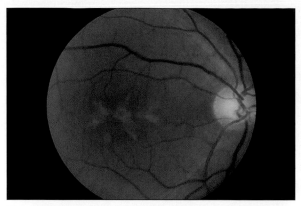

This patient had a characteristic "butterfly" pattern of yellowish deposits at the level of the retinal pigment epithelium.

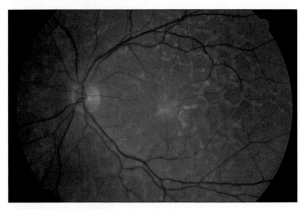

Reticular pattern dystrophy is characterized by coarse pigment deposits in the macula and posterior fundus.

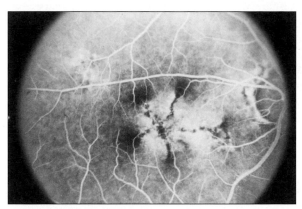

Fluorescein angiography reveals early hypofluorescence of the pigment patterns as a result of blockage. The vitelliform material may stain with fluorescein late.

PHOTIC RETINOPATHY

Light damage to the retina may arise from thermal or photochemical injuries. Photic retinopathy results from photochemical injuries.

Symptoms

Patients present with a reduction in central visual acuity and associated metamorphopsia. The degree of visual disability is variable. Patients with solar retinopathy typically have visual acuity in the 20/20 to 20/40 range.

Clinical Features

Photic retinopathy resulting from prolonged exposure to the operating microscope appears as an oval retinal lesion in the inferior macula that ranges from 0.5 to 2 disk diameters in size. Retinal edema and mild pigmentary changes are evident 24 to 48 hours after exposure. With time the lesion demonstrates more pigmentary mottling.

Solar retinopathy typically occurs in patients with psychiatric disorders or under the influence of psychotropic drugs. Exposures of greater than 90 seconds with a constricted pupil may be sufficient to cause photochemical damage. Acute injury produces a yellow-white foveolar lesion that fades after 1 to 2 weeks. The acute lesion resolves, leaving an outer lamellar macular hole approximately 100 μm to 200 μm in diameter.

Ancillary Testing

Fluorescein angiography in patients with solar maculopathy may demonstrate a focal window defect in the early period, but with long-term follow-up the angiogram often normalizes. Angiography in cases of iatrogenic photic injury demonstrates marked leakage in the early period with later development of a mottled transmission or "window" defect.

Pathology/Pathogenesis

The retina may be damaged by light as a result of thermal injury or photochemical injury. Thermal injury arises from exposure to light energy sufficient to raise the retinal temperature by at least 10°C. Photochemical injuries arise from prolonged light exposures at irradiances too low to produce photocoagulation. Energy from light exposure produces free radicals that lead to endothelial cell peroxidation and subsequent endothelial cell damage.

Iatrogenic light toxicity typically results from prolonged exposure to light from the operating microscope or endoilluminator.

Treatment/Prognosis

No specific therapy is available for photic retinopathy. Meticulous surgical technique and the appropriate use of microscope filters can limit intraoperative macular light exposure. Visual recovery is variable. Most patients with solar retinopathy retain stable but slightly reduced visual acuity over long-term follow-up.

Systemic Evaluation

Patients with solar retinopathy frequently suffer from major psychiatric disorders or abuse psychotropic medications.

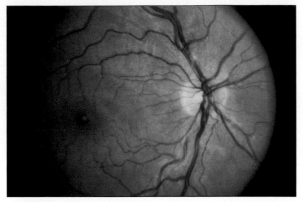

Acute solar retinopathy is observed in a patient following prolonged staring at the sun. The fundus photograph demonstrates the yellow-white lesions in the fovea.

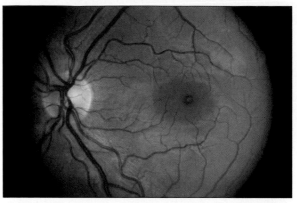

The fellow eye reveals the same finding. The yellow-white lesions of acute solar retinopathy in the fovea fade over 1 to 2 weeks.

Fundus photograph of a patient with outer lamellar macular defects characteristic of long-standing solar retinopathy.

The fellow eye of the same patient reveals similar findings. Patients may have normal visual acuity despite the retinal abnormalities.

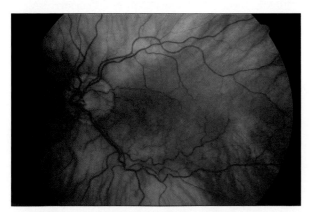

Postoperative photic retinopathy occurred in this patient as pigmentary mottling in the macular area after vitrectomy and membrane peeling.

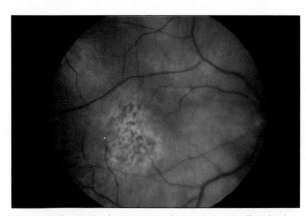

Photic retinopathy is seen as pigmentary mottling in the macula secondary to light toxicity during cataract extraction.

SELECTED REFERENCES

Age-Related Macular Degeneration: Nonexudative

1. Abdelsalam A, Del Priore L, Zarbin MA. Drusen in age-related macular degeneration: pathogenesis, natural course, and laser photocoagulation-induced regression. *Surv Ophthalmol.* 1999;44:1–29.

2. Age-Related Eye Disease Study Group. A randomized, placebo-controlled, clinical trial of high-dose supplementation with vitamins C and E, beta carotene, and zinc for age-related macular degeneration and vision loss. *Arch Ophthalmol.* 2001;119:1417–1436.

3. Gorin MB, Breitner JC, De Jong PT, Hageman GS, Klaver CC, Kuehn MH, et al. The genetics of age-related macular degeneration. *Mol Vis.* 1999;5:29.

4. Green WR, Enger C. Age-related macular degeneration histopathologic studies. *Ophthalmology.* 1993;100:1519–1535.

5. Ho AC, Maguire MG, Yoken J, Lee MS, Shin DS, Javornik NB, et al. Laser induced drusen reduction improves visual function at one year. *Ophthalmology.* 1999;106(7):1367–1374.

6. The Choroidal Neovascularization Prevention Trial Research Group. Laser treatment in eyes with large drusen. *Ophthalmology.* 1998;105:11–23.

7. Smiddy WE, Fine SL. Prognosis of patients with bilateral macular drusen. *Ophthalmology.* 1984;91:271–277.

8. Sunness JS, Gonzalez-Baron J, Applegate CA, Bressler NM, Tian Y, Hawkins B, et al. Enlargement of atrophy and visual acuity loss in the geographic atrophy form of age-related macular degeneration. *Ophthalmology.* 1999;106:1768–1779.

Age-Related Macular Degeneration: Exudative

1. Bressler NM. Photodynamic therapy of subfoveal choroidal neovascularization in age-related macular degeneration with verteporfin: two-year results of 2 randomized clinical trials—TAP report 2. *Arch Ophthalmol.* 2001;119:198–207.

2. Lewis H, Kaiser PK, Lewis S, Estafanous M. Macular translocation for subfoveal choroidal neovascularization in age-related macular degeneration: a prospective study. *Am J Ophthalmol.* 1999;128(2):135–146.

3. Macular Photocoagulation Study. Argon laser photocoagulation for neovascular maculopathy: five-year results. *Arch Ophthalmol.* 1991;109:1109–1114.

4. Macular Photocoagulation Study. Krypton laser photocoagulation for neovascular lesions of age-related macular degeneration. *Arch Ophthalmol.* 1990;108:816–824.

5. Macular Photocoagulation Study. Laser photocoagulation of subfoveal neovascular lesions in age-related macular degeneration. *Arch Ophthalmol.* 1991;109:1220–1231.

Angioid Streaks

1. Clarkson JG, Altman RD. Angioid streaks. *Surv Ophthalmol.* 1982;26:235–246.

2. Lim JI, Bressler NM, Marsh MJ, Bressler SB. Laser treatment of choroidal neovascularization in patients with angioid streaks. *Am J Ophthalmol.* 1993;116(4):414–423.

3. Mansour AM. Systemic associations of angioid streaks. *Int Ophthalmol Clin.* 1991;31:61–68.

4. Pece A, Avanza P, Galli L, Brancato R. Laser photocoagulation of choroidal neovascularization in angioid streaks. *Retina.* 1997;17(1):12–16.

5. Sickenberg M, Schmidt-Erfurth U, Miller JW, Pournaras CJ, Zografos L, Piguet B, et al. A preliminary study of photodynamic therapy using verteporfin for choroidal neovascularization in pathologic myopia, ocular histoplasmosis, angioid streaks and idiopathic causes. *Arch Ophthalmol.* 2000;118(3):327–336.

Central Serous Chorioretinopathy

1. Buruncek E, Mudun A, Karacorlu S, Arslan MO. Laser photocoagulation for persistent central serous choroidopathy. *Ophthalmology.* 1997;104:616–622.

2. Gelber GS, Schatz H, Loss of vision due to central serous chorioretinopathy following psychological stress. *Am J Psychiatry.* 1987;144:46–50.

3. Klein ML, Van Buskirk EM, Friedman E, Gragoudas E, Chandra S. Experience with nontreatment of central serous choroidopathy. *Arch Ophthalmol.* 1974;91:247–250.

4. Nagaroski K. Experimental study of choroidopathy with intravenous injection of adrenaline. *Acta Soc Ophthalmol Jpn.* 1971;75:1720–1727.

5. Quillen D, Gass DM, Brod RD, Gardner TW, Blankenship GW, Gottlieb JL. Central serous chorioretinopathy in women. *Ophthalmology.* 1996;103(1):72–79.

6. Tittl MK, Spaide RF, Wong D, Pilotto E, Yannuzzi LA, Fisher YL, et al. Systemic findings associated with central serous chorioretinopathy. *Am J Ophthalmol.* 1999;128(1):63–68.

Cystoid Macular Edema

1. Fung WE. Vitrectomy for chronic aphakic cystoid macular edema. *Ophthalmology.* 1985;92:1102–1111.

2. Harbour JW, Smiddy WE, Rubsamen PE, Murray TG, Davis JL, Flynn HW Jr. Pars plana vitrectomy for chronic pseudophakic cystoid macular edema. *Am J Ophthalmol.* 1995;120(3):302–307.

3. Katzen LE, Fleischman JA, Trokel S. YAG laser treatment of cystoid macular edema. *Am J Ophthalmol.* 1983;95:589–592.

4. Pendergast SD, Margherio RR, Williams GA, Cox MS Jr. Vitrectomy for chronic pseudophakic cystoid macular edema. *Am J Ophthalmol.* 1999(3);128:317–323.

5. Rocha G, Deschenes J. Pathophysiology and treatment of cystoid macular edema. *Can J Ophthalmol.* 1996;31:282–288.
6. Weisz JM, Bressler NM, Bressler SB, Schachat AP. Ketorolac treatment of pseudophakic cystoid macular edema identified more than 24 months after cataract surgery. *Ophthalmology.* 1999;106(9):1656–1659.

Epiretinal Membrane
1. Azzolini C, Patelli F, Codenotti M, Pierro L, Brancato R. Optical coherence tomography in idiopathic epiretinal macular membrane surgery. *Eur J Ophthalmol.* 1999;9(3):206–211.
2. de Bustros S, Thompson JT, Michels RG, Rice TA, Glaser BM. Vitrectomy for idiopathic epiretinal membranes causing macular pucker. *Br J Ophthalmol.* 1988;72(9):692–695.
3. Graham K, D'Amico DJ. Postoperative complications of epiretinal membrane surgery. *Int Ophthalmol Clin.* 2000;40:215–223.
4. Pournaras CJ, Donati G, Brazitikos PD, Kapetanios AD, Dereklis DL, Stangos NT. Macular epiretinal membranes. *Semin Ophthalmol.* 2000;15(2):100–107.

Hypotony Maculopathy
1. Costa VP, Wilson RP, Moster MR, Schmidt CM, Gandham S. Hypotony maculopathy following the use of topical mitomycin C in glaucoma filtration surgery. *Ophthalmic Surg.* 1993;24(6):389–394.
2. Delgado MF, Daniels S, Pascal S, Dickens CJ. Hypotony maculopathy: improvement of visual acuity after 7 years. *Am J Ophthalmol.* 2001;132:931–933.
3. Schubert HD. Post surgical hypotony: relationship to fistulization, inflammation, chorioretinal lesions and the vitreous. *Surv Ophthalmol.* 1996;41:97–125.
4. Suner IJ, Greenfield DS, Miller MP, Nicolela MT, Palmberg PF. Hypotony maculopathy after filtering surgery with mitomycin C: incidence and treatment. *Ophthalmology.* 1997;104(2):207–215.

Macular Hole
1. Freeman WR, Azen SP, Kim JW, et al. Vitrectomy for the treatment of full-thickness stage 3 or 4 macular holes. *Arch Ophthalmol.* 1997;115:11–21.
2. Gass JDM. Reappraisal of biomicroscopic classification of stages of development of a macular hole. *Am J Ophthalmol.* 1995;119:752–759.
3. Gaurdric A, Haouchine B, Massin P, Paques M, Blain P, Erginay A. Macular hole formation: new data provided by optical coherence tomography. *Arch Ophthalmol.* 1999;117(6):744–751.
4. Johnson MW, Van Newkirk MR, Meyer KA. Perifoveal vitreous detachment is the primary pathogenic event in idiopathic macular hole formation. *Arch Ophthalmol.* 2001;119:215–222.
5. Leonard RE II, Smiddy WE, Flynn HW Jr, Feuer W. Long-term visual outcomes in patients with successful macular hole surgery. *Ophthalmology.* 1997;104(10):1648–1652.

Myopic Degeneration
1. Bressler SB, Pieramici D, Marsh MJ, et al. Laser scar expansion in pathologic myopia and ocular histoplasmosis following treatment of choroidal neovascularization. *IOVS.* 1992;33:1207.
2. Curtin BJ, Karlin DB. Axial length measurements and fundus changes of the myopic eye. *Am J Ophthalmol.* 1971;71:42–53.
3. Fujikado T, Ohji M, Saito Y, Hayashi A, Tano Y. Visual function after foveal translocation with scleral shortening in patients with myopic neovascular maculopathy. *Am J Ophthalmol.* 1998;125(5):647–656.
4. Sickenberg M, Schmidt-Erfurth U, Miller JW, Pournaras CJ, Zografos L, Piguet B, et al. A preliminary study of photodynamic therapy using verteporfin for choroidal neovascularization in pathologic myopia, ocular histoplasmosis, angioid streaks and idiopathic causes. *Arch Ophthalmol.* 2000;118(3):327–336.
5. Soubrane G, Pison J, Bornert P, Perrenoud F, Coscas G. Neovaisseaux sous retiniens de la myopie degenerative: resultants de la photocoagulation. *Bull Soc Ophthalmol Fr.* 1986;86(3):269–272.
6. Uemura A, Thomas MA. Subretinal surgery in choroidal neovascularization in patients with high myopia. *Arch Ophthalmol.* 2000;118:344–350.
7. VIP Therapy Study Group. Photodynamic therapy of subfoveal choroidal neovascularization in pathologic myopia with verteporfin: one-year results of a randomized clinical trial—VIP report No. 1. *Ophthalmology.* 2001;108:841–852.

Pattern Dystrophy
1. Daniele S, Restagno G, Daniele C, Nardacchione A, Danese P, Carbonara A. Analysis of the rhodopsin and peripherin/RDS gene in two families with pattern dystrophy of the retinal pigment epithelium. *Eur J Ophthalmol.* 1996;6(2):197–200.
2. Moore AT, Evans K. Molecular genetics of central retinal dystrophies. *Austr N Z J Ophthalmol.* 1996;24:189–198.

Photic Retinopathy
1. McDonald HR, Irvine AR. Light induced maculopathy from the operating microscope in extracapsular cataract extraction and intraocular lens implantation. *Ophthalmology.* 1983;90:945.

chapter | 5

Retinal Vascular Diseases

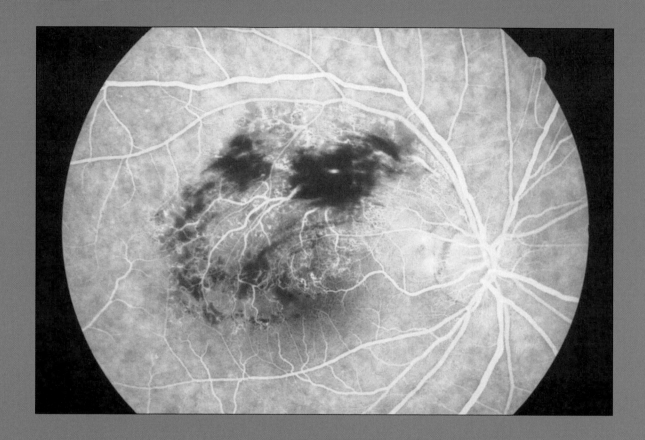

Kimberly A. Neely, MD, PhD

Thomas W. Gardner, MD, MS

Roy D. Brod, MD

David A. Quillen, MD

BRANCH RETINAL ARTERY OCCLUSION

Branch retinal artery occlusion (BRAO) most often occurs in older patients as an embolic complication of atherosclerosis. In younger patients, inflammatory (infectious and autoimmune) diseases, thrombotic states, cardiac valvular disorders, vasospastic conditions, and exogenous embolic sources must be considered in the differential diagnosis. Branch retinal artery occlusions are usually unilateral and unifocal but may be bilateral or multifocal in unusual cases.

Symptoms

Branch retinal artery occlusion is characterized by sudden, painless loss of visual field or visual acuity. Occasionally, episodes of transient visual loss lasting minutes (amaurosis fugax) precede permanent retinal arteriolar occlusion.

Clinical Findings

Funduscopic examination reveals opacification of the inner retina ("ischemic retinal whitening") in the distribution of the occluded branch retinal artery. In some patients, an embolus may be visible at an arterial bifurcation. The most common forms of emboli are fibrin-platelet, cholesterol, and calcific emboli. The ischemic retinal whitening usually clears within 3 weeks. Late funduscopic changes include segmental disc pallor and narrowing of the involved arteriole.

Multiple BRAOs may be observed in one or both eyes with or without associated systemic disease. Idiopathic recurrent BRAO is an unusual condition characterized by multiple BRAOs, hearing loss, and evidence of brain infarctions in otherwise healthy individuals. Multiple BRAOs may be seen in association with collagen vascular disorders (systemic lupus erythematosus), inflammatory conditions (toxoplasmosis, cat scratch neuroretinitis), and malignant hypertension. Branch retinal artery occlusions must be differentiated from cotton wool spots, Purtscher's-like retinopathy, and myelinated nerve fibers.

Ancillary Testing

Fluorescein angiography may demonstrate delay or absence of filling in the affected retinal arteriole. However, particularly with fibrin-platelet or cholesterol emboli, retinal blood flow may be restored by the time the patient seeks attention.

Pathology/Pathogenesis

Ischemic retinal whitening occurs secondary to denaturation of intracellular proteins. Retinal arteriolar emboli originate from various sites including the carotid artery (platelet, cholesterol, or calcific emboli), cardiac valves (calcific, platelet, or septic emboli), and exogenous sources (such as talc or steroidal suspensions injected intravascularly). Purtscher's-like retinopathy occurs in patients with long bone fractures, collagen vascular disease, acute pancreatitis, amniotic fluid embolism, incomplete central retinal artery occlusion, and other disorders. The multiple arteriolar occlusions in some patients with Purtscher's-like retinopathy are thought to result from emboli composed of leukocyte aggregates occurring in response to systemic complement activation.

Treatment/Prognosis

Treatment of BRAO has two components: first, to minimize the effects of the retinal arteriolar occlusion, and second, to address the underlying systemic cause, if known. As with central retinal artery occlusion, the treating physician may attempt to move or dislodge the embolus by anterior chamber paracentesis, having the patient rebreathe into a paper bag, or having the patient inhale carbogen. However, treatment is not effective in most cases. If the occlusion is thought to be secondary to a systemic inflammatory disorder, treatment with systemic corticosteroids or immunosuppressive drugs, managed in cooperation with an internist, may be indicated.

The visual prognosis for BRAO is generally favorable, with most eyes retaining vision of 20/40 or better, provided the fovea is not involved. Visual field defects corresponding to the distribution of the BRAO are permanent.

Systemic Evaluation

Patients with atherosclerotic risk factors such as diabetes or hypertension require an embolic workup including carotid Doppler studies and echocardiography (transthoracic or transesophageal, depending on the recommendation of the cardiologist performing the study). Review of systems may direct further evaluation for coagulopathy, systemic or ocular inflammatory disorder, or embolic source.

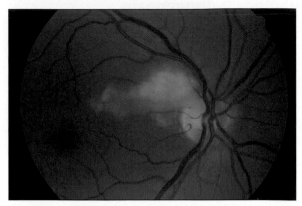

A 64-year-old man with ischemic retinal whitening in the distribution of a small branch retinal arteriole. The ischemic retinal whitening results from infarction of the inner retinal layers.

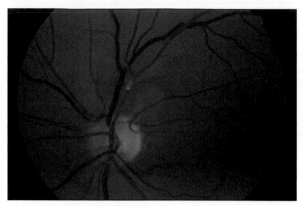

An intra-arterial embolus (Hollenhorst plaque) is observed at the first branching site of the superotemporal arteriole in the fellow eye of the same patient.

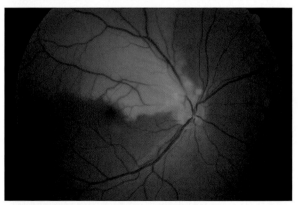

A 36-year-old woman presented with a prominent superotemporal branch retinal artery occlusion. She had a history of migraines and was taking oral contraceptive medication. Her systemic evaluation was negative.

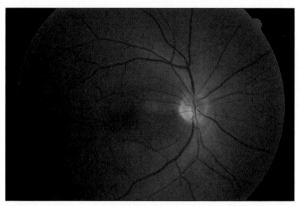

Fundus photograph 1 year after an inferotemporal branch retinal artery occlusion. Note the segmental disc pallor, nerve fiber layer dropout, and marked attenuation of the inferotemporal retinal arteriole.

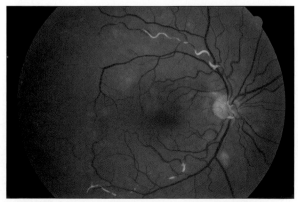

Idiopathic recurrent multifocal branch retinal artery occlusions in a 59-year-old man. There were unusual fibrin-platelet aggregates within multiple branch retinal arterioles. The periphery had a featureless, ischemic appearance.

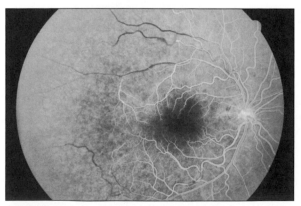

Fluorescein angiography of the same patient demonstrates multifocal branch retinal artery occlusions and midperipheral retinal ischemia.

BRANCH RETINAL VEIN OCCLUSION

Branch retinal vein occlusion (BRVO) is a common retinal vascular disease. Branch retinal vein occlusion appears most frequently between the sixth and eighth decades and affects men and women equally. Branch retinal vein occlusion is unilateral, with a 5% to 10% risk to the fellow eye. Risk factors for BRVO include hypertension, cardiovascular disease, increasing age, elevated body mass, glaucoma, and possibly diabetes mellitus.

Symptoms

Symptoms of BRVO include blurred vision, metamorphopsia, visual field loss, and floaters. Individuals may be asymptomatic, depending on the location of the BRVO.

Clinical Features

Occlusion of a retinal vein occurs almost invariably at an arteriovenous crossing site where the artery lies anterior to the vein. Acute retinal findings include venous dilation and tortuosity, superficial and deep retinal hemorrhages, cotton wool spots, and retinal edema. Chronic retinal findings are variable. The retinal hemorrhages may resolve in weeks to months. Dilated capillaries and microaneurysms may be seen in the territory of the vein occlusion. Macular edema may be associated with lipid exudation and blood-filled cysts. Small, tortuous venous collateral vessels may cross the horizontal raphe or "bridge" the site of venous occlusion. There may be sheathing of retinal arteries and veins in the region of the BRVO. The major complications of BRVO are macular edema and retinal neovascularization with vitreous hemorrhage.

Ancillary Testing

Fluorescein angiography reveals delayed venous filling and prolonged venous circulation time of the involved vein. The retinal vascular bed may show microvascular abnormalities such as microaneurysms, telangiectasis, and macroaneurysm formation. Leakage of fluorescein from microvascular abnormalities is common. Capillary nonperfusion and disruption of the foveal capillary ring may be seen in cases of macular ischemia. Areas of neovascularization are characterized by intense hyperfluorescence and are usually located at the junction of perfused and nonperfused retina.

Pathology/Pathogenesis

At an arteriovenous crossing site, the vein and artery share a common advential sheath. Atherosclerosis and hypertension may result in increased rigidity of the artery wall and contraction of the common advential sheath. This, in turn, results in compression of the venous lumen and predisposes the venule to thrombosis and venous occlusion.

Treatment/Prognosis

In general, BRVOs are followed up for 3 to 4 months for spontaneous improvement prior to consideration of laser surgery. The Branch Retinal Vein Occlusion Study provides clear guidelines for the treatment of BRVO. Macular grid photocoagulation to areas of macular edema increases the likelihood of visual recovery and reduces the risk of visual loss. If retinal neovascularization develops, scatter photocoagulation to the ischemic retina reduces the risk of vitreous hemorrhage and further visual loss. Long-term visual loss is usually related to chronic macular edema and macular ischemia.

Systemic Evaluation

It is important for individuals to have a systemic evaluation to identify potentially treatable risk factors for BRVO including hypertension. In atypical cases, investigation for coagulopathy or inflammatory disease is also considered.

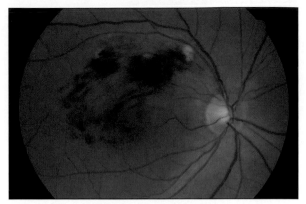

Acute branch retinal vein occlusion produces intraretinal hemorrhages in the distribution of the occluded branch retinal vein. Flame-shaped hemorrhages are in the nerve fiber layer, whereas dot/blot hemorrhages are in the deeper retinal layers. The white lesions are cotton wool spots.

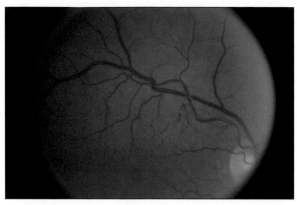

An arteriovenous crossing site, where the artery lies anterior to the vein, is where branch vein occlusions occur. Note the prominent venous narrowing at the proximal crossing site along the superotemporal arcade.

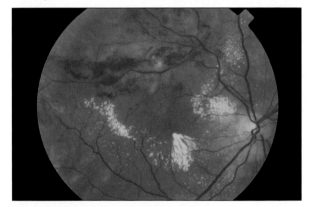

Macular edema is the most common complication following a branch retinal vein occlusion (BRVO). This BRVO is characterized by marked macular edema and lipid exudation.

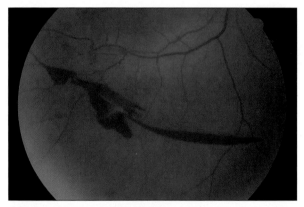

Preretinal/vitreous hemorrhage and neovascularization may occur in branch retinal vein occlusions associated with retinal ischemia.

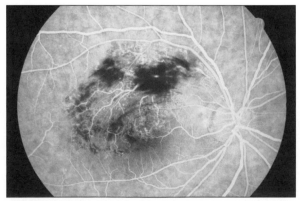

Fluorescein angiography in branch retinal vein occlusion (BRVO) shows a delay in the venous circulation time as well as capillary nonperfusion in the distribution of the BRVO. The capillaries are dilated and tortuous and leak throughout the study.

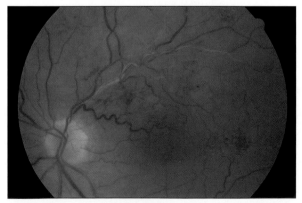

This chronic branch retinal vein occlusion reveals sheathing of the involved vein. There are retinal pigment epithelial alterations in the fovea as a result of chronic macular edema. The capillaries in the involved area are dilated and tortuous.

CENTRAL RETINAL ARTERY OCCLUSION

Central retinal artery occlusion (CRAO) occurs in older patients as a complication of atherosclerosis. Rarely, CRAO in the elderly may be related to giant cell arteritis. When CRAO occurs in younger patients, other etiologies such as coagulopathy, cardiac emboli, or collagen vascular disease with vasculitis must be considered.

Symptoms

Sudden, severe, painless loss of vision characterizes the onset of CRAO. Episodes of transient visual loss lasting minutes (amaurosis fugax) may precede permanent visual loss. If eye pain is associated with CRAO, unusual causes such as carotid dissection or orbital cellulitis must be considered. Symptoms of giant cell arteritis including jaw claudication, scalp tenderness, headache, fatigue, and myalgias may occur in some patients.

Clinical Findings

In the majority of eyes with CRAO, visual acuity is 20/200 or worse. Retention of good central acuity may be seen in individuals with a cilioretinal artery. An afferent pupillary defect is invariably present. The characteristic funduscopic lesion in CRAO is a cherry red spot. The cherry red spot refers to the macular appearance of a central red spot surrounded by superficial retinal whitening. Occlusion of the central retinal artery results in ischemia and infarction of the inner retina, including the nerve fiber and ganglion cell layers. This occlusion is manifest by whitening and edema of the inner retina in the macular area where the nerve fiber and ganglion cell layers are thickest. The foveola retains its reddish color because the inner retinal layers are displaced laterally and the underlying choroidal circulation remains intact. Blood flow within retinal arterioles may appear slow and segmented, a finding referred to as "box-car" or "cattle-truck" formation. Iris neovascularization may be seen in up to 20% of patients with CRAO.

Ancillary Testing

Fluorescein angiography may demonstrate delay or absence of filling in the retinal arteries. Retrograde filling of retinal veins or arteries may be noted. Retinal blood flow may be restored by the time the patient seeks attention, in which case fluorescein angiographic findings may appear normal.

Pathology/Pathogenesis

Occlusion of the central retinal artery by embolism or thrombosis results in ischemic retinal whitening secondary to infarction of the inner retinal layers and denaturation of intracellular proteins. Irreversible damage to the neurosensory retina occurs after 90 minutes of complete CRAO.

Treatment/Prognosis

Central retinal artery occlusion typically results in severe visual loss in the range of 20/200 to light perception. For embolic CRAO of less than 24 hours' duration, the treating physician may attempt to improve perfusion pressure and/or "dislodge" the embolus. This may be accomplished by lowering the intraocular pressure (anterior chamber paracentesis, ocular massage, or administration of aqueous suppressants) or dilation of retinal arterioles (having the patient rebreathe into a paper bag or inhale carbogen). Treatment rarely alters the visual outcome. Systemic anticoagulation therapy and the use of fibrinolytic agents (given systemically or by selective catherization of the ophthalmic or supraorbital artery) have been tried with variable success. Systemic corticosteroids may be appropriate for CRAO related to vasculitis to protect the fellow eye and limit systemic complications. Prompt panretinal photocoagulation is indicated for eyes that develop iris or anterior chamber angle neovascularization.

Systemic Evaluation

In older patients, the major risk factors for CRAO include hypertension (up to two thirds of patients in one series), diabetes mellitus, carotid artery disease, and coronary artery disease. In patients with atherosclerotic risk factors or evidence of retinal embolization, carotid Doppler studies and echocardiography (either transthoracic or transesophageal) are indicated. If systemic symptoms of vasculitis or collagen vascular disease are present, a sedimentation rate and urgent rheumatological consultation are indicated.

Younger patients require the above embolic workup, with additional consideration given to coagulopathies (sickle cell disease, oral contraceptive use, pregnancy, protein S or antithrombin III deficiency, antiphospholipid antibody syndrome, or homocysteinuria).

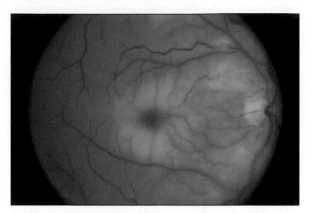

An acute embolic central retinal artery occlusion produces sudden vision loss in a 68-year-old man. Visual acuity was 20/400. A prominent cherry red spot was present.

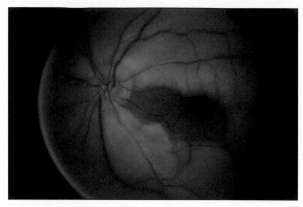

Acute central retinal artery occlusion with cilioretinal artery sparing is seen in this fundus photograph. Diffuse ischemic retinal whitening of the inner retina is observed. The inferior macula is spared as a result of the cilioretinal artery.

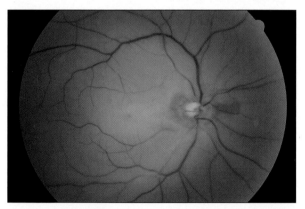

Acute central retinal artery occlusion. Ischemic retinal whitening is present throughout the macula. A very small cherry red spot is visible.

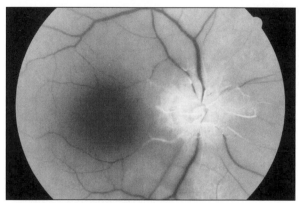

The fluorescein angiogram of the same patient demonstrates nonperfusion of the major retinal arterioles. Only the optic disc and peripapillary vessels fill with fluorescein. The normal choroidal fluorescence is present.

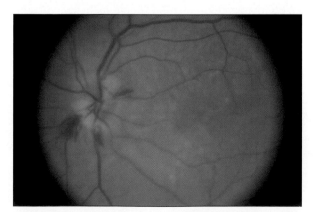

Central retinal artery occlusion (CRAO) in a 72-year-old woman with combined CRAO and anterior ischemic optic neuropathy as a result of giant cell arteritis.

CENTRAL RETINAL VEIN OCCLUSION

Central retinal vein occlusion (CRVO) is a common retinal vascular disease that is usually seen in adults over age 50 years. Men may be more commonly affected than women, especially in younger age groups. Risk factors for CRVO include systemic vascular disease (hypertension, cardiovascular disease, diabetes mellitus) and primary open-angle glaucoma. Central retinal vein occlusions are classified as perfused or nonperfused, based on the extent of retinal ischemia.

Symptoms

Individuals with CRVO may be asymptomatic or present with profound visual loss. Loss of vision may be sudden or gradual. Other symptoms include central scotoma, photopsias, transient visual obscurations, pain, and eye redness.

Clinical Features

Visual acuity of less than 20/200 and the presence of an afferent pupillary defect suggest ischemia. It is also important to measure intraocular pressure and perform an undilated slit lamp examination and gonioscopy to examine for iris or anterior chamber angle neovascularization. Acute retinal findings include dilated and tortuous veins, scattered intraretinal hemorrhages in all four quadrants of the retina, cotton wool spots, macular edema, and optic disc edema. Late findings include collateral vessels on the optic disc, persistent venous dilation and tortuosity, perivascular sheathing, arterial narrowing, and macular abnormalities (chronic macular edema and retinal pigment epithelial alterations).

The major complications of CRVO are macular edema and neovascular glaucoma. Macular edema may range from mild retinal thickening to frank cystoid macular edema. Approximately one third of eyes with CRVO are classified as nonperfused or ischemic. Of those ischemic eyes, one third to one half will develop neovascular glaucoma as a result of iris and anterior chamber angle neovascularization.

Ancillary Testing

Fluorescein angiography demonstrates a marked delay in the filling of the retinal veins with prolongation of the arteriovenous transit time. Leakage is routinely observed from the optic disc and retinal vessels. Varying degrees of macular ischemia and leakage occur. Central retinal vein occlusions also vary in the extent of peripheral retinal nonperfusion. Eyes with areas of at least 10 disc diameters (DD) of retinal nonperfusion are classified as nonperfused or ischemic.

In addition to fluorescein angiography, the extent of retinal ischemia can be estimated by electrophysiologic testing. Inner retinal ischemia is associated with a reduction in the b-wave amplitude on the electroretinogram. A b-wave to a-wave ratio of less than 1 is associated with significant retinal ischemia and an increased risk for neovascular glaucoma.

Pathology/Pathogenesis

Histopathologic study of autopsy eyes with CRVO reveals thrombosis of the central retinal vein at the level of the lamina cribrosa. Obstruction of the central retinal vein leads to varying degrees of fluid and lipid exudation, red cell extravasation, and ischemia in all quadrants of the retina.

Treatment/Prognosis

The CRVO Study examined the natural history of perfused CRVOs, the effect of macular grid laser photocoagulation for macular edema, and the timing of panretinal photocoagulation (PRP) in eyes with significant nonperfusion. Approximately one third of eyes initially judged as perfused progressed to the nonperfused group by 3 years (most rapidly within the first 4 months). These results indicated that even those patients with initially perfused CRVOs require close follow-up and careful examination for neovascularization of the iris or anterior chamber angle at each visit. Macular grid-pattern photocoagulation reduced the extent of macular edema but did not result in significant visual improvement. Prophylactic PRP in eyes with significant retinal ischemia offered no advantage over prompt PRP when iris or angle neovascularization was detected. The CRVO Study recommended patients be examined monthly for the first 6 months. Examination should include undilated slit lamp examination and gonioscopy to detect iris or anterior chamber angle neovascularization. If iris or angle neovascularization is found, PRP should be initiated promptly.

Systemic Evaluation

Common systemic associations with CRVO include hypertension, cardiovascular disease, and diabetes mellitus. Evaluation for a hyperviscosity syndrome is indicated for patients with bilateral simultaneous CRVO. Review of systems in younger patients with CRVO may direct systemic evaluation for hypertension, diabetes, or hypercoagulable states.

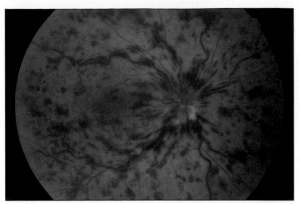

Acute central retinal vein occlusion produces optic disc edema and hemorrhage, venous dilation and tortuosity, intraretinal hemorrhages in all four quadrants, and varying degrees of macular edema.

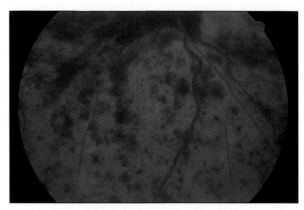

Acute central retinal vein occlusion at a higher magnification demonstrates diffuse dot/blot hemorrhages in the midperipheral retina.

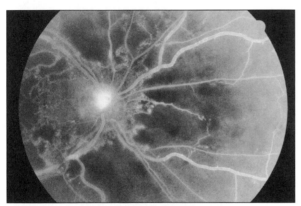

Fluorescein angiogram of an ischemic central retinal vein occlusion reveals widespread retinal capillary nonperfusion. The patient had 20/400 vision and a relative afferent pupillary defect.

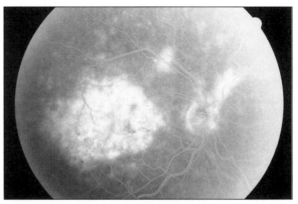

Fluorescein angiogram demonstrates chronic macular edema in central retinal vein occlusion. Cystic macular edema is seen with diffuse vascular leakage throughout the macula.

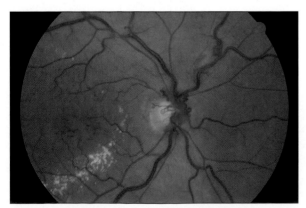

Collateral vessels on the optic disc become apparent within months after the onset of the central retinal vein occlusion. Also note the macular edema associated with lipid exudation.

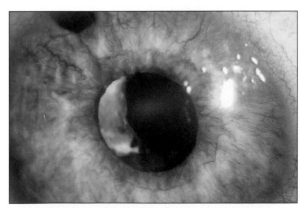

Iris neovascularization results from widespread retinal ischemia and requires prompt panretinal photocoagulation.

COATS' DISEASE

Coats' disease is an idiopathic, developmental retinal vascular abnormality usually affecting one eye of male patients. No genetic predisposition is known. Coats' disease primarily affects children and young adults; the majority of cases present prior to age 20 years.

Symptoms

The degree of visual loss is variable and usually related to the degree of macular involvement. Infants and children commonly have a more severe variant of the disease and often present with severe visual loss. At the other end of the spectrum, Coats' disease may be identified on a routine examination in an asymptomatic patient.

Clinical Features

Infants and young children may present with a severe exudative detachment as a result of leakage from telangiectatic changes and aneurysmal dilations of most or all of the retinal vessels. These eyes are at great risk for developing neovascular glaucoma and phthisis bulbi. A less severe variant, usually occurring in young to middle-aged adults, can present with either macular or peripheral telangiectasia and aneurysmal dilation with varying degrees of leakage and exudation. Juxtafoveal telangiectasia can result in cystoid macular edema and/or macular exudation. Visual loss is usually mild to moderate. Macular telangiectasia may be isolated or associated with peripheral telangiectasia. Peripheral telangiectasia and aneurysmal dilation may also occur as an isolated finding. In such a case, visual loss is due to gravitational deposition of exudate into the macula from the peripheral retinal telangiectasia. The telangiectatic vessels may be associated with retinal capillary nonperfusion and vascular sheathing.

Ancillary Testing

Fluorescein angiography is important in confirming the diagnosis of Coats' disease. It clearly demonstrates the aneurysmal dilation of the capillary bed, the retinal arteries, and veins. Retinal capillary nonperfusion is often present and more prominent in patients with large aneurysmal dilations. The later phases of the angiogram demonstrate leakage from the telangiectatic vessels.

Pathology/Pathogenesis

The pathogenesis of Coats' disease is unknown. Histopathologic information derived from eyes enucleated with severe variants of the disease demonstrates irregular dilation of capillaries, arteries, and veins with leakage of periodic acid Schiff (PAS)-positive exudate into the retina and subretinal space. Lipid-engorged macrophages are present in the subretinal space and usually seen remote from the telangiectatic vessels. Electron microscopy demonstrates retinal vascular endothelial abnormalities.

Treatment/Prognosis

Treatment varies according to the severity of disease. Asymptomatic patients with either juxtafoveal or peripheral telangiectasia may not require treatment. These patients should be followed up periodically for progression and instructed to report any changes in vision due to retinal thickening or macular exudation. When vision is threatened or affected, treatment is indicated. Photocoagulation and/or cryotherapy are used to destroy the telangiectatic vessels. Multiple treatment sessions may be necessary. When extensive exudative retinal detachment is present, surgery to drain the subretinal fluid prior to destruction of the telangiectatic vessels may be necessary. A temporary increase in exudation may occur shortly after treatment. If it involves the macula, it may be associated with further loss of vision. Macular distortion secondary to epiretinal membrane formation may follow treatment. The visual prognosis is variable and relates to the degree of macular involvement. Extensive macular lipid deposition may result in permanent changes in the retina and retinal pigment epithelium.

Systemic Evaluation

A systemic workup is usually not indicated in patients presenting with features typical of Coats' disease. Coats' disease has been associated with several systemic diseases, including Alport's disease, tuberous sclerosis, Turner's syndrome, and Senior-Loken syndrome, as well as muscular dystrophy and fascioscapulohumeral dystrophy. Coats' disease has also been reported in association with retinitis pigmentosa.

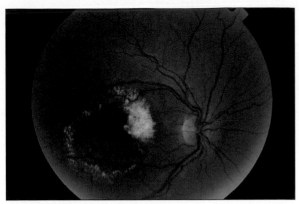

Fundus photograph demonstrates a circinate ring of lipid surrounding the fovea from macular telangiectasia in a 16-year-old boy with a limited variant of Coats' disease.

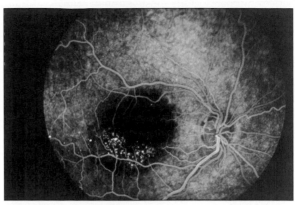

Venous-phase fluorescein angiogram of the same patient demonstrates retinal telangiectasia inferior and temporal to the fovea.

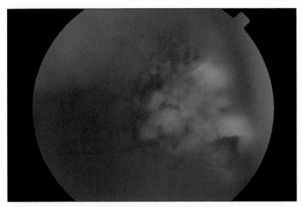

Peripheral retinal telangiectasia with associated intra- and subretinal lipid and hemorrhage simulating a peripheral retinal mass in a 12-year-old boy with Coats' disease.

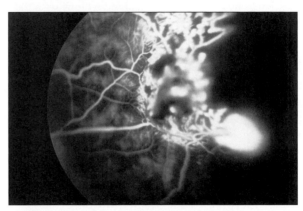

Fluorescein angiogram of the same patient demonstrates leaking telangiectatic vessels. Note the associated retinal capillary nonperfusion adjacent to retinal telangiectasia.

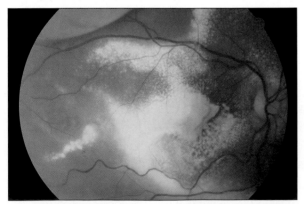

A 17-year-old female patient presented with visual loss related to marked submacular lipid exudation. She had extensive peripheral retinal telangiectasis.

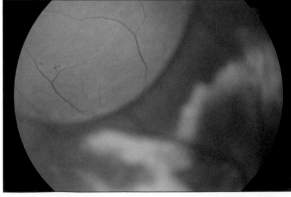

In the same patient peripheral areas of exudative retinal detachment are observed.

DIABETIC RETINOPATHY: NONPROLIFERATIVE

Diabetic retinopathy is the most common retinal vascular disease. It is the leading cause of new blindness in adults during the third through sixth decades of life. The risk of diabetic retinopathy is related to many factors, including the duration of diabetes and the level of diabetes control. Additional factors, including uncontrolled hypertension, hyperlipidemia, intravascular fluid overload states, renal disease, anemia, pregnancy, and intraocular surgery may aggravate the risk and severity of diabetic retinopathy. Nonproliferative diabetic retinopathy (NPDR) is the most common form of diabetic retinopathy.

Symptoms

Most persons with NPDR have no or minimal symptoms through the preclinical phase prior to the onset of ophthalmoscopically visible vascular lesions. In fact, patients usually do not complain of vision loss until moderate nonproliferative retinopathy develops with the onset of macular edema or ischemia.

Clinical Features

In the preclinical phase, the standard clinical evaluations of ophthalmoscopy and fluorescein angiography are normal. However, patients may have impaired retinal function as indicated by electroretinography, contrast sensitivity, or color vision testing. Nonproliferative diabetic retinopathy is characterized by the presence of microaneurysms, intraretinal hemorrhages, lipid exudate, and cotton wool spots. As the condition progresses, most patients have increased vasodilation and tortuosity. The retinal circulation normally autoregulates the blood supply to match the metabolic demands, as does the brain. However, with progressive retinopathy the autoregulatory mechanisms are overwhelmed, especially by elevated systemic blood pressure, intravascular fluid overload, or hypoalbuminemia. Then the vessels leak, and edema collects in the macula (macular edema), as noted by cystic spaces, retinal thickening, and lipoprotein ("hard" exudate) deposits.

Macular edema is associated with most cases of visual loss in NPDR. The term clinically significant macular edema (CSME) is used to describe those eyes at risk for visual loss related to macular edema. Clinically significant macular edema is defined as any of the following: retinal thickening at or within 500 μm of the center of the macula, lipid exudates at or within 500 μm of the center of the macula associated with adjacent retinal thickening, and retinal thickening greater than 1 disc diameter (DD) in area within 1 DD of the center of the macula.

The severity of NPDR can be estimated by using the 4-2-1 rule. Eyes with severe NPDR have any one of the following features: 4 quadrants of dot/blot hemorrhage, 2 quadrants of venous beading, or 1 quadrant of intra-retinal microvascular abnormality (IRMA).

Ancillary Testing

Fluorescein angiography is performed to determine the degree of macular perfusion and identify the location and extent of treatable lesions in patients with clinically significant macular edema. Treatable lesions include discrete points of retinal hyperfluorescence or leakage (microaneurysms); areas of diffuse leakage (microaneurysms, IRMA, and capillary bed leakage); and areas of retinal capillary nonperfusion (except for the normal foveal avascular zone).

Pathology/Pathogenesis

The clinical features of diabetic retinopathy result from a combination of ocular and systemic factors. The retinal features derive from damage to retinal glial cells, neurons, and retinal vascular cells. For example, the factors that contribute to vascular leakage (such as vascular endothelial growth factor) arise from neurons and glial cells. Loss of vision results from direct or indirect insults to neurons. In addition, systemic factors such as hypertension or fluid overload increase the hydrostatic pressure and aggravate the tendency for the blood vessels to leak.

Treatment/Prognosis

The physiologic features described above serve as principles of therapy. First, the primary systemic metabolic control must be optimized. The Diabetes Control and Complications Trial (DCCT) confirmed the benefit of intensive blood glucose control in reducing the development and progression of diabetic retinopathy in individuals with type 1 diabetes mellitus. Similar results have been demonstrated for those with type 2 diabetes. Second, other cardiovascular risk factors (hypertension, fluid overload, hyperlipidemia, anemia) must be treated. Third, local ocular processes of vascular leakage are treated by focal laser photocoagulation. In eyes with CSME, the Early Treatment Diabetic Retinopathy Study demonstrated that macular laser photocoagulation reduced the risk of moderate visual loss by greater than 50%. Macular photocoagulation for CSME involves both focal laser treatment for leaking microaneurysms and grid-pattern laser photocoagulation for areas of diffuse macular edema.

Systemic Evaluation

The development and progression of diabetic retinopathy is influenced by many factors. Patients with diabetes should undergo regular examination and treatment by their primary care provider or endocrinologist to optimize control of their diabetes and improve their overall medical status.

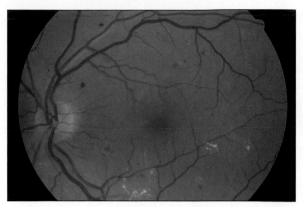

Clinical findings of nonproliferative diabetic retinopathy include microaneurysms, intraretinal hemorrhages, and lipid exudate. Many patients in the early stages of diabetic retinopathy are asymptomatic.

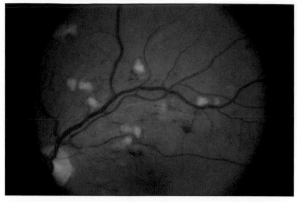

Cotton wool spots are common in patients with diabetic retinopathy. They result from microinfarctions in the nerve fiber layer.

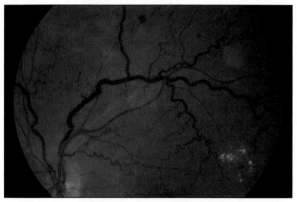

As diabetic retinopathy progresses, patients develop vasodilation and tortuosity of the retinal vessels. Venous beading is characterized by an irregular dilation of the retinal veins.

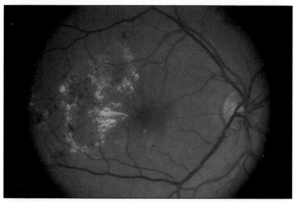

The most common cause of visual loss in patients with nonproliferative diabetic retinopathy is macular edema. Macular edema results from retinal vascular leakage and ischemia.

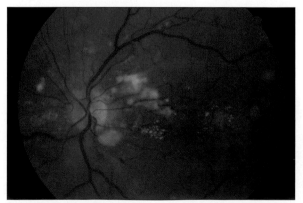

The development and progression of diabetic retinopathy are influenced by many factors including duration of diabetes, quality of diabetes control, and coexisting medical problems. This patient had exacerbation of her diabetic retinopathy related to hypertension.

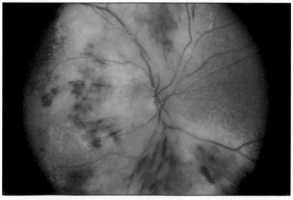

Hyperlipidemia is a common finding in patients with diabetes. Hyperlipidemia may be associated with a significant increase in the presence of retinal lipid exudate and visual loss, as seen in this patient.

DIABETIC RETINOPATHY: NONPROLIFERATIVE (CONT'D)

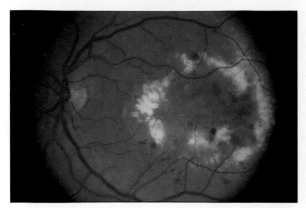

Clinically significant macular edema is determined by the location and extent of the edema. This patient had retinal thickening and lipid exudate involving the center of the macula.

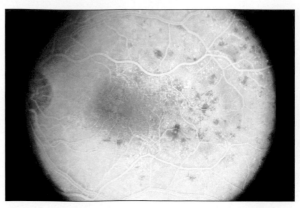

The same patient also had retinal thickening greater than 1 disc diameter in size. Her fluorescein angiogram revealed numerous microaneurysms in the temporal macula.

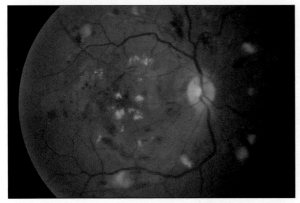

Clinically significant macular edema (CSME) is a clinical diagnosis based on careful fundus contact lens ophthalmoscopic examination. This patient had CSME with retinal thickening and lipid exudate within 500 μm of the center of the macula.

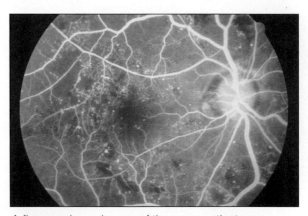

A fluorescein angiogram of the same patient was obtained to identify treatable lesions before laser photocoagulation. The numerous hyperfluorescent spots are consistent with microaneurysms.

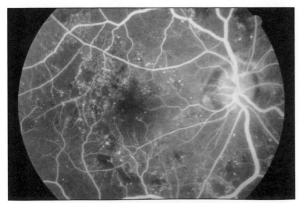

The fluorescein angiogram of the same patient reveals enlargement of the foveal avascular zone, along with areas of capillary nonperfusion.

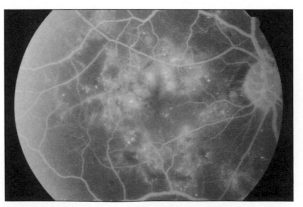

Throughout the study, fluorescein leaks from the microaneurysms resulting in increased hyperfluorescence.

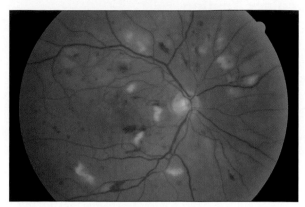

Macular edema results not only from vascular leakage but also from retinal ischemia. This 64-year-old man had clinically significant macular edema with diffuse retinal thickening in his right eye.

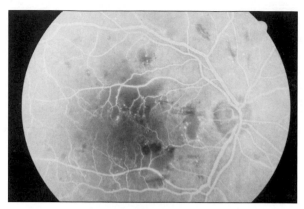

Fluorescein angiography of the same patient reveals hypofluorescence throughout the macula related to capillary nonperfusion.

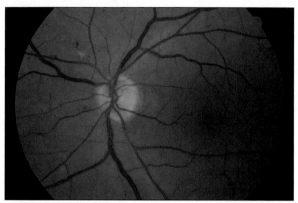

The severity of diabetic retinopathy can be estimated using the 4-2-1 rule. Eyes with severe nonproliferative diabetic retinopathy have any one of the following features: 4 quadrants of dot/blot hemorrhage, 2 quadrants of venous beading, or 1 quadrant of intraretinal microvascular abnormalities.

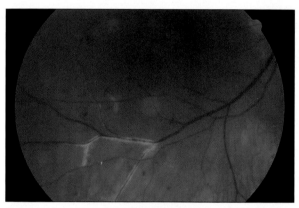

Patients with diabetic retinopathy rarely may develop a pseudovasculitis. The perivascular sheathing is likely the result of lipid exudate along the vessel wall.

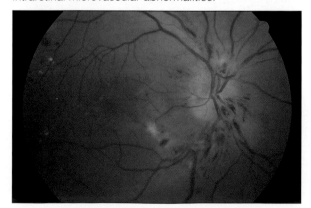

Diabetic papillopathy is a cause of temporary visual loss in patients with type 1 diabetes. Patients present with sudden visual loss in one eye. The optic disc is swollen and hyperemic with superficial optic disc and retinal hemorrhages.

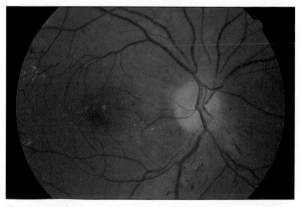

The disc edema and hemorrhages in the same patient resolved over weeks to months. Visual acuity returned to normal.

DIABETIC RETINOPATHY: PROLIFERATIVE

Diabetic retinopathy is the most common retinal vascular disease. It is the leading cause of new blindness in adults during the third through sixth decades of life. Proliferative diabetic retinopathy (PDR) is an advanced form of diabetic retinopathy characterized by the proliferation of new vessels on the optic disc, retina, or iris as a result of widespread retinal ischemia. Complications of PDR include vitreous hemorrhage, fibrovascular proliferation, traction retinal detachment, and neovascular glaucoma.

Symptoms

Individuals with PDR may be asymptomatic or complain of visual loss and floaters related to vitreous hemorrhage. In cases of neovascular glaucoma, patients may present with eye pain and redness in addition to loss of vision.

Clinical Features

Individuals with PDR exhibit the same findings as patients with nonproliferative diabetic retinopathy: microaneurysms, retinal hemorrhages, cotton wool spots, lipid exudates, and macular edema. In addition, neovascularization arises on the optic disc, retina, and/or iris. Neovascularization of the optic disc (NVD) appears as fine, lacy vessels on the surface of the optic disc. Neovascularization elsewhere (NVE) is retinal neovascularization located at sites other than on or within 1 disc diameter (DD) of the optic disc. Neovascularization elsewhere is observed most commonly along or just anterior to the temporal retinal vascular arcades. Neovascularization of the optic disc and neovacularization elsewhere are associated with a variable amount of fibrosis.

The vitreous plays a critical role in the development of PDR. It appears that the vitreous provides a scaffold for the growth of new vessels. The strong interaction between the vitreous and the neovascular tissue contributes to the development of vitreous hemorrhage and traction retinal detachment.

Iris neovascularization is characterized by the proliferation of fine, lacy vessels on the iris surface or anterior chamber angle. Frank neovascular glaucoma may present with conjunctival injection, corneal edema, anterior chamber flare, iris and angle neovascularization, and intraocular pressure elevation.

Ancillary Testing

Fluorescein angiography reveals significant midperipheral capillary nonperfusion. Neovascularization of the optic disc or neovascularization elsewhere hyperfluoresces early and leaks throughout the study. Neovascularization elsewhere usually is observed at the junction of the perfused and nonperfused retina.

Pathology/Pathogenesis

The risk of PDR is related to the extent of retinal ischemia. Vascular endothelial growth factor (VEGF) is a leading candidate linking retinal ischemia and intraocular neovascularization. This growth factor is an angiogenic peptide, the expression of which is markedly increased by retinal hypoxia. Conversely, VEGF levels decline significantly after successful panretinal photocoagulation (PRP).

Treatment/Prognosis

The Diabetic Retinopathy Study identified four retinopathy risk factors for severe visual loss: new vessels present, NVD, preretinal or vitreous hemorrhage, and severe new vessels (NVD greater than one-third disc area, or in the absence of NVD, NVE greater than one-half DD). The presence of three or four risk factors indicates "high risk" for severe visual loss and requires prompt PRP. Panretinal photocoagulation is successful in reducing the risk of severe visual loss by more than 50%. A favorable response to PRP is associated with a regression of retinopathy risk factors, which in turn is associated with a favorable visual prognosis. The beneficial effects of PRP are long standing. In eyes with nonclearing vitreous hemorrhage or traction retinal detachment, pars plana vitrectomy may be performed. Iris neovascularization and neovascular glaucoma are treated with prompt PRP.

Systemic Evaluation

The development and progression of diabetic retinopathy are influenced by many factors. Patients with diabetes should undergo regular examination and treatment by their primary care provider or endocrinologist to optimize their diabetes control and improve their overall medical status. Particular attention should be directed to the treatment of hypertension and renal failure or other fluid overload states.

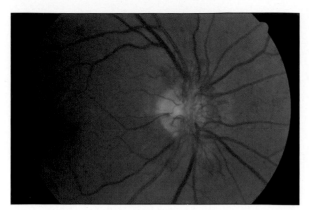

Optic disc neovascularization (NVD) is characterized by the growth of fine, lacy vessels from the optic disc. If NVD is larger than one-third disc area in size, it is classified as high-risk proliferative diabetic retinopathy.

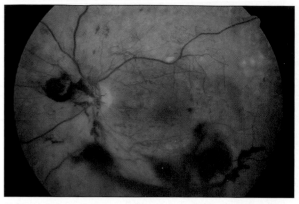

Patients with neovascularization of the optic disc may be asymptomatic early in the course of proliferative diabetic retinopathy. Visual loss is related to the development of vitreous hemorrhage or traction retinal detachment.

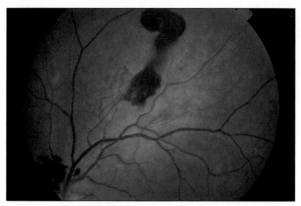

Neovascularization elsewhere is found along the major vascular arcades or in the midperipheral retina.

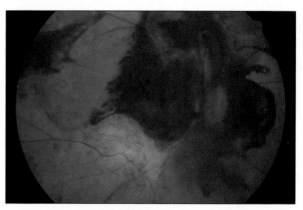

Fibrovascular proliferation causes areas of adhesion between the optic disc or retina and the posterior vitreous. Contraction of the fibrovascular tissue results in vitreous hemorrhage or traction retinal detachment.

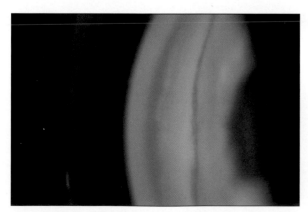

Iris and angle neovascularization is a severe complication of proliferative diabetic retinopathy. Secondary closure of the anterior chamber angle leads to neovascular glaucoma. Prompt panretinal photocoagulation is required for patients with iris or angle neovascularization.

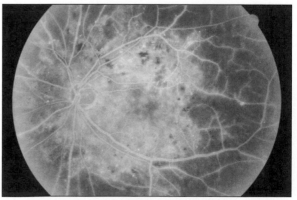

The development of proliferative diabetic retinopathy is a result of widespread retinal ischemia. This fluorescein angiogram demonstrates peripheral hypofluorescence as a result of retinal capillary nonperfusion.

DIABETIC RETINOPATHY: PROLIFERATIVE (CONT'D)

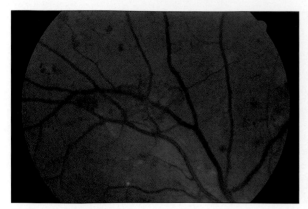

Neovascularization elsewhere is found most commonly along the temporal vascular arcades.

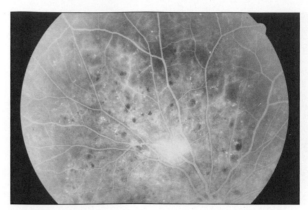

The new vessels are located at the junction of the perfused and nonperfused retina. The abnormal vessels hyperfluoresce intensely with fluorescein angiography.

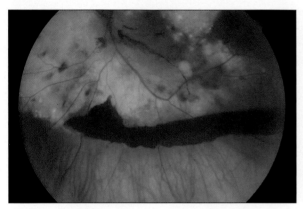

Preretinal hemorrhage may assume a boat-shaped pattern. This patient also had hyperlipidemia with extensive lipid exudation.

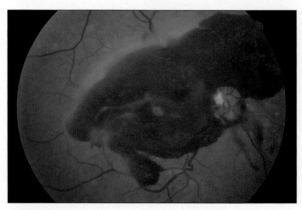

The hemorrhage obscures the macula and retinal blood vessels, confirming the preretinal location. This preretinal hemorrhage is associated with a smoky rim of fibrin along the superior margin.

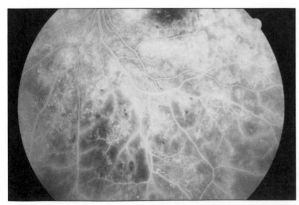

Fluorescein angiogram of a 24-year-old woman with proliferative diabetic retinopathy. Extensive peripheral capillary nonperfusion is evident.

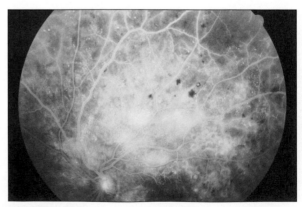

The areas of intense hyperfluorescence on the optic disc and along the vascular arcades are suggestive of neovascularization.

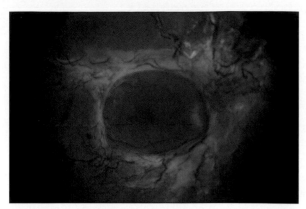

Untreated proliferative diabetic retinopathy may result in extensive fibrovascular proliferation, as shown in this patient. Fibrovascular proliferation may lead to vitreous hemorrhage and traction retinal detachment.

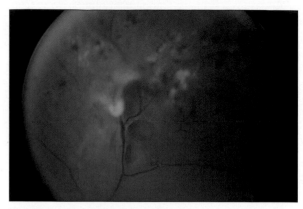

Patients with traction retinal detachments may occasionally develop retinal holes and secondary rhegmatogenous retinal detachments. The white area is the point of vitreoretinal traction.

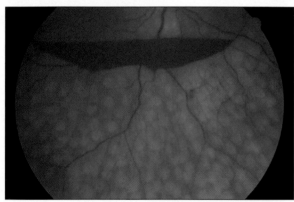

Panretinal photocoagulation (PRP) is indicated for the treatment of high-risk proliferative diabetic retinopathy. This fundus photograph was taken immediately after PRP. The white burns are visible inferior to the preretinal, boat-shaped hemorrhage.

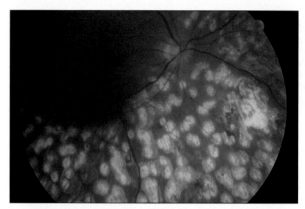

Fundus photograph of a patient successfully treated with panretinal photocoagulation approximately 6 months previously for high-risk proliferative diabetic retinopathy.

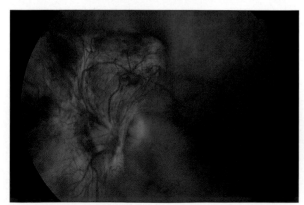

This 24-year-old woman had high-risk proliferative diabetic retinopathy that did not respond to standard panretinal photocoagulation. She developed extensive fibrovascular proliferation with vitreous hemorrhage.

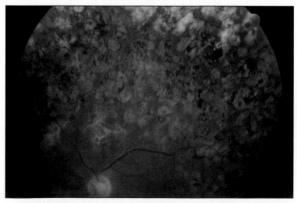

She did well after pars plana vitrectomy and supplemental laser photocoagulation.

EALES' DISEASE

Eales' disease is a primary, idiopathic obliterative vasculopathy that most often affects young adults between 20 and 30 years of age. Men are affected more commonly than women. Eales' disease is characterized by perivascular sheathing, peripheral retinal nonperfusion, neovascularization, and recurrent vitreous hemorrhages. The disease is bilateral but may be asymmetric.

Symptoms

Most patients present with symptoms related to recurrent vitreous hemorrhage, including floaters and reduced vision. Others may complain of blurred vision not associated with floaters.

Clinical Features

Patients with Eales' disease typically have evidence of retinal venous and/or arterial sheathing, telangiectatic changes in the midperipheral retina, and optic disc or peripheral retinal neovascularization. Preretinal or vitreous hemorrhage is common. Fibrovascular proliferation may lead to traction retinal detachment. Macular abnormalities include cystoid macular edema and epiretinal membrane formation. Some patients have vitreous cells but anterior segment inflammation is uncommon.

The major differential diagnostic considerations include other causes of peripheral retinal neovascularization such as peripheral branch retinal vein occlusion, sickle cell retinopathy, multiple sclerosis, and sarcoidosis.

Ancillary Testing

Fluorescein angiography shows midperipheral retinal nonperfusion with well-demarcated borders between areas of perfused and nonperfused retina. Leakage of fluorescein from areas of neovascularization may be observed from the optic disc or located at the junction of perfused and nonperfused retina.

Pathology/Pathogenesis

Little is understood of the pathogenesis. Peripheral retinal inflammation may incite an obliterative vasculitis leading to subsequent ischemia and neovascularization.

Treatment/Prognosis

Laser photocoagulation to the ischemic peripheral retina is the treatment of choice, but cryotherapy may used if the vitreous is opaque. The inflammatory component and macular edema may respond to periocular or systemic corticosteroids. Most patients have a good prognosis, but rare patients develop macular ischemia or traction retinal detachment.

Systemic Evaluation

Most patients diagnosed with Eales' disease in the United States are healthy and without associated systemic disease. However, there is an association with tuberculosis, especially in the Middle East, so tuberculin skin testing is recommended.

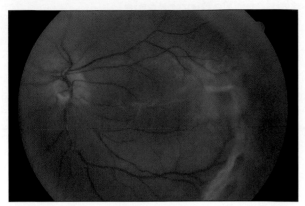

This 31-year-old man with Eales' disease had a history of intermittent vision loss. He had vitreous opacities consistent with old hemorrhage and areas of vasculitis involving the retinal veins (periphlebitis).

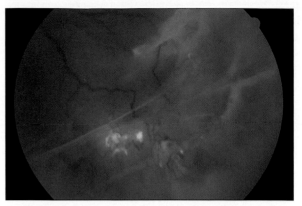

Peripheral retinal examination of the same patient revealed retinal neovascularization with fibrovascular proliferation and traction retinal detachment.

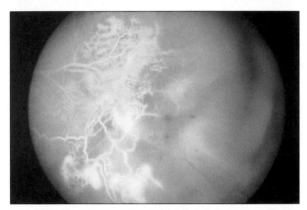

Fluorescein angiography of the same patient demonstrates peripheral retinal ischemia with large areas of capillary nonperfusion. The hyperfluorescence corresponds to the areas of peripheral neovascularization.

HYPERTENSIVE RETINOPATHY

Arterial hypertension is a major risk factor for cardiovascular disease, which is a leading cause of morbidity and mortality. The effects of arterial hypertension can be directly visualized in the fundus. These changes may involve the retinal arterioles, the choroid, and the optic nerve. Observation of these fundus changes may lead to a diagnosis of hypertension in a previously undiagnosed patient.

Symptoms

Mild to moderate degrees of hypertension often result in asymptomatic fundus changes. Severe or malignant hypertension may produce fundus changes resulting in blurred or distorted vision. These fundus changes include central macular thickening or lipid deposition from retinal vascular or optic disc leakage. Serous macular detachment secondary to choroidal ischemia may occur also. In addition, transient obscurations of vision may result from hypertension-induced optic disc edema.

Clinical Features

The clinical features of hypertensive retinopathy are categorized as retinal vascular changes, choroidopathy, and optic neuropathy. The large retinal arterioles may be focally or difusely narrowed. The arterial walls become thickened due to leakage of blood elements into the wall, which may lead to focal ischemic whitening of the retina, producing the classic cotton wool spot. The focal ischemia may also lead to surrounding microvascular abnormalities in addition to retinal hemorrhages and intraretinal serous exudation and lipid deposition. Hypertensive choroidopathy results from choroidal ischemia, leading to necrosis of the overlying retinal pigment epithelium (RPE) and often resulting in serous retinal detachments. Changes in the pigment epithelium (Elschnig spots) and larger choroidal vessels (Segrist streaks) remain after resolution of the serous detachment. Severe or malignant hypertension often leads to bilateral optic disc edema presumed to be due to ischemia. Lipid deposition may result in formation of a macular star.

Pathology/Pathogenesis

Pathogenesis of hypertensive retinopathy probably begins with failure of retinal vascular autoregulation, leading to endothelial cell alterations and breakdown of the blood-retinal barrier, resulting in leakage of fluid, blood, and macromolecules into the retina. Also, occlusion of terminal retinal arterioles can lead to nerve fiber layer infarction. The choroidopathy results from acute multifocal areas of fibrin-platelet occlusion and necrosis of choroidal arteries and choriocapillaris which leads to necrosis of overlying RPE.

Treatment/Prognosis

The primary treatment for hypertensive retinopathy is systemic arterial blood pressure control. The visual prognosis is excellent in mild to moderate cases of hypertensive retinopathy. When there is foveal edema and/or lipid deposition, a variable degree of permanent visual loss may occur due to structural changes in the retina and RPE. The presence of associated retinal vascular conditions, including arterial macroaneurysms and branch retinal vein obstruction (BRVO) also may affect the prognosis.

Systemic Evaluation

The systemic evaluation should focus on the etiology of the hypertension. As many as 85% to 90% of cases are classified as essential hypertension. Secondary causes should be ruled out in selected patients.

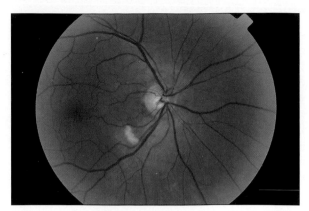

Fundus photograph of a 48-year-old man with a recent diagnosis of hypertension. He had diffuse and focal arterial narrowing, arterial-venous crossing changes, and cotton wool spots.

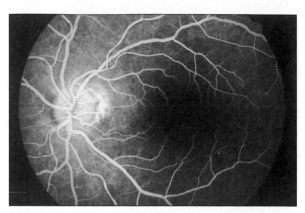

Fluorescein angiogram of a 60-year-old woman with newly onset hypertension reveals areas of focal attenuation of the proximal arterioles.

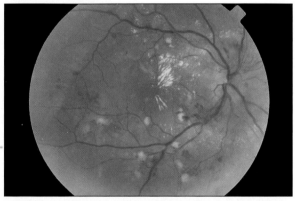

A 22-year-old woman was admitted to the hospital with severe headaches. Her blood pressure was 240/150 mm Hg. She had bilateral optic disc edema, macular stars, cotton wool spots, and intraretinal hemorrhages.

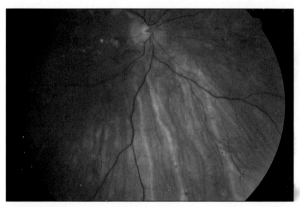

This fundus photograph demonstrates the late sequelae of hypertensive choroidopathy: Elschnig spots (areas of focal hyperpigmentation) and Segrist streaks (areas of choroidal sclerosis).

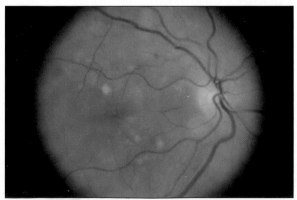

A 32-year-old woman with severe hypertension and seizures complained of visual loss during her third trimester of pregnancy. She had serous detachment of the macula, with patchy white areas, indicating infarction of the retinal pigment epithelium.

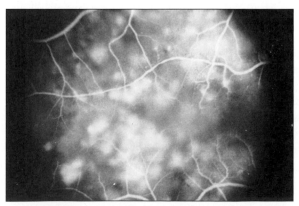

The fluorescein angiogram of the same patient revealed multiple areas of leakage at the level of the retinal pigment epithelium resulting from choroidal ischemia.

IDIOPATHIC JUXTAFOVEOLAR RETINAL TELANGIECTASIS

Idiopathic juxtafoveolar retinal telangiectasis (the terms parafoveal telangiectasis and juxtafoveal telangiectasis are also used) refers to a group of retinal vascular disorders in which a portion of the parafoveal capillary network develops dilated and tortuous blood vessels. Patients with idiopathic juxtafoveolar retinal telangiectasis (IJRT) may be categorized into three subgroups that have distinct retinal findings, but all are located in the parafoveal retina. In all groups, the telangiectasis is a primary condition rather than a finding secondary to a retinal disorder such as diabetic retinopathy or venous occlusion.

Symptoms

The primary visual symptom of IJRT is blurred central vision in one or both eyes. Patients with group 1 IJRT have blurred vision in one eye only. Group 2 patients, which includes both women and men, have bilateral, mild to moderate central visual loss that typically begins in the fifth or sixth decade of life. In group 3 IJRT, a rare condition, patients have bilateral visual loss that is associated with central nervous system symptoms.

Clinical Findings

Group 1 patients have unilateral retinal telangiectasis in the parafoveal region that may consist of a single aneurysm or a large cluster of aneurysms. The telangiectatic vessels and aneurysms are easily visible and are accompanied by retinal edema. Cystoid macular edema and lipid exudate also may be present. These patients, who are predominantly male, tend to have mild-to-moderate visual loss beginning in their 30s and 40s.

In group 2 IJRT, the retina has a subtle gray appearance, with loss of the normal retinal transparency, and bilateral thickening of the parafoveal retina. Superficial retinal crystals may form in the early or late stage of the disease. Telangiectatic vessels, foveal cysts, and lipid exudate are clinically absent. Early in the disease, group 2 patients may develop "right angle venules," which are dilated and blunted in appearance. With time, pigmentary plaques may form in the neurosensory retina. Group 2 patients may have visual loss due to retinal pigment epithelial atrophy or subretinal new vessels.

Group 3 patients demonstrate progressive central macular capillary nonperfusion in addition to aneurysmal dilation of the parafoveal capillary bed.

Ancillary Testing

Fluorescein angiography is the most useful test in demonstrating juxtafoveolar telangiectasia. In group 1 IJRT, filling of the telangiectatic vessels is prompt, with late leakage in only one eye. Group 2 IJRT is characterized by bilateral telangiectasis involving the temporal portion of the juxtafoveolar retina (usually confined to 1 disc diameter of the center of the fovea). Subretinal neovascularization may be detected. Patients in group 3 have occlusion of the juxtafoveolar capillary network in both eyes.

Pathology/Pathogenesis

The underlying cause of IJRT is not known. Group 1 IJRT is most likely a congenital retinal telangiectasis. Group 2 IJRT may be the result of a low-grade, chronic venous stasis in the macula. Electron microscopic findings reveal changes in the retinal capillaries similar to those found in diabetic retinopathy.

Treatment/Prognosis

Photocoagulation to leaking microaneurysms is the treatment of choice in group 1 IJRT. In group 2 IJRT, subretinal neovascularization may be treated with confluent photocoagulation. Although grid photocoagulation has been advocated by some retinal experts to treat intraretinal edema in group 2 patients, laser treatment does not appear to reverse the retinal pigment epithelial alterations that are the ultimate cause of visual loss. Laser therapy may be effective in rare cases of extrafoveal subretinal neovascularization. The role of photodynamic therapy is unclear.

Systemic Evaluation

No definitive systemic associations occur with group 1 or group 2 IJRT. Controversy exists as to whether there is a link between group 2 IJRT and diabetes mellitus. Group 3 IJRT has been associated with central nervous system disease.

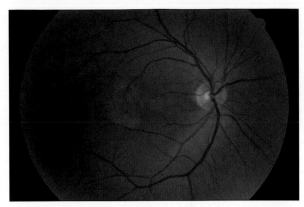

Group 2 idiopathic juxtafoveolar retinal telangiectasis is the most common type of parafoveal retinal telangiectasis. It is characterized by subtle abnormalities of the parafoveal capillary system.

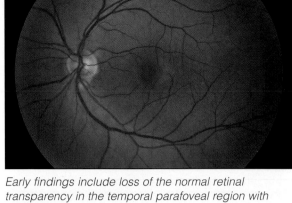

Early findings include loss of the normal retinal transparency in the temporal parafoveal region with irregular, telangiectatic vessels. Group 2 IJRT is bilateral but may be asymmetric.

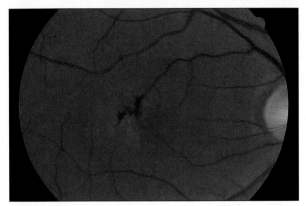

Other findings in patients with group 2 idiopathic juxtafoveolar retinal telangiectasis include "right angle venules" and intraretinal pigment accumulation.

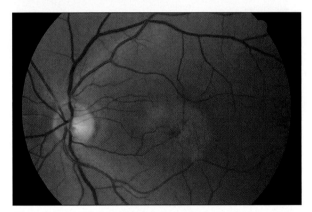

Superficial retinal crystals may be seen in addition to the retinal vascular and pigmentary alterations.

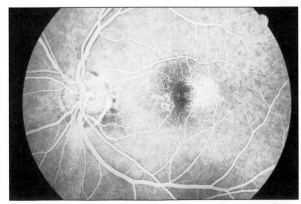

Fluorescein angiography reveals irregularities of the parafoveal capillary network. Telangiectatic vessels are more commonly observed temporal to the fovea.

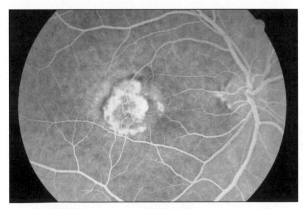

Some patients with group 2 idiopathic juxtafoveolar retinal telangiectasis develop subretinal neovascularization. It has been proposed that the subretinal new vessels originate from the retinal circulation rather than the choroid. Fluorescein angiography reveals a lacy vascular network that leaks throughout the fluorescein study.

LEUKEMIC RETINOPATHY

Ocular involvement in leukemia occurs in approximately 80% of cases, although many are asymptomatic. The ocular manifestations of leukemia may be divided into three categories: leukemic infiltrates; secondary complications related to anemia, thrombocytopenia, and hyperviscosity; and opportunistic infections. The term "leukemic retinopathy" typically refers to the secondary manifestations of leukemia.

Symptoms

Individuals with leukemic retinopathy may be asymptomatic or complain of abrupt visual loss related to preretinal or intraretinal hemorrhage involving the macula. Occasionally, patients will report decreased vision as the initial manifestation of their leukemia.

Clinical Features

Preretinal and intraretinal hemorrhages are the most common retinal findings in patients with leukemia. A strong correlation exists between the level of thrombocytopenia and the presence of retinal hemorrhages. White-centered hemorrhages, cotton wool spots, and dilation of retinal veins may be manifestations of hyperviscosity and leukostasis. A minority of patients may develop venous stasis retinopathy and peripheral retinal neovascularization. Other findings include vitreous infiltration, optic nerve swelling, orbital inflammation with proptosis, and cranial neuropathies.

Opportunistic infections are common in patients who have become immunosuppressed as a result of leukemia or chemotherapy. Some of the more common infections involving the retina and choroid include cytomegalovirus, herpes simplex virus, toxoplasmosis, and various fungal organisms.

Ancillary Testing

The diagnosis of leukemic retinopathy is based on clinical examination.

Pathology/Pathogenesis

Leukemic infiltration may occur in the vitreous, optic disc, retina, and choroid (most common). The secondary manifestations of leukemia are related to the hematologic abnormalities induced by the leukemia—namely anemia, thrombocytopenia, and hyperviscosity. White-centered hemorrhages are commonly observed. Although it has been speculated that the white center may represent collections of abnormal white blood cells, it most likely is a fibrin-platelet aggregate that develops during the normal physiologic healing process after localized capillary rupture.

Treatment/Prognosis

The ocular manifestations of leukemia typically resolve with improvement of hematologic parameters after chemotherapy and/or radiation therapy. Primary ocular therapy is seldom required. Ocular radiation may be considered for ocular infiltrates that do not respond to systemic therapy. Treatment with use of the Nd:YAG laser may be performed in cases of persistent preretinal hemorrhage obscuring the macula.

Systemic Evaluation

Hematologic evaluation for hematocrit, leukocyte and platelet counts, and bone marrow biopsy for clinical staging and classification are mandatory.

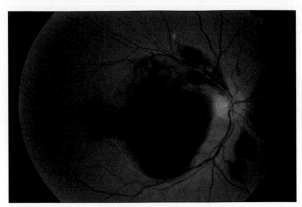

Leukemic retinopathy with preretinal hemorrhage was observed in this 19-year-old man who presented with loss of vision in each eye. Examination revealed bilateral preretinal hemorrhages overlying the macula.

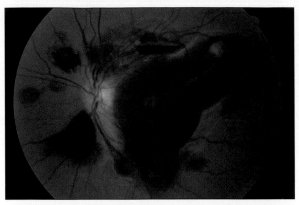

He also had scattered intraretinal hemorrhages and a few white-centered hemorrhages. He subsequently was diagnosed with acute myelogenous leukemia.

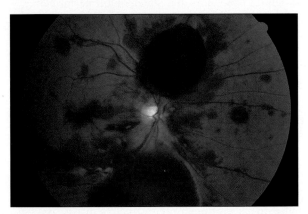

White-centered hemorrhages are commonly observed in patients with leukemia. White-centered hemorrhages have been described in association with anemia and thrombocytopenia.

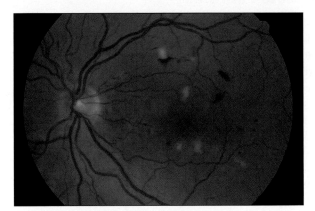

Additional findings in patients with leukemia include cotton wool spots and venous dilation and tortuosity.

OCULAR ISCHEMIC SYNDROME

The ocular ischemic syndrome occurs when there is significant obstruction of blood flow to the eye. A 90% or greater stenosis in the carotid system is the most common cause, although ophthalmic artery obstruction may be responsible for a minority of cases. Men are affected twice as often as women, and the mean age is 65 years. Atherosclerosis involving the carotid artery is the major cause of the ocular ischemic syndrome.

Symptoms

The most common symptom is gradual onset of visual loss. Slow recovery of vision after light exposure may also occur. Patients may report amaurosis fugax. A dull ache in or around the eye occurs in about 40% of patients.

Clinical Features

Visual acuity at presentation is variable and may range from 20/20 to no light perception. Rubeosis iridis is visible at presentation in two thirds of eyes. Elevation of intraocular pressure may be present, if there is angle involvement, but elevated intraocular pressure is not invariable due to associated reduced aqueous production from ciliary body ischemia. Mild anterior chamber inflammation is common. The retinal arteries may be narrowed and the veins slightly dilated but not tortuous. Spontaneous arterial pulsations may be present. Retinal hemorrhages are common and usually observed in the midperiphery. Microaneurysms and cotton wool spots are seen less commonly. Optic disc neovascularization is present in 35% of eyes, and neovascularization elsewhere (NVE) in about 8%.

Ancillary Testing

Fluorescein angiography is helpful in making the diagnosis by demonstrating delayed and patchy choroidal filling and prolongation of the retinal arterial venous transit time. Angiography may also show staining of retinal vessels and leakage from microvascular abnormalities. Electroretinography demonstrates reduction or absence of the a- and b-wave amplitudes.

Pathology/Pathogenesis

The ocular ischemic syndrome is caused by reduced blood flow to the eyeball, producing both anterior and posterior segment ischemia. Retinal ischemia leads to endothelial cell and pericyte damage, resulting in hemorrhage, macular edema, and retinal capillary nonperfusion.

Treatment/Prognosis

Panretinal photocoagulation is indicated in most cases when either anterior or posterior segment neovascularization is present. Glaucoma medication should be used to treat elevated intraocular pressure, and topical steroids and cycloplegics may be helpful when there is a significant anterior segment inflammatory response. The role of carotid endarterectomy is controversial and probably most helpful from an ocular standpoint if performed before the onset of rubeosis. It may also be helpful in reducing the risk of subsequent stroke. Visual prognosis is variable. Approximately 60% of patients have counting fingers or worse vision at the end of the 1-year follow-up. About 25% of patients retain better than 20/50 vision. The 5-year mortality rate for patients with ocular ischemic syndrome is 40%, with the leading cause of death being cardiovascular disease.

Systemic Evaluation

A complete cardiovascular evaluation, with particular attention to causes of carotid obstructive disease, is recommended for all patients presenting with the ocular ischemic syndrome. A dissecting aneurysm of the carotid artery and temporal arteritis have been reported to cause ocular ischemic syndrome and should be included in the workup.

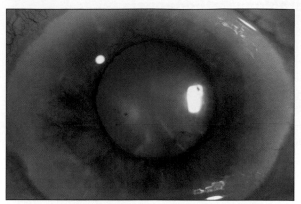

Ocular ischemic syndrome is caused by insufficient blood flow to the eye. Many patients present with iris neovascularization. Patients with anterior chamber angle involvement may develop neovascular glaucoma.

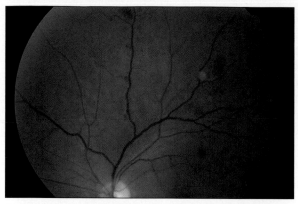

Funduscopic examination usually reveals intraretinal hemorrhages. The retinal arteries are narrowed, and the veins may be slightly dilated.

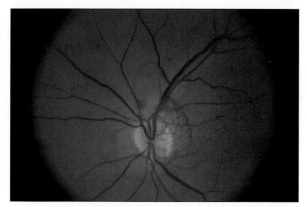

Optic disc neovascularization develops in approximately one third of patients.

PREGNANCY-RELATED RETINAL DISEASE

Pregnancy may affect the specific findings present in otherwise common disorders such as central serous retinopathy or it may alter preexisting problems such as diabetic retinopathy. The treatment of otherwise common problems such as toxoplasmic retinochoroiditis may be made more problematic because of concern for the fetus. Systemic complications of pregnancy, including preeclampsia, toxemia of pregnancy, and amniotic fluid embolism, may cause chorioretinal disease more specific to pregnancy.

Symptoms

In the pregnant woman, visual symptoms such as blurred vision, photopsias, or visual field defects may be related not only to retinal disease but also to refractive changes, optic nerve disease, or cerebrovascular alterations.

Clinical Findings

Central serous chorioretinopathy (CSC) is characterized by localized serous neurosensory retinal detachments in the macula. It typically develops in the third trimester of pregnancy. The finding of subretinal fibrin is more common in pregnant women than in nonpregnant patients.

Diabetic retinopathy is characterized by nonproliferative changes, including microaneurysms, retinal hemorrhages, cotton wool spots, venous beading, intraretinal lipid, and retinal thickening (edema). Proliferative changes include neovascularization of the optic disc and retina.

Preeclampsia and toxemia produce retinal changes that are, in part, secondary to systemic hypertension that may cause vasospasm of the retinal and choroidal circulations. Hypertension-associated retinal findings in pregnancy range from arteriolar narrowing to central retinal artery occlusion. Choroidal vasospasm or infarction may result in retinal pigment epithelial changes (Elschnig spots) and exudative retinal detachments (which resolve after delivery).

Ancillary Testing

Usually, the ophthalmoscopic examination is sufficient to ascertain the diagnosis of retinal disorders in pregnant patients. Fluorescein angiography may be performed without harm to the mother or fetus but is used sparingly. Fluorescein angiography demonstrates choroidal nonfilling, leakage of dye from the optic disc and deep retinal lesions, and retinal pigment epithelial window defects. Indocyanine green angiographic findings in patients with preeclampsia include nonperfusion in the early phases of the angiogram and staining of the choroidal vasculature with subretinal leakage in the late phases.

Pathology/Pathogenesis

It is not known whether CSC in pregnancy is coincidental to or secondary to pregnancy. It has been linked to various hypercortisolemic states. Serum cortisol levels increase dramatically throughout pregnancy and peak in the third trimester.

Pregnancy is a risk factor for progression of diabetic retinopathy. Women with longer duration of diabetes, hypertension, or rapid tightening of blood glucose control at the onset of pregnancy are more likely to have progression of retinopathy.

Hypertension, hypercoagulability, and, in patients with toxemia of pregnancy, disseminated intravascular coagulopathy play a role in the formation of exudative retinal detachments and in retinal/choroidal infarction.

Treatment/Prognosis

In those with CSC, the visual prognosis is generally good, with resolution of subretinal fluid and recovery of vision shortly after delivery. Central serous retinopathy may or may not recur in subsequent pregnancies. Pregnant patients with diabetes should have regular dilated funduscopic examinations to screen for diabetic retinopathy. Laser treatment is applied with the same criteria used in nonpregnant patients. The primary treatment for women with preeclampsia/toxemia is delivery and management of hypertension.

Systemic Evaluation

Hypertension is a common association of CSC. Pregnant patients are usually under tight control of their diabetes, but the ophthalmologist should keep the obstetrician informed of the patient's retinal status. Occasionally, the ophthalmologist may be the first physician contacted by a preeclamptic patient with visual symptoms. The obstetrician should be notified urgently.

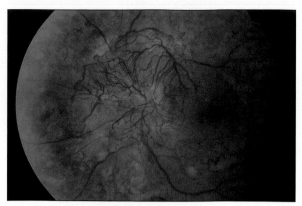

Fundus photographs of a 24-year-old woman who developed high-risk proliferative diabetic retinopathy in her first trimester of pregnancy. She had massive optic disc neovascularization despite extensive panretinal photocoagulation and required pars plana vitrectomy.

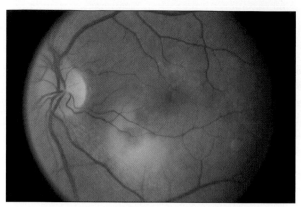

Central serous chorioretinopathy may develop during pregnancy, usually in the third trimester. The presence of subretinal fibrin suggests very active leakage.

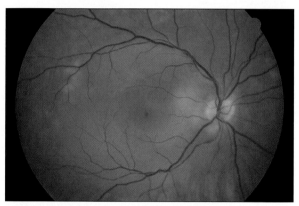

This 21-year-old woman with preeclampsia/toxemia of pregnancy reported a sudden loss of vision of her right eye. She had a large exudative neurosensory retinal detachment of her right macula.

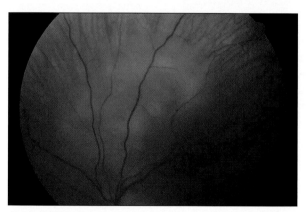

Subretinal fluid and fibrin were found superior to the optic disc in the left eye of the same patient.

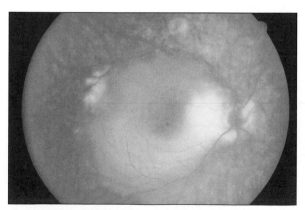

Fluorescein angiogram of the same patient reveals intense hyperfluorescence in the right macula.

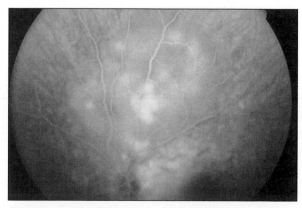

The left eye had numerous hyperfluorescent spots in the region of the exudative retinal detachment superior to the optic disc. The hyperfluorescence was due to increased choroidal permeability and breakdown of the outer blood-retinal barrier as a result of choroidal vasospasm and ischemia.

RADIATION RETINOPATHY

Ionizing radiation from external beam radiography or local sources (radioactive eyewall plaques) can induce a retinopathy that closely resembles diabetic retinopathy clinically and pathologically. Treatment for intracranial, orbital, nasopharyngeal, and cutaneous tumors may lead to radiation retinopathy. The radiation doses associated with retinopathy range from 11 to 35 Gy. The onset of radiation retinopathy ranges from 1 to 8 years following the exposure to radiation.

Symptoms

Patients may have few symptoms in the early stages of radiation retinopathy. Reduced vision is usually associated with macular hemorrhages, edema, ischemia, or vitreous hemorrhage.

Clinical Features

The earliest clinical signs are those related to capillary occlusion: cotton wool spots, microaneurysms, retinal telangiectasis, lipid exudation, and intraretinal hemorrhages. Neovascularization develops on the disc and/or retinal surface, and may involve the iris if untreated. Some patients may also have optic disc edema indicative of associated radiation optic neuropathy.

Ancillary Testing

Fluorescein angiography confirms the presence of capillary occlusion and neovascularization. Foveal capillary dropout suggests a poor visual prognosis.

Differential diagnosis includes diabetic retinopathy, leukemia, sickle cell retinopathy, and branch retinal vein occlusion.

Pathology/Pathogenesis

Radiation retinopathy results from damage to the endothelial cells of the retinal blood vessels. As in diabetes, capillary occlusion in the inner retina is the predominant finding. Inner retinal neurons are also lost. Radiation induces DNA damage that leads to progressive retinal cell death.

Treatment/Prognosis

The treatment for radiation retinopathy is virtually the same as for diabetic retinopathy. Laser photocoagulation is applied for macular edema and neovascularization, and vitrectomy is useful for nonclearing vitreous hemorrhage. Two thirds of eyes maintain visual acuity of 20/200 or better. Visual loss is related to macular edema and ischemia, vitreous hemorrhage, and neovascular glaucoma.

Systemic Evaluation

A history of ocular or head and neck radiation is necessary to make the diagnosis of radiation retinopathy. The oncologist should be notified when radiation retinopathy is detected.

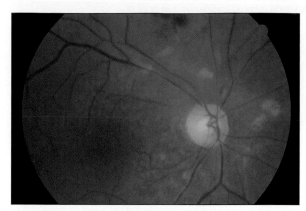

Radiation retinopathy demonstrates ischemia-related findings that include optic disc pallor, cotton wool spots, and retinal arteriolar occlusion.

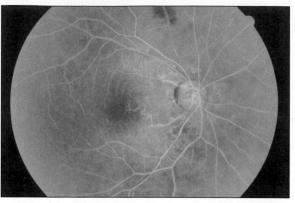

Fluorescein angiography in radiation retinopathy reveals retinal capillary nonperfusion and "pruning" of several branches of the temporal retinal arterioles.

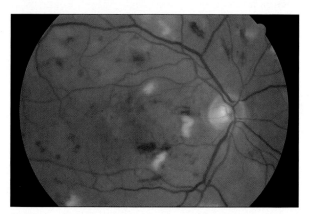

Radiation retinopathy may be more severe in patients with diabetic retinopathy or other retinal vascular disease. This patient had progression of diabetic retinopathy following orbital radiation.

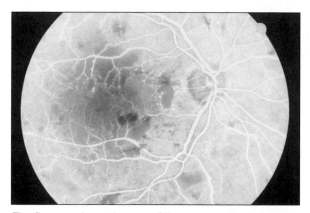

The fluorescein angiogram of the same patient shows marked enlargement of the foveal avascular zone with significant ischemia. A few scattered microaneurysms are noted.

RETINAL ARTERIAL MACROANEURYSMS

Retinal arterial macroaneurysms are round or oval arteriolar dilations, usually seen in the posterior pole. They occur more commonly in women than men, in the sixth or seventh decade of life. Typically, they are solitary and unilateral. An estimated 50% to 75% of patients have a history of systemic hypertension.

Symptoms

Macroaneurysms may be found in asymptomatic patients when there is no foveal involvement. Symptoms associated with macroaneurysms include blurred or distorted vision, a blind spot in the vision, or, less commonly, floaters resulting from vitreous hemorrhage.

Clinical Features

Macroaneurysms occur within the first three orders of retinal arterial bifurcation. They are usually located superotemporally and often occur at an arterial bifurcation or arteriovenous crossing site. They may be obscured or surrounded by hemorrhage or a circinate pattern of proteinaceous and lipid exudates. Also, a serous detachment of the retina may be associated. A distinguishing feature of a ruptured macroaneurysm is the presence of blood in multiple layers (subretinal, intraretinal, and preretinal). Visual loss may occur when fluid, lipid, or hemorrhage involves the fovea. Visual loss may also occur from vitreous hemorrhage.

Ancillary Testing

Fluorescein angiography is helpful in delineating the macroaneurysm. If not obscured by blood, it is evident as a focal area of hyperfluorescence early in the study, with or without associated late leakage of dye. There may be an associated partial or complete obstruction of the affected artery at the site of the macroaneurysm, and, in some cases, microvascular abnormalities are seen surrounding the aneurysm. Indocyanine green angiography has been used to identify macroaneurysms obscured by intra- or preretinal hemorrhage.

Pathology/Pathogenesis

Histopathologically, macroaneurysms represent linear breaks in the arterial wall surrounded by laminar-fibrin platelet clot, hemorrhage, lipid-laden macrophages, hemosiderin, and a fibroglial reaction.

Treatment/Prognosis

Treatment is indicated when visual loss results from accumulation of fluid or exudate in the macula. Since the majority of macroaneurysms heal spontaneously, treatment is usually not indicated in the absence of central visual loss. Recommended treatment is photocoagulation, with either the green or yellow wavelength applied directly to or surrounding the macroaneurysm. A low-intensity, longer-duration burn is recommended.

Complications of treatment may include arterial obstruction and vitreous hemorrhage. Visual prognosis is directly related to the degree and duration of foveal involvement with either hemorrhage or exudate. Controversy exists regarding the efficacy of surgical evacuation of large macular hemorrhages.

Systemic Evaluation

Because of the strong association between arterial macroaneurysms and hypertension, patients with arterial macroaneurysms should be evaluated for hypertension.

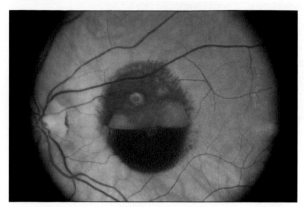

A 68-year-old woman had sudden loss of vision in her right eye following rupture of a retinal arterial macroaneurysm. Note the presence of preretinal, intraretinal, and subretinal hemorrhage.

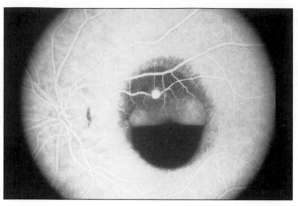

Fluorescein angiogram demonstrates hyperfluorescence of the macroaneurysm. Hypofluorescence is caused by preretinal and subretinal blood.

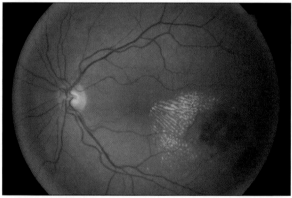

Visual loss from a retinal arterial macroaneurysm may also result from macular edema. This patient had a macular star pattern of lipid exudate originating from an inferotemporal macroaneurysm.

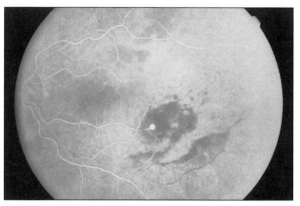

Fluorescein angiography demonstrates the hyperfluorescent macroaneurysm. This patient suffered a branch retinal arterial occlusion following rupture of the macroaneurysm.

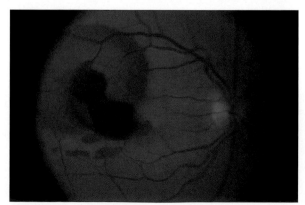

The presence of hemorrhage in multiple layers (preretinal, subretinal, and intraretinal) suggests the possibility of a ruptured macroaneurysm. In general, the visual prognosis is favorable.

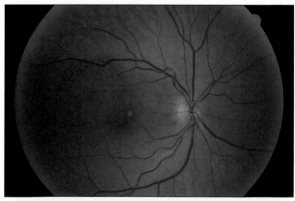

However, pigmentary alterations following prolonged subretinal hemorrhage may limit the recovery.

RETINOPATHY OF PREMATURITY

Retinopathy of prematurity (ROP), known in the past as retrolental fibroplasia, is a neovascular disorder of the developing retina that occurs in premature infants. The disease tends to occur bilaterally but may be asymmetric in its severity. In some infants with ROP, especially those of very low birth weight and early gestational age, macular distortion (dragging) or traction retinal detachment may occur, resulting in profound visual loss.

Symptoms

Premature infants with early-stage ROP exhibit no observable symptoms. The diagnosis of ROP must be made by careful screening examinations. If macular distortion or detachment occurs, the infant will fail to exhibit normal visual behavior (such as fixing on faces or objects).

Clinical Findings

Detection of ROP requires indirect ophthalmoscopic examination with scleral depression. The funduscopic findings are classified into five stages, and the fundus is divided into three zones.

A normal premature infant's fundus has retinal vessels extending from the optic disc outward into the retina with peripheral featureless, avascular retina. In stage 1 ROP, a flat white "demarcation line" develops between the vascular and avascular retina. In stage 2 ROP, this line has visible height and is called a ridge. Stage 3 ROP denotes the development of pink to red fibrovascular proliferations emanating from the surface of the ridge into the overlying vitreous. Stages 4 and 5 ROP denote retinal detachment, with stage 4 being subtotal and stage 5 being total retinal detachment. Stage 4 ROP is further subdivided into 4A (macula on) and 4B (macula off).

The zone designation indicates the anterior to posterior location of disease in the fundus. All zones are centered on the optic disc, not the fovea, because the retinal vessels grow out from the disc. Zone 1 is a circle with a radius of twice the distance between the optic disc and the center of the macula. Zone 2 has a radius equal to the distance between the optic disc and the nasal ora serrata. Zone 3 is the remaining temporal crescent of retina.

The designation "plus disease" indicates that the retinal vessels appear dilated and tortuous (thought to be due to high blood flow through peripheral neovascular tissue and arteriovenous shunts). Other features include iris vascular engorgement, pupillary rigidity, and vitreous haze.

Ancillary Testing

Aside from careful ophthalmoscopic examination, no other testing is necessary. However, visual evoked potentials may be of use in evaluating infants with total retinal detachment before attempted surgical repair.

Treatment/Prognosis

The treatment of stage 3 ROP consists of ablation of the peripheral avascular retina by either cryotherapy or indirect laser photocoagulation. In general, treatment is not instituted until the degree of stage 3 reaches threshold and until plus disease develops. Threshold is defined as more than 5 contiguous clock hours of stage 3 disease or as less than 8 noncontiguous clock hours of stage 3 disease.

The beneficial effects of cryotherapy were well documented in the CRYO-ROP study. Since the study, which was performed in the mid-1980s, diode (infrared) indirect laser photocoagulation has become available and is the generally accepted mode of treatment. Infants with retinal detachment may be treated with either scleral buckling or vitrectomy.

Systemic Evaluation

The CRYO-ROP study demonstrated that infants with birth weights less than 1250 g have a higher risk of developing stage 3 ROP than do those infants with higher birth weights. The risk of neovascular ROP rises with lower birth weight, such that infants with birth weights less than 750 g have at least a 15% risk of developing threshold ROP.

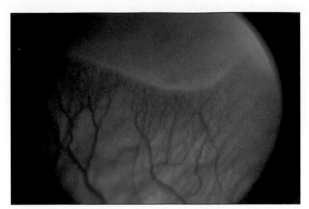

Stage 1 retinopathy of prematurity demonstrates a demarcation line that develops between the vascularized and avascular retina. (Photograph reproduced with permission from the CRYO-ROP Study Group.)

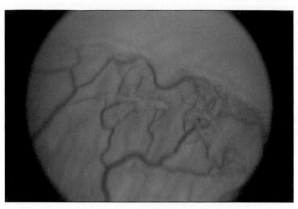

Stage 2 retinopathy of prematurity exhibits the demarcation line after it develops thickness and height, forming a ridge. (Photograph reproduced with permission from the CRYO-ROP Study Group.)

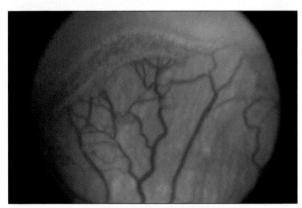

Stage 3 retinopathy of prematurity (ROP) shows fibrovascular proliferations that extend from the ridge to the vitreous. Threshold ROP is defined. (Photograph reproduced with permission from the CRYO-ROP Study Group.)

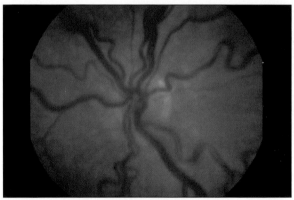

Plus disease indicates that the retinal vessels are dilated and tortuous. Other features include iris vascular engorgement, pupillary rigidity, and vitreous haze. (Photograph reproduced with permission from the CRYO-ROP Study Group.)

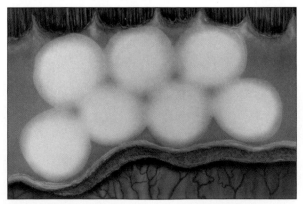

Treatment for retinopathy of prematurity involves applying cyrotherapy or laser photocoagulation to the peripheral avascular retina. This schematic from the CRYO-ROP study demonstrates the near confluent application of cyrotherapy. (Photograph reproduced with permission from the CRYO-ROP Study Group.)

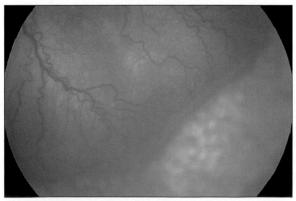

RetCam image immediately following laser photocoagulation for threshold retinopathy of prematurity. Laser treatment is applied to the peripheral avascular retina.

SICKLE CELL RETINOPATHY

Sickle cell retinopathy is the general term applied to retinal vascular lesions resulting from hemoglobin (Hb) mutations SS, SC, and Sthal. Ocular manifestations of sickle cell disease are most commonly observed in SC disease. The Hb AS and AC mutations rarely cause ocular changes. Sickle cell retinopathy is characterized by an occlusive vasculopathy as a result of intravascular sickling, hemolysis, hemostasis, and thrombosis. Both nonproliferative and proliferative features occur.

Symptoms

The symptom complex in sickle cell retinopathy resembles that of diabetic retinopathy and radiation retinopathy: patients have reduced central vision due to macular ischemia or vitreous floaters due to neovascularization and vitreous hemorrhage. In all of these disorders, patients can have substantial lesions before symptoms develop.

Clinical Features

Vascular beds throughout the eye can be involved from the conjunctiva to the retina. The retinal lesions include salmon patch hemorrhages, black sunburst pigmentation, and iridescent deposits or "spots," and the retinal depression sign. Salmon patch hemorrhages are intraretinal hemorrhages following retinal arteriolar occlusion. Black sunburst lesions represent localized areas of retinal pigment epithelial hypertrophy and hyperplasia. Iridescent spots are areas of hemosiderin deposition within the retina in acquired schisis cavities beneath the internal limiting membrane following intraretinal hemorrhage resorption. Capillary occlusion in the macula may result in visual loss. Capillary occlusion in the midperipheral and peripheral fundus may lead to neovascularization. The neovascularization often assumes a "sea fan" appearance. Neovascular sea fans often undergo spontaneous autoinfarction; they may be associated with vitreous hemorrhage and traction retinal detachment. Patients may develop central or branch retinal artery occlusions. Angioid streaks may be observed in individuals with Hb SS disease.

Ancillary Testing

Fluorescein angiography reveals areas of macular and peripheral retinal nonperfusion. Areas of neovascularization hyperfluorescence intensely and may be seen at the junction of perfused and nonperfused retina.

Pathology/Pathogenesis

In sickle cell hemoglobin, the valine is substituted for glutamic acid at the sixth position in the β-polypeptide chain. The single amino acid substitutions alter the hemoglobin conformation and the deformability of erythrocytes, thus impeding migration through capillaries. The gene is located on 11p15 in the β-globulin complex.

Treatment/Prognosis

Laser photocoagulation may be applied peripheral to areas of retinal neovascularization to reduce the risk of vitreous hemorrhage and traction retinal detachment. Spontaneous regression or autoinfarction of retinal neovascularization may occur, reducing the need for laser treatment. Vitrectomy can be performed to clear vitreous hemorrhages or repair traction retinal detachments. Scleral buckling surgery may be associated with a risk of anterior segment ischemia. The systemic hematologic condition should be stabilized preoperatively.

The visual prognosis is variable but generally favorable. The visual prognosis is worse in patients with Hb SC and Sthal disease compared to those with SS mutations. Sickle SS disease is associated with angioid streaks and has more systemic complications.

Patients with traumatic hyphema and sickle hemoglobinopathies have a greater risk of rebleeding, glaucoma, and optic nerve damage than do normal subjects. Therefore, patients with African or Mediterranean heritage should undergo hemoglobin electrophoresis in the setting of hyphema.

Systemic Evaluation

Hemoglobin electrophoresis is indicated to obtain a correct genetic diagnosis.

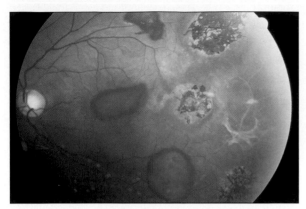

This fundus photograph demonstrates several of the characteristic findings of sickle cell retinopathy: salmon patch hemorrhages, black sunbursts, and iridescent crystals.

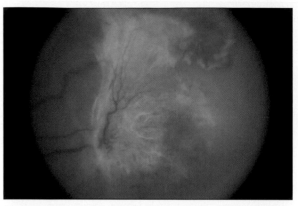

Proliferative sickle cell retinopathy is characterized by the presence of retinal neovascularization that assumes a "sea fan" appearance.

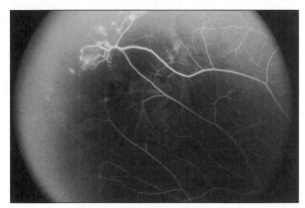

Fluorescein angiography demonstrates a frond of retinal neovascularization. The new vessels are found at the junction between the perfused and nonperfused retina.

SELECTED REFERENCES

Branch Retinal Artery Occlusion

1. Brown GC. Retinal arterial obstruction. *Focal Points.* 1994;12:1–11.

2. Greven CM, Slusher MM, Weaver RG. Retinal arterial occlusion in young adults. *Am J Ophthalmol.* 1995;120:776–783.

3. Johnson MW, Thomley ML, Huang SS, Gass JDM. Idiopathic recurrent branch retinal artery occlusion: natural history and laboratory evaluation. *Ophthalmology.* 1994;101:480–489.

Branch Retinal Vein Occlusion

1. Branch Vein Occlusion Study Group. Argon laser photocoagulation for macular edema in branch vein occlusion. *Am J Ophthalmol.* 1984;98:271–282.

2. Branch Vein Occlusion Study Group. Argon laser photocoagulation for prevention of neovascularization and vitreous hemorrhage in branch vein occlusion. *Arch Ophthalmol.* 1986;104:34–41.

3. Christoffersen NL, Larsen M. Pathophysiology and hemodynamics of branch retinal vein occlusion. *Ophthalmology.* 1999;106:2054–2062.

4. Sperduto RD, Hiller R, Chew E, Seigel D, Blair N, Burton TC, et al. Risk factors for hemiretinal vein occlusion: comparison with risk factors for central and branch retinal vein occlusion: the eye disease case-control study. *Ophthalmology.* 1998;105:765–771.

Central Retinal Artery Occlusion

1. Atebara NH, Brown GC, Cater J. Efficacy of anterior chamber paracentesis and carbogen in treating acute nonarteritic central retinal artery occlusion. *Ophthalmology.* 1995;102:2029–2035.

2. Greven CM, Slusher MM, Weaver RG. Retinal arterial occlusions in young adults. *Am J Ophthalmol.* 1995;120:776–783.

Central Retinal Vein Occlusion

1. The CRVO Study Group. Evaluation of grid pattern photocoagulation for macular edema in central retinal vein occlusion. *Ophthalmology.* 1995;102:1425–1433.

2. The CRVO Study Group. Natural history and clinical management of central retinal vein occlusion. *Arch Ophthalmol.* 1997;115:486–491.

3. Fong ACO, Schatz H. Central retinal vein occlusion in young adults. *Surv Ophthalmol.* 1993;37:393–417.

Coats' Disease

1. Char DH. Coats' syndrome: long-term follow-up. *Br J Ophthalmol.* 1999;84:37–39.

2. Haik BG. Advanced Coats' disease. *Trans Am Ophthalmol Soc.* 1991;89:371–476.

3. Kirath H, Eldem B. Management of moderate-to-advanced Coats' disease. *Ophthalmologica.* 1998;212:19–22.

4. Ridley ME, Shields JA, Brown GL. Coats' disease: evaluation and management. *Ophthalmology.* 1982;89:1381–1387.

Diabetic Retinopathy: Nonproliferative

1. Aiello LP, Gardner TW, King GL, Blankenship G, Cavallerano JD, Ferris FL, Klein R. Diabetic retinopathy (technical review). *Diabetes Care.* 1998;21:143–156.

2. Barber AJ, Lieth E, Khin SA, Antonetti DA, Buchanan AG, Gardner TW. The Penn State Retina Research Group. Neural apoptosis in the retina during experimental and human diabetes: early onset and effect of insulin. *J Clin Invest.* 1998;102:783–791.

3. Early Treatment Diabetic Retinopathy Study Research Group. Photocoagulation for diabetic macular edema. ETDRS Report No. 1. *Arch Ophthalmol.* 1985;103:1796–1806.

4. Flynn HF, Smiddy W, eds. *Diabetes and Ocular Disease: Past, Present, and Future Therapies.* San Francisco: American Academy of Ophthalmology; 2000.

5. Molyneaux LM, Constantino MI, McGill M, Zilkens R, Yue DK. Better glycaemic control and risk reduction of diabetic complications in Type 2 diabetics: comparison with the DCCT. *Diabetes Res Clin Pract.* 1998;42:77–83.

6. The Diabetes Control and Complications Trial Research Group. The effect of intensive treatment of diabetes on the development and progression of long-term complications in insulin-dependent diabetes mellitus. *N Engl J Med.* 1993;329:977–986.

Diabetic Retinopathy: Proliferative

1. Blankenship GW. Fifteen-year argon laser and xenon photocoagulation results of Bascom Palmer Eye Institute's patients participating in the Diabetic Retinopathy Study. *Ophthalmology.* 1991;98:125–128.

2. Flynn HF, Smiddy W, eds. *Diabetes and Ocular Disease: Past, Present, and Future Therapies.* San Francisco: American Academy of Ophthalmology; 2000.

3. Quillen DA, Gardner TW, Blankenship GW. Proliferative diabetic retinopathy. In: Guyer DR, Yannuzzi LA, Chang S, Shields JA, Green RL, eds. *Retina-Vitreous-Macula.* Philadelphia: WB Saunders Co; 1999:1407–1431.

4. The Diabetic Retinopathy Study Research Group. Four risk factors for severe visual loss in diabetic retinopathy: the third report from the Diabetic Retinopathy Study. *Arch Ophthalmol.* 1979;97:654–655.

5. The Diabetic Retinopathy Study Research Group. Preliminary report on the effects of photocoagulation therapy. *Am J Ophthalmol.* 1976;81:383–396.

Eales' Disease

1. Madhavan HN, Therese KL, Gunisha P, Jayanthi U, Biswas J. Polymerase chain reaction for detection of *Mycobacterium tuberculosis* in epiretinal membrane in Eales' disease. *Invest Ophthalmol Vis Sci.* 2000;41:822–825.
2. Renie WA, Murphy RP, Anderson KC, Lippman SM, McKusick VA, Proctor LR, et al. The evaluation of patients with Eales' disease. *Retina.* 1983;3:243–248.

Hypertensive Retinopathy

1. Hayreh SS. Classification of hypertensive fundus changes and their order of appearance. *Ophthalmologica.* 1989;98:247–260.
2. Hayreh SS. Systemic arterial blood pressure and the eye. *Eye.* 1996;10:5–28.
3. Liang EI, Wong SW. Hypertension and the eye. *Curr Concepts Ophthalmol.* 1999;41–44.
4. Walsh JB. Hypertensive retinopathy: description, classification, and prognosis. *Ophthalmology.* 1982;89: 1127–1131.

Idiopathic Juxtafoveal Retinal Telangiectasis

1. Eliassi-Rad B, Green WR. Histopathologic study of presumed parafoveal telangiectasis. *Retina.* 1999;19: 332–335.
2. Gass JDM, Blodi BA. Idiopathic juxtafoveolar retinal telangiectasis. *Ophthalmology.* 1993;100:1536–1546.
3. Gass JDM. *Stereoscopic Atlas of Macular Diseases, Diagnosis and Treatment,* 4th ed. St. Louis: Mosby, Inc; 1997:501–503.
4. Park DW, Schatz H, McDonald HR, Johnson RN. Grid laser photocoagulation for macular edema in bilateral juxtafoveal telangiectasis. *Ophthalmology.* 1997;104:1838–1846.

Leukemic Retinopathy

1. Gordon KB, Rugo HS, Duncan JL, Irvine AR, Howes EL Jr, O'Brien JM, et al. Ocular manifestations of leukemia: leukemic infiltration versus infectious process. *Ophthalmology.* 2001;108:2293–2300.
2. Guyer DR, Schachat AP, Vitale S, Markowitz JA, Braine H, Burke PJ, et al. Leukemic retinopathy: relationship between fundus lesions and hematologic parameters at diagnosis. *Ophthalmology.* 1989;96:860–864.
3. Kincaid MC, Green WR. Ocular and orbital involvement in leukemia. *Surv Ophthalmol.* 1983;27:211–232.
4. Schachat AP, Markowitz JA, Guyer DR, Burke PJ, Karp JE, Graham ML. Ophthalmic manifestations of leukemia. *Arch Ophthalmol.* 1989;107:697–700.

5. Zaman F, Irwin R, Godley BF. Nd:YAG laser treatment for macular preretinal hemorrhage. *Arch Ophthalmol.* 1999;117:694–695.

Ocular Ischemic Syndrome

1. Brown GC, Magargal LE. The ocular ischemic syndrome: clinical, fluorescein angiographic and carotid angiographic features. *Int Ophthalmol.* 1988;11:239–251.
2. Mizner JB, Podhajsky P, Hayreh SS. Ocular ischemic syndrome. *Ophthalmology.* 1997;104:859–864.
3. Sivalingam A, Brown GC, Magargal LE. The ocular ischemic syndrome, III: visual prognosis and the effect of treatment. *Int Ophthalmol.* 1991;15:15–20.

Pregnancy-Related Retinal Disease

1. Fastenberg DM, Fetkenhour CL, Choromokos E, Shoch DE. Choroidal vascular changes in toxemia of pregnancy. *Am J Ophthalmol.* 1980;89:362–368.
2. Gass JDM. Central serous chorioretinopathy and white subretinal exudation during pregnancy. *Arch Ophthalmol.* 1991;109:677–681
3. Klein BE, Moss SE, Klein R. Effect of pregnancy on progression of diabetic retinopathy. *Diabetes Care.* 1990;13:34–40.
4. Valluri S, Adelberg DA, Curtis RS, Olk RJ. Diagnostic indocyanine green angiography in preeclampsia. *Am J Ophthalmol.* 1996;122:672–677.

Radiation Retinopathy

1. Archer DB, Amoaku WMK, Gardiner TA. Radiation retinopathy: clinical, histopathological, ultrastructural and experimental correlations. *Eye.* 1991;5:239–251.
2. Brown GC, Shields JA, Sanborn G, Augsburger JJ, Savino PJ, Schatz NJ. Radiation retinopathy. *Ophthalmology.* 1982;89:1494–1501.
3. Kinyoun JL, Chittum ME, Wells CG. Photocoagulation treatment of radiation retinopathy. *Am J Ophthalmol.* 1988;105:470–478.
4. Thorne JE, Maguire AM. Good visual outcome following laser therapy for proliferative radiation retinopathy. *Arch Ophthalmol.* 1999;117:125–126.

Retinal Arterial Macroaneurysms

1. Brown DM, Sobol WM, Folk JC, Weingeist TA. Retinal arteriolar macroaneurysms: long-term visual outcome. *Br J Ophthalmol.* 1994;78:534–538.
2. Panton RW, Goldberg MF, Farber MD. Retinal artery macroaneurysms: risk factors and natural history. *Br J Ophthalmol.* 1990;74:595–600.
3. Rabb MF, Gagliano DA, Teske MP. Retinal arterial macroaneurysms. *Surv Ophthalmol.* 1988;33:73–96.

Retinopathy of Prematurity

1. DeJonge MH, Ferrone PJ, Trese MT. Diode laser ablation for threshold retinopathy of prematurity: short-term structural outcome. *Arch Ophthalmol.* 2000;118:365–367.
2. The International Committee for the Classification of the Late Stages of Retinopathy of Prematurity. An international classification of retinopathy of prematurity; II: the classification of retinal detachment. *Arch Ophthalmol.* 1987;105:906–912.

Sickle Cell Retinopathy

1. Al-Abdulla NA, Haddock TA, Kerrison JB, Goldberg MF. Sickle cell disease presenting with extensive peri-macular arteriolar occlusions in a nine-year-old boy. *Am J Ophthalmol.* 2001;131:275–276.
2. Clarkson JG. The ocular manifestations of sickle-cell disease: a prevalence and natural history study. *Trans Am Ophthalmol Soc.* 1992;90:481–504.
3. Goldberg MF. Classification and pathogenesis of proliferative sickle cell retinopathy. *Am J Ophthalmol.* 1971;71:649–665.
4. Nagpal KC, Goldberg MF, Rabb MF. Ocular manifestations of sickle hemoglobinopathies. *Surv Ophthalmol.* 1977;21:391–411.

chapter 6

Hereditary Retinal Disorders

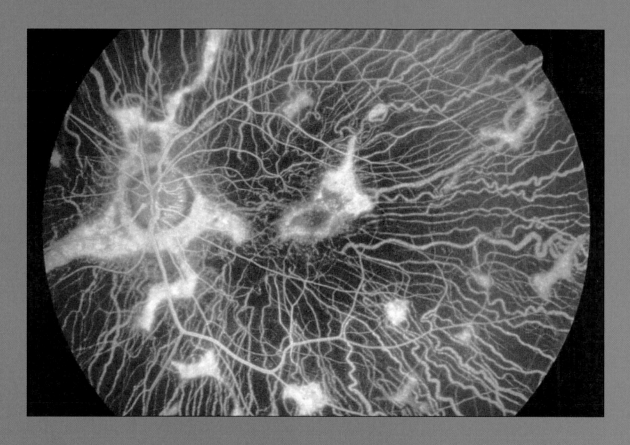

Vanessa Cruz-Villegas, MD

Philip J. Rosenfeld, MD, PhD

ALBINISM

Albinism is caused by an inborn error of metabolism and is classified as oculocutaneous albinism and ocular albinism. Oculocutaneous albinism is usually an autosomal recessive condition. However, autosomal dominant transmission can occur. Ocular albinism is commonly an X-linked disease.

Symptoms

Patients affected with albinism typically experience subnormal visual acuity and photophobia.

Clinical Features

Individuals with oculocutaneous and ocular albinism show nystagmus, iris transillumination defects, hypopigmented fundus, and foveal hypoplasia. Other ocular findings include strabismus, myopia, and astigmatism. In addition to the ocular features, persons affected with oculocutaneous albinism show decreased pigmentation in hair and skin. Tyrosinase-negative patients lack pigmentation entirely, while tyrosinase-positive patients have variable pigmentation.

Ancillary Testing

Tyrosinase hair bulb testing helps to classify oculocutaneous albinism as tyrosinase positive and tyrosinase negative. However, there are several subtypes among both tyrosinase-negative and tyrosinase-positive oculocutaneous albinism. The majority of patients with oculocutaneous albinism and ocular albinism have normal electroretinographic findings.

Pathology/Pathogenesis

In albinism the production of melanin is affected. Histopathologic reports demonstrate absence of the foveal pit. In oculocutaneous albinism the quantity of melanin in the melanosomes is reduced. Ocular albinism has a diminished amount of melanosomes.

Treatment/Prognosis

There is no known treatment for albinism.

Systemic Evaluation

Oculocutaneous albinism can be associated with several systemic findings. Impairment of the reticuloendothelial system, with subsequent susceptibility to infections and an increased risk of development of lymphoreticular malignancies, is seen in Chédiak-Higashi syndrome. This form of oculocutaneous albinism is inherited as an autosomal recessive trait and can be fatal. Hermansky-Pudlak syndrome is characterized by abnormal platelets and bleeding, and easy bruising can occur as a result. The majority of these patients are from Puerto Rico. Due to the potential mortality associated with these conditions, it is extremely important to consult a hematologist if any of these syndromes is suspected.

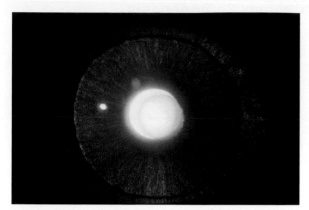

Oculocutaneous albinism is characterized by iris transillumination. The outlines of the lens and ciliary processes are visible through this nondilated pupil.

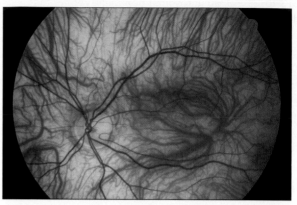

Ophthalmoscopic examination reveals a hypopigmented fundus. The larger choroidal vessels are visible through the hypopigmented retinal pigment epithelium.

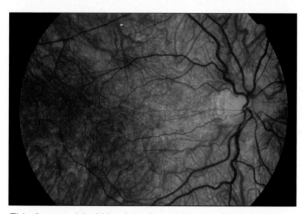

This 9-year-old girl had oculocutaneous albinism with nystagmus, high myopia, and visual acuity of 20/400.

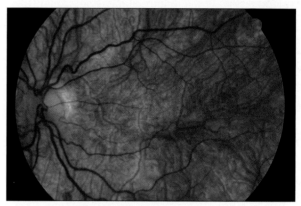

Both eyes demonstrated hypopigmentation of the fundus and foveal hypoplasia, with lack of the normal foveal reflex.

BEST'S DISEASE

Best's disease is an autosomal dominantly inherited macular dystrophy. Patients with Best's disease usually retain reading vision during adult life in at least one eye.

Symptoms

Individuals with Best's disease or vitelliform macular dystrophy experience mild visual loss. This visual loss occurs slowly throughout the years. Other complaints include metamorphopsia and central scotomas.

Clinical Features

Best's macular dystrophy is characterized by a yellow, egg yolk-like lesion at the level of the retinal pigment epithelium. This lesion is usually detected in infancy or childhood. Vitelliform lesions are typically bilateral and symmetric, ranging from 0.5 disc diameter (DD) to 2 DD in dimension. It is not unusual to visualize multifocal vitelliform lesions in this dystrophy. The vitelliform lesion becomes disrupted and reabsorbs with time, producing the pseudohypopyon and scrambled egg stages. Eventually, an area of atrophy develops. Some patients develop choroidal neovascularization and experience further decrease in visual acuity.

Ancillary Testing

Fluorescein angiography reveals a blockage of the choroidal fluorescence by the vitelliform lesion. As the condition progresses, evolving into the atrophic stage, retinal pigment epithelial atrophic areas develop. These areas appear as hyperfluorescent window defects by fluorescein angiography.

A normal electroretinogram (ERG) in conjunction with an abnormal electro-oculogram (EOG) characterizes Best's disease. The EOG light to dark ratio (Arden ratio) is usually below 1.5. This electrophysiologic test plays an important role in the diagnosis of this condition, as patients without the characteristic fundus lesion can have abnormal EOG findings.

Pathology/Pathogenesis

The genetic defect causing Best's disease has been mapped to chromosome 11q13. The gene causing Best's disease has been designated vitelliform macular dystrophy type 2 gene (VMD2). VMD2 encodes a transmembrane protein of RPE cells, known as bestrophin, involved in the transport of polyunsaturated fatty acids in the retina. Best's disease is characterized by an underlying retinal pigment epithelial abnormality. Histopathologic reports show accumulation of lipofuscin within retinal pigment epithelial cells However, no histopathologic studies have described the vitelliform stage.

Treatment/Prognosis

There is no treatment for Best's disease. Nevertheless, if choroidal neovascularization develops, certain therapeutic regimens such as laser photocoagulation, photodynamic therapy, and submacular surgery may be considered.

Systemic Evaluation

There are no known systemic findings associated with Best's disease.

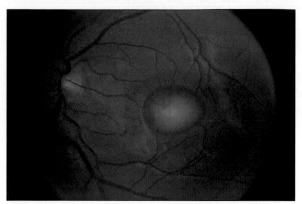

Best's disease is characterized by a "sunny side up," yellow egg yolk-like lesion at the level of the retinal pigment epithelium. Visual acuity in this stage is usually normal or only mildly reduced.

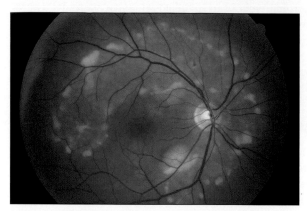

Most cases of Best's disease have a solitary lesion in the center of the macula of each eye, as shown in the previous figure. However, the disease may be asymmetric or have mutifocal lesions, as demonstrated here.

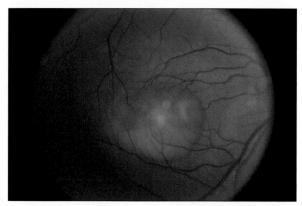

The "pseudohypopyon" stage of Best's disease is characterized by liquefaction of the vitelliform material, producing a boat-like lesion in the macula.

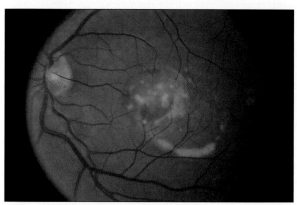

As the retinal pigment epithelium atrophies, the lesion develops a "scrambled egg" appearance.

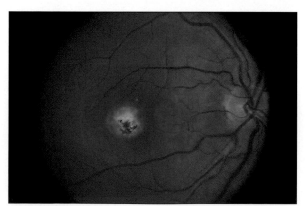

Visual loss is related to atrophy or the development of choroidal neovascularization. This fundus photograph demonstrates atrophy and retinal pigment epithelial hyperplasia.

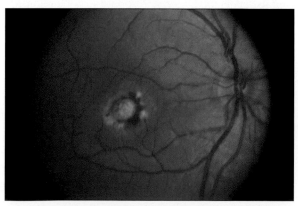

Patients with Best's disease may develop choroidal neovascularization. Signs of choroidal neovascularization include subretinal blood and subretinal fluid.

CHOROIDEREMIA

Choroideremia is an X-linked recessive choroidal dystrophy. It is characterized by a progressive degeneration of the retinal pigment epithelium (RPE), choroid, and choriocapillaris. Typically, most male patients experience the onset of symptoms in the first or second decade of life.

Symptoms

Affected males experience night blindness and peripheral visual field loss. Central vision becomes affected later in the course of the disease. Color vision is usually unaffected. Female carriers are commonly asymptomatic.

Clinical Features

Early in the disease course, the fundus shows pigment mottling near the equator. As the disease progresses, areas of choroidal and retinal pigment epithelial atrophy develop in the midperiphery and spread toward the macula and toward the periphery. In female carriers, the fundus appearance shows generalized or localized pigment mottling.

Ancillary Testing

Fluorescein angiography reveals loss of the retinal pigment epithelium and choriocapillaris. Fluorescein angiography also shows a delayed filling of the choroidal vasculature. However, there may be a relative sparing of the RPE and choriocapillaris in the central macular region.

The electroretinogram (ERG) is abnormal in the early stages of the disease and becomes extinguished later. If recordable, the scotopic response is markedly reduced, whereas the photopic response may be reduced but with delayed implicit times. Female carriers have normal ERG responses.

Pathology/Pathogenesis

The genetic defect in choroideremia is a deletion in Rab escort protein (REP-1) gene. The locus of this gene has been mapped to Xq21.1-21.3. This gene product is a component of Rab geranylgeranyl transferase, which regulates intracellular protein transport. Histopathologic studies reveal atrophy of the RPE, choroid, choriocapillaris, and outer retina. However, the pathogenesis of this atrophy is not understood.

Treatment/Prognosis

There is no known treatment for choroideremia. Usually, central vision becomes poor in the later stages of the disease.

Systemic Evaluation

No systemic associations have been reported in choroideremia.

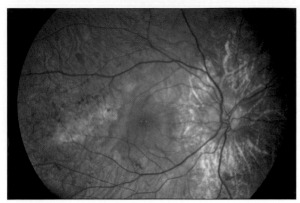

Choroideremia is an X-linked recessive disorder characterized by atrophy of the retinal pigment epithelium and choroid. This atrophy unmasks the larger choroidal vessels.

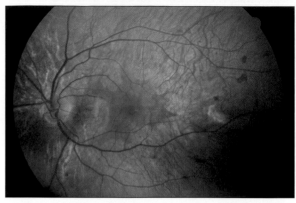

Focal areas of atrophy are first visualized in the midperipheral and posterior fundus. The center of the macula is spared until the late stages of the disease.

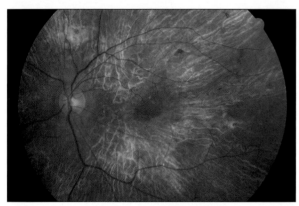

This patient with choroideremia demonstrates atrophy of the retinal pigment epithelium and choroid.

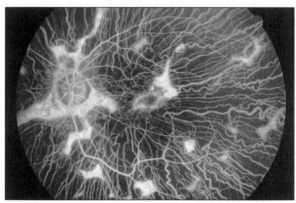

A fluorescein angiogram of the patient in the previous figure demonstrates marked hypofluorescence as the result of choroidal atrophy. Only the larger choroidal vessels remain.

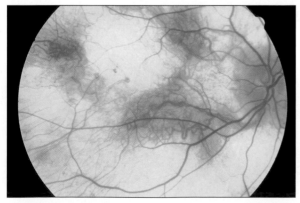

Advanced choroideremia, with marked atrophy of the retinal pigment epithelium and choroid, reveals the underlying sclera.

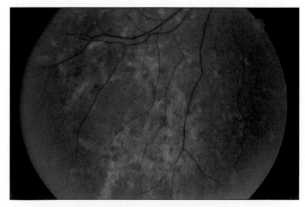

In female carriers, the fundus appearance shows generalized or localized pigment mottling. This woman's son had advanced choroideremia.

CONE DYSTROPHIES/CONE-ROD DYSTROPHIES

Cone dystrophies consist of a group of disorders characterized by cone dysfunction. Cone dystrophies can be congenital and nonprogressive in nature, such as in rod monochromatism (autosomal recessive) and blue-cone monochromatism (X-linked recessive). Noncongenital progressive cone dystrophies may be autosomal recessive, autosomal dominant, or X-linked recessive.

Symptoms

Patients with rod monochromatism or achromatopsia and blue-cone monochromatism usually experience nyctalopia, poor vision, abnormal color vision, and photoaversion. Affected males with X-linked blue-cone monochromatism are typically myopic. Individuals with progressive cone dystrophies present with progressive central visual loss, poor color vision, and aversion to light. The age at onset of symptoms of these hereditary progresssive cone dystrophies ranges from the first to the sixth decade of life.

Clinical Features

Patients with congenital nonprogressive cone dystrophies may have a normal-appearing fundus, while others show minimal pigmentary disturbances or bull's eye macular changes. Affected patients with progressive cone dystrophies present initially with a normal-appearing fundus; as the disease progresses, a bull's eye maculopathy develops. Some patients can develop macular staphylomas. If rod photoreceptors become involved, optic disc atrophy, attenuated vessels, and bone spicule-like pigmentation may evolve with time.

Ancillary Testing

In rod monochromatism, the electroretinogram (ERG) is characteristic, showing an absent or markedly reduced cone response and normal rod response. Rod monochromatism also has typical findings on dark adaptation. There is no cone segment or cone-rod break in the dark-adapted curve. Blue-cone monochromatism reveals a blue-cone response on ERG. Progressive cone or cone-rod dystrophies have a marked reduction of the ERG cone response. Rod response may be affected later in the course of the disease.

Pathology/Pathogenesis

Rod monochromatism has been mapped to 2q11, 8q21-22, and 14. Histopathologic studies have shown a diminution of extrafoveal cones and ultrastructural abnormalities of foveal cones. Blue-cone monochromatism has been mapped to Xq28. This condition occurs secondarily to a functional defect on the red and green cone pigments. Progressive cone dystrophies have been mapped to different loci (chromosomes 1, 6, 8, 12, 17, 19, X). Functional abnormalities of cone pigments and impairment in processing by bipolar cells have been proposed as possible etiologies. Mutations in the guanylate cyclase activator 1A gene, which encodes guanylate cyclase activating protein-1, have been determined to be responsible for some cases of dominant cone-rod dystrophy. Histopathologic studies have shown loss of the outer nuclear layer and pigmentary changes as well.

Treatment/Prognosis

This heterogeneous group of conditions has no known treatment. Rod monochromatism and blue-cone monochromatism tend to be stationary, while cone or cone-rod dystrophies are progressive, with variability in onset, severity, and rate of progression.

Systemic Evaluation

No known systemic associations have been reported.

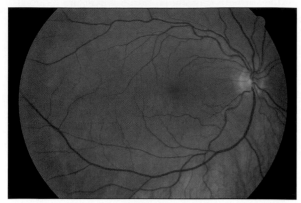

In some patients with cone dystrophy, the fundus may appear normal or have mild mottling of the retinal pigment epithelium.

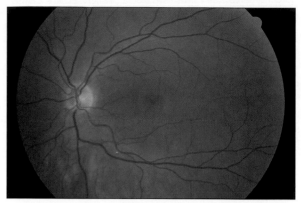

The fellow eye of the patient in the previous figure demonstrates a slightly more noticeable pattern of retinal pigment epithelial atrophy. Note the subtle temporal disc pallor.

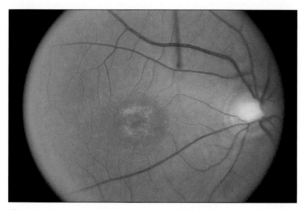

The classic fundus finding in a patient with cone dystrophy is a bull's eye maculopathy.

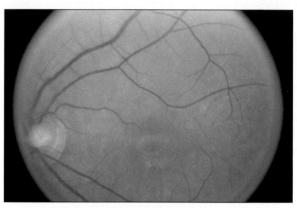

Bull's eye maculopathy refers to a pattern of retinal pigment epithelial alterations in the macula characterized by a central region of hyperpigmentation surrounded by a zone of hypopigmentation reminiscent of an aiming target.

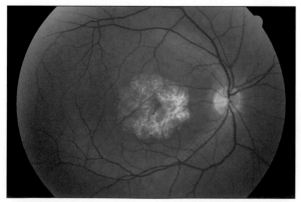

Occasionally, patients with cone dystrophy may develop central geographic atrophy.

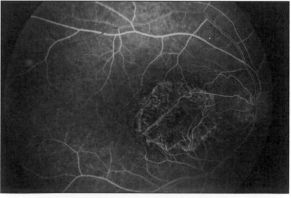

A fluorescein angiogram of the patient in the previous figure reveals a "window" defect corresponding to the region of atrophy.

CONGENITAL STATIONARY NIGHT BLINDNESS

Congenital stationary night blindness (CSNB) is a group of diseases characterized by nonprogressive night blindness. The diseases are classified as CSNB with normal fundus and CSNB with fundus abnormality. The CSNB with normal fundus can be further divided in three subtypes based on hereditary patterns: autosomal recessive, autosomal dominant, and X-linked. The CSNB variety with fundus abnormality includes Oguchi disease (autosomal recessive), fundus albipunctatus (autosomal recessive), and the flecked retina of Kandori.

Symptoms

Vision in autosomal dominant CSNB usually is normal, while in the autosomal recessive form of CSNB it may be normal or moderately decreased. Individuals with the X-linked form of CSNB may have poor vision; nevertheless, they usually do not complain of nyctalopia. In Oguchi disease and fundus albipunctatus, affected persons have normal vision and problems with dark adaptation. Flecked retina of Kandori is characterized by normal visual acuity and less impairment of night vision.

Clinical Features

Autosomal dominant CSNB, autosomal recessive CSNB, and X-linked CSNB are characterized by a normal-appearing fundus. Patients with the autosomal recessive and X-linked forms are likely to be myopic. Nystagmus is part of the clinical findings of X-linked CSNB. The retinal appearance of individuals with Oguchi disease shows a yellowish sheen after light exposure. After several hours of dark adaptation, the retina looks normal (Mizuo-Nakamura phenomenon). The retinal findings of fundus albipunctatus consist of white-yellow dots scattered in the posterior pole (sparing the macula) and radiating toward the midperiphery and retinal vessels of normal caliber. The flecked retina of Kandori shows large flecks in the equatorial zone.

Ancillary Testing

Dark adaptometry studies reveal delayed or poor rod adaptation and elevated final thresholds. The CSNB with normal fundus demonstrates two electroretinogram (ERG) patterns. The negative ERG (Schubert-Bornschein), which is the most common pattern, consists of a normal scotopic a-wave and a reduced or absent scotopic b-wave. This pattern can be seen in autosomal recessive and X-linked CSNB. The negative ERG pattern can be further classified into a complete type (rod function is almost absent) or incomplete type (moderate rod function). In the second ERG pattern (Riggs), the amplitudes of both scotopic a- and b-waves are reduced. This ERG pattern is usually characteristic of autosomal dominant CSNB. The ERG in Oguchi disease has a normal a-wave and a reduced b-wave under scotopic conditions with persistence of this abnormal response after prolonged dark adaptation. Fundus albipunctatus has elevated dark adaptation thresholds, and the ERG becomes normal with dark adaptation.

Pathology/Pathogenesis

Several mutational defects have been identified as the cause of CSNB. For autosomal dominant CSNB, three loci have been mapped: 3p22 (gene product is an alpha subunit of rod transducin), 3q21-q24 (rhodopsin gene), and 4p16.3 (beta subunit of rod cyclic guanosine monophosphate [cGMP] phosphodiesterase). The complete type of x-linked CSNB has been mapped to Xp11.4. The gene encodes nyctalopin (leucine-rich protein expressed in the retina and brain). The incomplete type has been mapped to Xp11.23. A defect in the process of pigment regeneration is the underlying etiology of fundus albipunctatus, whereas in Oguchi disease the pigment regeneration is not affected. Oguchi disease has a mutation in 2q37.1 (arrestin gene), and prolonged stimulation of photoreceptors by light is a possible explanation of the clinical findings.

Treatment/Prognosis

There is no known treatment for this group of disorders. Fortunately, these conditions are stationary.

Systemic Evaluation

No systemic associations have been described with CSNB.

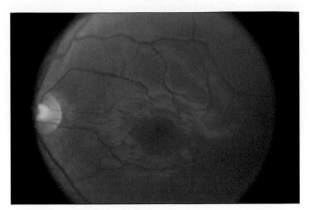

Individuals with congenital stationary night blindness may have a normal-appearing fundus.

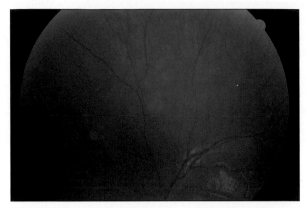

The scotopic electroretinogram in those with congenital stationary night blindness may demonstrate a normal a-wave and a reduced or absent b-wave.

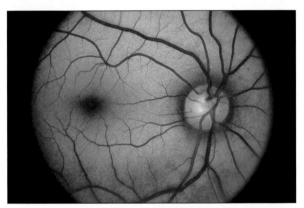

Oguchi disease is characterized by an unusual yellowish sheen of the fundus following light exposure.

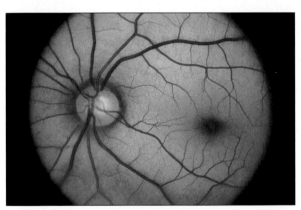

Fundus photograph of the fellow eye of the patient in the previous figure demonstrates the same yellowish sheen. After several hours of dark adaptation, the retina may appear normal (Mizuo-Nakamura phenomenon).

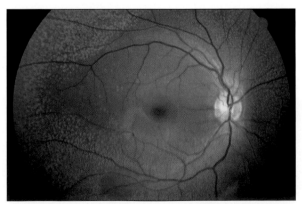

Fundus albipunctatus is characterized by numerous white-yellow dots scattered throughout the retina. The macula is usually spared.

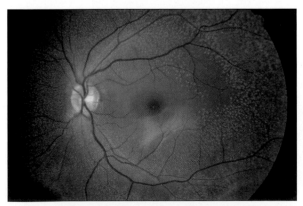

Patients with fundus albipunctatus have normal-appearing optic discs and retinal vessels (in contrast to patients with retinitis punctata albescens).

DOMINANT DRUSEN

Dominant drusen, also known as Doyne's honeycomb dystrophy, malattia leventinese, Hutchinson-Tay choroiditis, and Holthouse-Batten superficial chorioretinitis, is a dominantly inherited macular disorder. The onset of macular drusen occurs in the second to third decades.

Symptoms

Affected patients usually have good visual acuity despite the presence of multiple drusen. Drusen are initially evident during the third decade of life. In the late stages of the disease, the central vision becomes affected. Patients may complain of metamorphopsia and central scotomas.

Clinical Features

This disorder is characterized by multiple, small round or elongated drusen in the posterior pole extending beyond the arcades and involving retina nasal to the optic nerve head. As the disease progresses, the drusen may become confluent. Subretinal fibrous metaplasia and retinal pigment epithelial (RPE) and choriocapillaris atrophy may be observed. Choroidal neovascularization rarely may occur.

Ancillary Testing

Fluorescein angiography shows hyperfluorescent dots corresponding to drusen. Often fluorescein angiography reveals more drusen and RPE atrophy than are evident clinically. Findings of electroretinogram, dark adaptation, and electro-oculogram are usually normal. Visual field testing may reveal central scotomas. In the late stages of the disease a red-green dyschromatopsia may be evident.

Pathology/Pathogenesis

Dominant drusen is inherited as an autosomal dominant disorder. The genetic defect causing dominant drusen (EFEMP1) has been mapped to 2p16-p21. A single mutation (Arg345Trp) has been identified in all affected patients. The genetic defect is a defective extracellular matrix protein that leads to a defective basement membrane. Histopathologic studies reveal thickening of the basement membrane of the RPE. In the late stages of the condition, the retina and choroid may be atrophied.

Treatment/Prognosis

Patients affected with dominant drusen usually have good visual acuity in spite of their clinical findings. Central vision may become affected gradually as the disease progresses. Nevertheless, visual loss may occur as a result of choroidal neovascularization. Fortunately, this complication is rare.

Systemic Evaluation

Certain hereditary renal conditions with underlying basement membrane anomalies like Alport's syndrome and glomerulonephritis type II may be associated with drusen-like deposits in the retina.

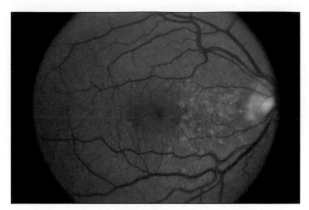

Dominant drusen is characterized by multiple, small round or oval deposits at the level of the retinal pigment epithelium.

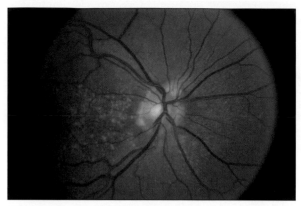

The drusen are most common in the posterior pole but may extend beyond the vascular arcades and involve the retina nasal to the optic nerve head.

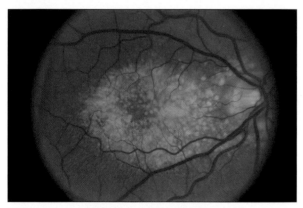

This young man had confluent macular drusen surrounded by a radial pattern of fine drusen deposits.

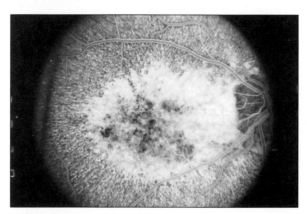

Fluorescein angiography reveals innumerable hyperfluorescent spots corresponding to the drusen.

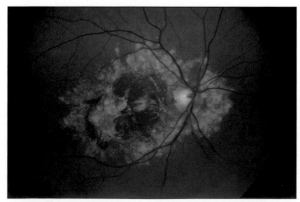

Some patients with dominant drusen may develop subretinal fibrous metaplasia.

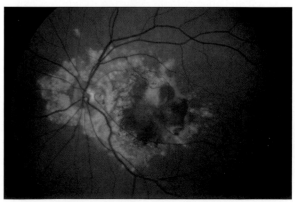

The fellow eye of the patient in the previous figure demonstrates the symmetric nature of dominant drusen.

GYRATE ATROPHY

Gyrate atrophy is an autosomal recessive chorioretinal dystrophy. Most patients become aware of symptoms in the second or third decade of life.

Symptoms

Affected patients present with night blindness and progressive peripheral visual loss in their second or third decade. Central vision is preserved until later in life. Color vision remains unaffected until the later stages of the condition. This dystrophy is characterized by a slowly progressive course.

Clinical Features

Fundus findings consist of focal areas of midperipheral chorioretinal atrophy. These areas eventually enlarge and coalesce, spreading toward the macula and peripherally. These atrophic regions have characteristic scalloped borders, creating a contrast between normal and abnormal retinal pigment epithelium. Extensive choroidal atrophy and pigment clumping as well as optic disc pallor and narrowing of the retinal vessels are evident in the late stages of the disease. Most individuals with gyrate atrophy have high myopia, astigmatism, and posterior subcapsular cataracts.

Ancillary Testing

Fluorescein angiography reveals absence of the choriocapillaris in the affected zones. The junction between choriocapillaris atrophy and normal choriocapillaris flush of unaffected tissues is hypofluorescent because of pigment accumulation.

The electro-oculogram (EOG) is abnormal in gyrate atrophy. The electroretinogram (ERG) demonstrates reduced rod and cone responses during the early stages in spite of minimal findings. With further progression of the condition, the ERG becomes extinguished.

Patients with gyrate atrophy have high levels of ornithine in serum, urine, and cerebrospinal fluid.

Pathology/Pathogenesis

The genetic mutation of this condition involves a deficiency of the enzyme ornithine aminotransferase. This pyridoxal phosphate-dependent enzyme is involved in ornithine metabolism. The gene coding for ornithine aminotransferase has been mapped to 10q26. Histopathologic study of eyes of a patient with vitamin B_6-responsive gyrate atrophy revealed areas of focal atrophy of the retinal pigment epithelium (RPE) and photoreceptors in the posterior pole. There was an abrupt transition from normal retina to almost absolute atrophy of the retina, RPE, and choroid.

Treatment/Prognosis

Some studies have shown a slower progression of the condition, with treatment aimed toward reducing ornithine levels. Lowering of plasma ornithine levels can be accomplished with a restricted intake of arginine as well as with vitamin B_6 administration. Nonetheless, different results have been reported with these treatment modalities.

Systemic Evaluation

Several associated systemic findings have been reported. These include ultrastructural changes in skeletal muscle fibers, enlarged mitochondria in hepatic cells, atrophic white matter lesions detected on brain magnetic resonance imaging, and abnormal findings on electroencephalography.

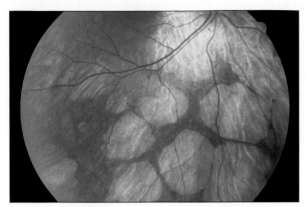

The fundus findings in patients with gyrate atrophy include midperipheral chorioretinal atrophy that spreads toward the macula and periphery.

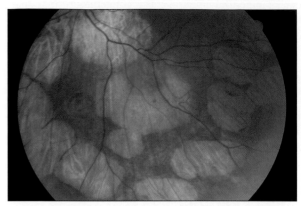

The atrophic areas have well-defined, scalloped borders. The areas between the atrophic patches may be hyperpigmented. Serum ornithine levels are elevated as a result of ornithine aminotransferase deficiency.

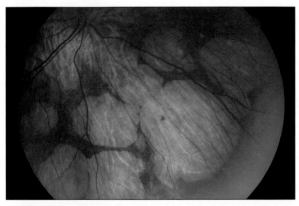

The stage of chorioretinal atrophy in patients with gyrate atrophy is relatively uniform in all affected areas.

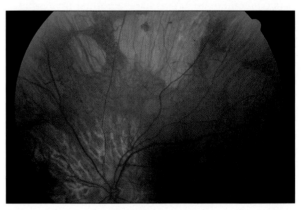

Pigment clumps may be visible within areas of chorioretinal atrophy.

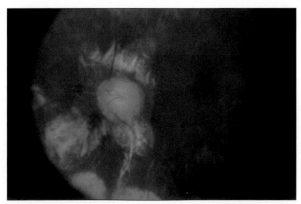

In the late stages of gyrate atrophy, the optic discs are pale and the retinal vessels are attenuated.

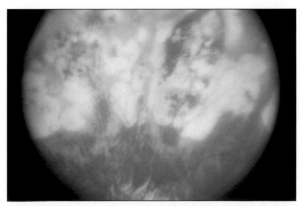

Extensive chorioretinal atrophy reveals the underlying sclera in advanced cases.

LEBER'S CONGENITAL AMAUROSIS

Leber's congenital amaurosis is a congenital retinal disorder inherited as an autosomal recessive trait. Patients affected with this condition usually present with the clinical picture at birth.

Symptoms

Children affected with Leber's congenital amaurosis experience poor vision and photophobia. Most patients have nystagmus. It is not unusual for patients to continuously push or rub their eyes (oculodigital sign or reflex).

Clinical Features

The clinical picture of patients with Leber's congenital amaurosis includes very poor visual acuity, nystagmus, sluggish pupillary reflexes, hyperopia, and a positive oculodigital reflex. The majority of children with Leber's congenital amaurosis have a normal-appearing fundus. However, some patients may present with pigmentary changes, optic nerve pallor, and vessel attenuation. Keratoconus and cataracts can be associated findings in older children with this condition.

Ancillary Testing

Electroretinographic testing plays a pivotal role in establishing the diagnosis. Patients affected with this disorder have a severely abnormal or undetectable electroretinogram. This feature is helpful to distinguish Leber's congenital amaurosis from other conditions that can mimic it in certain ways.

Pathology/Pathogenesis

Mutations in different genes have been associated with Leber's congenital amaurosis. Mutational defects at locus 1p31, which gene product is a 65-kD retinal pigment epithelium (RPE) protein, can be associated with this disorder. Mutations in a gene encoding for a retinal-specific guanylate cyclase (17p13.1), which is involved in the phototransduction process, can be associated with Leber's congenital amaurosis (LCA). Defects in the arylhydrocarbon-interacting receptor protein-like 1 gene at 17p13.1, at 6q11-q16, and at 14q24 loci may account for some LCA cases. Histopathologic studies have shown loss of photoreceptors, gliosis, degeneration of retina and RPE, and intraretinal pigment migration.

Treatment/Prognosis

Unfortunately, there is no treatment for Leber's congenital amaurosis. This disease is a retinal dysgenesis in which a progression of retinal changes is unlikely to greatly affect the level of visual acuity. Decrease of visual acuity can result from keratoconus, macular colobomas, or cataract formation.

Systemic Evaluation

The term *Leber's congenital amaurosis* implies no associated systemic findings. Some cases of mental or psychomotor retardation have been reported in association with the disease. Nevertheless, some authors have argued that this feature is secondary to visual deprivation.

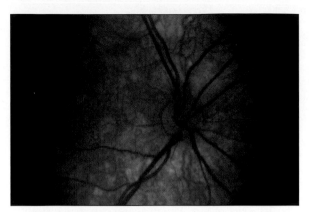

The majority of patients with Leber's congenital amaurosis have normal-appearing retinas. However, extensive pigmentary abnormalities may be observed.

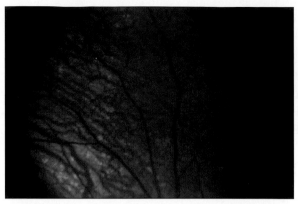

This patient has extensive retinal pigmentary alterations but normal-appearing optic discs and retinal vessels.

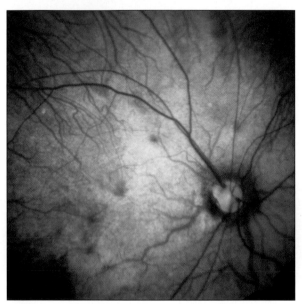

This 6-year-old boy had a history of poor vision since birth. Fundus photograph of his right eye reveals diffuse mottling of the retinal pigment epithelium with a "salt and pepper" stippling of the retina.

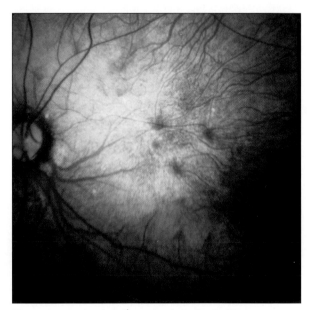

The same patient's left eye had similar findings, demonstrating the symmetric nature of the retinal alterations in Leber's cogenital amaurosis.

NORTH CAROLINA MACULAR DYSTROPHY

North Carolina macular dystrophy is inherited as an autosomal dominant trait. The onset of this condition is usually early in life.

Symptoms

Patients usually present with progressive central visual loss. Symptoms start very early, typically becoming stabilized at the end of the first decade of life.

Clinical Features

The clinical presentation of North Carolina macular dystrophy is highly variable. At the earlier stages of the condition, the visual acuity may be good, with drusen in the macular area. As the disease progresses, the drusen increase in number and become confluent. The condition may show a further progression to an end-stage state characterized by macular staphylomas.

Ancillary Testing

Individuals affected with this condition may show a central scotoma on visual field testing. However, peripheral visual fields, color vision, electroretinogram, and electro-oculogram are typically normal.

Fluorescein angiography shows window defects that correspond to the drusen. The staphylomatous lesion in the end stage of the condition is hypofluorescent on fluorescein angiography due to chorioretinal atrophy.

Pathology/Pathogenesis

No histopathologic studies have been reported. The condition has been mapped to the 6q14-q16.2 locus. A recent histopathologic examination of an eye of a patient with North Carolina macular dystrophy showed loss of photoreceptors and retinal pigment epithelium as well as choriocapillaris atrophy localized to the macula.

Treatment/Prognosis

There is no known treatment for North Carolina macular dystrophy. It is a hereditary condition that usually stabilizes by 10 years of age. Visual acuity may range from 20/20 to 20/200.

Systemic Evaluation

There are no known systemic associations of North Carolina macular dystrophy.

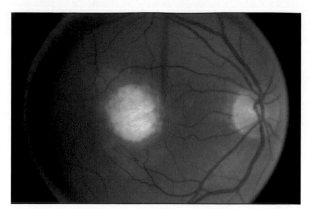

North Carolina macular dystrophy is an autosomal dominant disorder, as demonstrated by this series of fundus photographs of a mother and her two sons.

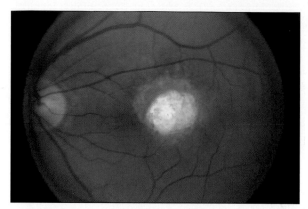

Fundus photographs of a 57-year-old woman demonstrate macular atrophy. In some cases, the macular lesions have a staphylomatous-like appearance.

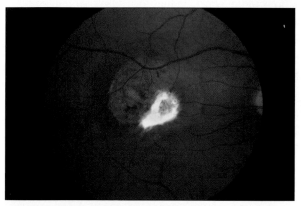

The 34-year-old son of the woman shown in the previous figure had extensive retinal pigment epithelial alterations and chorioretinal atrophy. Pigment clumping may be observed in the macula and peripheral retina.

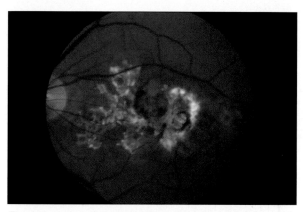

The fellow eye of the patient shown in the previous figure revealed prominent retinal pigment epithelial hyperplasia in addition to the chorioretinal atrophy.

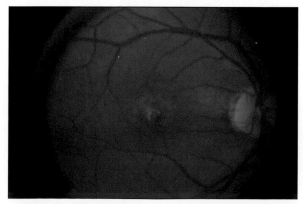

The 20-year-old son of the same woman had mild macular changes consisting of central drusen and mild pigmentary changes.

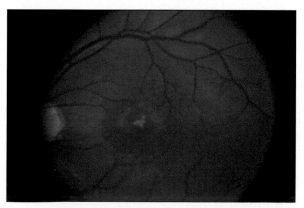

Some of the macular drusen were confluent. No significant retinal pigment epithelial abnormalities were noted.

RETINITIS PIGMENTOSA (ROD-CONE DYSTROPHIES)

Retinitis pigmentosa (RP; rod-cone dystrophies) includes a diverse group of inherited retinal dystrophies characterized by a progressive degeneration of the photoreceptor cells. The majority of cases of RP are sporadic and have no clear identifiable family history. However, some hereditary patterns have been described: autosomal dominant (20%); autosomal recessive (15%); and X-linked recessive (10%). The age at onset varies, depending on the inheritance pattern. X-linked cases usually have an earlier onset and autosomal dominant cases tend to have a later onset of the condition.

Symptoms

The typical symptoms of RP include nyctalopia and progressive peripheral visual loss. Central vision is usually spared in the initial stages of the condition. Eventually, the peripheral visual loss increases, leaving a tunnel of central vision.

Clinical Features

The typical fundus appearance of RP consists of peripheral atrophy of the retina, retinal pigment epithelium (RPE), and choriocapillaris, optic disc pallor, arteriolar narrowing, and retinal pigment migration. These pigmentary changes may be manifested as a diffuse granularity, pigment clumping, or bone spicule-like deposits. Other findings may be cystoid macular edema, wrinkling of the internal limiting membrane, vitreous cells or opacities, posterior subcapsular cataracts, and optic nerve drusen.

There are several presentations of RP. Retinitis pigmentosa sine pigmento is a variant of RP (probably an early stage of RP) in which the typical pigment changes are absent or minimal. Retinitis punctata albescens presents the typical findings of RP in addition to many small white dots at the level of RPE.

Ancillary Testing

Fluorescein angiography shows patches of hyperfluorescence resulting from RPE atrophy, choriocapillaris non-filling defects, and an increase in the retinal circulation time. Patients with cystoid macular edema often show the typical staining pattern on fluorescein angiography, while in others, only minimal staining can be detected. Visual field testing reveals a midperipheral ring scotoma in the earlier stages that progresses into a constricted visual field with a remaining central tunnel of vision in the late stages of the condition. Dark-adaptation studies show an elevated adaptation curve of the rod segments and a delayed cone-rod break. The electroretinogram is essential in the evaluation of RP patients. It shows reduced and prolonged a- and b-waves and becomes unrecordable with time.

Pathology/Pathogenesis

Histopathologic studies have revealed photoreceptor degeneration, atrophy of the retina and RPE, migration of RPE cells into the retina, thickening and hyalinization of vessel walls and atrophy, and gliosis of the optic nerve.

A wide spectrum of genotypes exist in this condition. Approximately 26 RP genes have been identified and mapped to different loci (chromosomes 1, 2, 3, 4, 5, 6, 7, 8, 9,10, 11, 14, 15, 16, 17, 19, X). More than 70 mutations in the rhodopsin gene have been identified as responsible for autosomal dominant RP. Defects in the peripherin gene also have been recognized as the etiology in some cases of autosomal dominant RP. Mutations in the genes coding for ROM1 protein and cGMP phosphodiesterase have also been identified in some RP patients.

Treatment/Prognosis

This condition is characterized by a slowly progressive course. Total blindness is unusual. Patients with RP should be followed up on a yearly basis. If present, cystoid macular edema may be treated with acetazolamide. Cataracts can be extracted if they are visually significant. Therapy for autosomal dominant RP with high doses of vitamin A palmitate (15 000 IU/day) may show a slightly slower rate of progression of the condition. This finding, however, is controversial, as is the reported slightly adverse effect of vitamin E on RP.

Systemic Evaluation

Several systemic diseases are associated with RP or RP-like fundus patterns, such as Usher syndrome (RP and congenital sensorineural hearing loss), Laurence Moon and Bardet-Biedl syndromes, neuronal ceroid lipofuscinosis, Refsum's disease, abetalipoproteinemia, Kearns-Sayre syndrome, Alström's disease, and others.

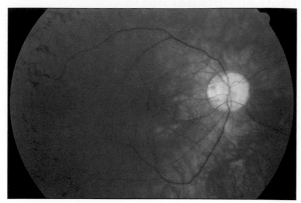

The classic findings of retinitis pigmentosa include waxy pallor of the optic discs, retinal vessel attenuation, and peripheral pigmentary alterations.

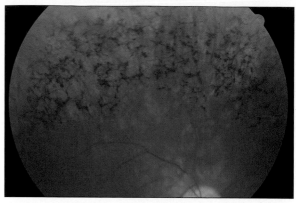

Although the extent of optic disc pallor and peripheral pigmentary alterations may vary, patients with retinitis pigmentosa invariably have retinal vascular attenuation. The presence of mild vitreous cells is common.

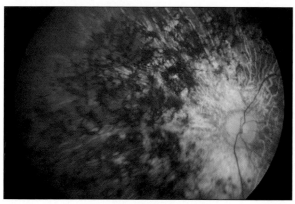

The peripheral pigmentary alterations vary from mild stippling of the retinal pigment epithelium to extensive retinal pigmentary derangement.

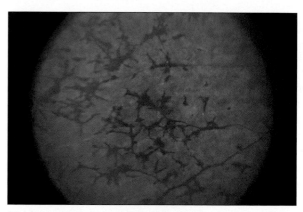

The characteristic peripheral pigmentary changes are described as "bone spicules." The bone spicules are most prominent in the midperipheral retina.

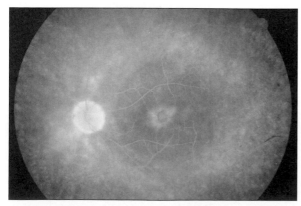

Loss of visual acuity may result from posterior subcapsular cataracts or cystoid macular edema (CME). The CME is characterized by a petaloid pattern of hyperfluorescence in the fovea.

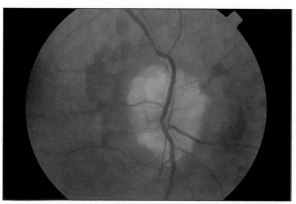

Optic nerve drusen may be observed in patients with retinitis pigmentosa.

SORSBY'S FUNDUS DYSTROPHY

Sorsby's fundus dystrophy is a progressive maculopathy inherited as an autosomal dominant trait. Patients usually experience the onset of symptoms in the third or fourth decade of life.

Symptoms

Persons affected typically experience loss of central vision and nyctalopia.

Clinical Features

During the early stages of this progressive maculopathy, confluent plaques are observed at the posterior pole beneath the retinal pigment epithelium (RPE). As the disease progresses, choroidal neovascularization develops. The maculopathy evolves into geographic atrophy, subretinal fibrosis, and pigment clumping.

Ancillary Testing

Color vision testing may reveal a tritan color defect in the early stages of the disease. This feature is useful for identifying individuals with this condition but with a normal-appearing fundus. Visual field testing typically shows a central scotoma that may increase as a result of progression of atrophy into the peripheral retina. Fluorescein angiography reveals a delay in choroidal filling. Choroidal neovascularization is manifested by hyperfluorescence and leakage in fluorescein angiography. The electroretinogram and electro-oculogram findings are typically normal in the initial stages of this maculopathy. Dark adaptation becomes affected in the late stages, showing a delayed or absent cone-rod break.

Pathology/Pathogenesis

Histopathologic studies have shown thickening of Bruch's membrane secondary to lipid deposition between the RPE basement membrane and the inner collagenous zone. The gene for Sorsby's fundus dystrophy has been mapped to 22q12.1-q13.2, which codes for a tissue inhibitor of metalloproteinase-3. This gene product is necessary for the extracellular matrix remodeling process. Hence, mutations in this gene lead to changes in the extracellular matrix milieu affecting Bruch's membrane.

Treatment/Prognosis

Sorsby's fundus dystrophy has a poor prognosis, because atrophy and scarring may extend into the periphery as the condition evolves. Patients may have severely affected nonambulatory vision. In a clinical study, administration of high doses of vitamin A was associated with an improvement of symptoms and retinal functional tests in affected patients. However, no treatment has been established for this condition, and further investigations are necessary.

Systemic Evaluation

There are no known systemic associations with Sorsby's fundus dystrophy.

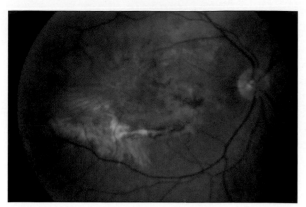

Sorsby's fundus dystrophy is associated with subretinal fibrosis, retinal pigment epithelial atrophy, and pigment clumping throughout the macula.

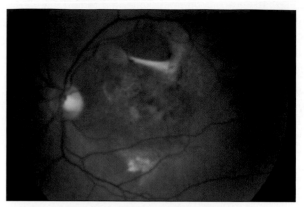

This patient had bilateral, symmetric macular abnormalities, which is characteristic of Sorsby's fundus dystrophy.

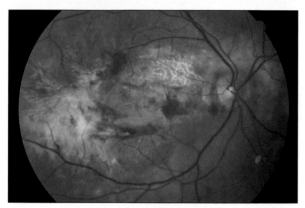

Seven years later, the patient shown in the previous figures had more extensive subretinal fibrosis, retinal pigment epithelial atrophy, and pigment plaques. Subretinal hemorrhage and fluid were also observed.

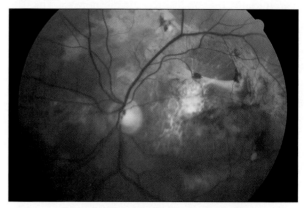

The progression of her macular abnormalities was evident bilaterally. Her left eye showed extensive abnormalities extending beyond the macula to the superior and nasal retina.

STARGARDT DISEASE

Stargardt disease is a common inherited retinal disorder. It typically affects young, healthy individuals in the first or second decade of life. Stargardt disease is usually autosomal recessive, but autosomal dominant and mitochondrial pedigrees have been described.

Symptoms

Individuals with Stargardt disease experience bilateral visual loss in childhood or young adulthood. Visual complaints may be disproportionate to the clinical findings—particularly early in the course of the disease. Other symptoms include dyschromatopsia, central scotomas, or photophobia.

Clinical Features

There is a wide spectrum of clinical findings in Stargardt disease. Initially, the fundus may appear normal. The macula may have a vermilion discoloration as the heavily pigmented retinal pigment epithelium (RPE) obscures the underlying choroidal details. Yellowish "flecks" may be visualized at the level of the RPE. The flecks are variable in size, shape, and distribution but are usually symmetric between eyes. The flecks have a triradiate or pisciform (fish-tail) configuration. The flecks tend to fade over time, often replaced by RPE atrophy. Macular alterations range from mild RPE mottling to marked geographic atrophy. The fovea may develop a "beaten metal" appearance or a "bull's eye" pattern of atrophy. Rarely, choroidal neovascularization and midperipheral RPE hyperplasia are seen.

Ancillary Testing

The classic fluorescein angiographic finding is a "silent choroid" distinguished by blockage of choroidal fluorescence. Hyperfluorescence in the macula is variable, depending on the degree of RPE atrophy. Flecks usually do not hypo- or hyperfluoresce; however, when the flecks are associated with RPE atrophy, an irregular pattern of hyperfluorescence may be seen.

Electrophysiologic testing is usually normal but may be abnormal in advanced cases with more widespread flecks or RPE abnormalities. Abnormalities in the pattern electroretinogram are common.

Pathology/Pathogenesis

Mutations in the adenosine triphosphate (ATP)-binding cassette transporter gene (ABCA4, formerly known as ABCR) have been identified in Stargardt disease. Stargardt disease is characterized by accumulation of lipofuscin-like material in the RPE. Lipofuscin accumulation may result from abnormal photoreceptor degradation. Other histopathologic findings include heterogeneity of RPE cells, loss of photoreceptors, and Müller cell hypertrophy.

Treatment/Prognosis

There is no known treatment for Stargardt disease. The visual prognosis depends on the degree of macular involvement. Vision usually stabilizes in the 20/200 range when affected. Low-vision aids are very effective. Laser therapy may be helpful for those rare cases of choroidal neovascularization.

Systemic Evaluation

There are no known systemic associations of Stargardt disease.

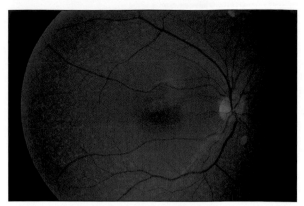

Stargardt disease is characterized by the presence of numerous yellowish "flecks" located at the level of the retinal pigment epithelium. The flecks are variable in size, shape, and distribution but are usually symmetric between eyes.

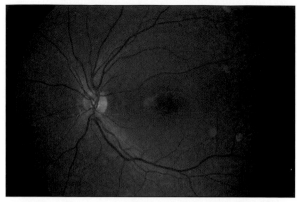

The flecks have a triradiate or pisciform (fish-tail) configuration. They may be widespread or concentrated in the macula. The flecks tend to fade over time, often replaced by retinal pigment epithelium atrophy.

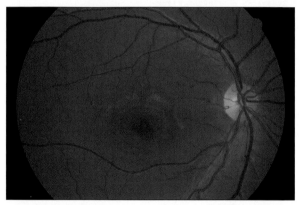

Macular alterations range from mild retinal pigment epithelial mottling to marked geographic atrophy. In some patients, the macula has a "beaten metal" appearance.

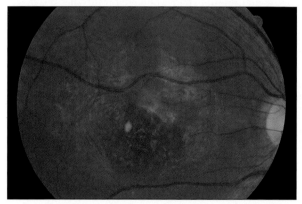

Stargardt disease must be considered in patients with a bull's eye maculopathy. The bull's eye maculopathy results from atrophy of the retinal pigment epithelium.

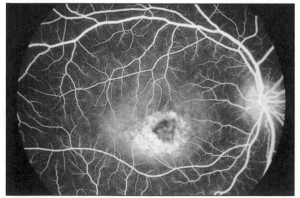

Fluorescein angiogram of 6-year-old girl with Stargardt disease. The characteristic "silent choroid" is observed in the peripheral macula. This relative hypofluorescence is the result of the lipofuscin-laden retinal pigment epithelial cells blocking the underlying choroidal fluorescence.

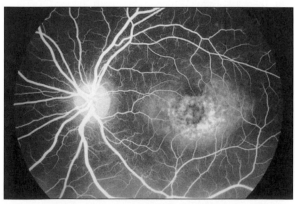

The central hyperfluorescence observed in each eye is the result of retinal pigment epithelial atrophy.

X-LINKED JUVENILE RETINOSCHISIS

X-linked juvenile retinoschisis is a vitreoretinal dystrophy that occurs in the male population. Patients affected with this X-linked recessive condition present with symptoms in early childhood.

Symptoms

Individuals with X-linked retinoschisis usually experience mild or moderate visual loss. Progression of the condition occurs mainly in the first years of life and then stabilizes or progresses at a much slower rate. Visual acuity may range from 20/50 to 20/400.

Clinical Features

X-linked retinoschisis is characterized by a stellate maculopathy. This foveal schisis is found in almost all patients. However, adult patients may have atrophic retinal pigment epithelial (RPE) changes following the disappearance of this classic foveal cystic appearance. Peripheral retinoschisis occurs in about 50% of affected patients. The most common location for this peripheral schisis is the inferotemporal quadrant. This retinal splitting occurs at the nerve fiber layer level. Other findings include holes in the inner retinal layer, retinal dragging, vitreous strands, and sheathing of vessels. The clinical course of these patients could be complicated by the development of vitreous hemorrhage and rhegmatogenous retinal detachments. Hypermetropia, strabismus, nystagmus, and cataracts may be present in this dystrophy.

Ancillary Testing

X-linked retinoschisis may present a fluorescein angiographic pattern similar to that of cystoid macular edema. However, the late phases do not reveal leakage of dye. In some patients, the retinal vessels from the peripheral schisis areas may leak on fluorescein angiography.

Visual field testing demonstrates an absolute scotoma that corresponds to the areas of peripheral schisis. The electroretinogram (ERG) shows a reduced b-wave amplitude in photopic and scotopic conditions. The oscillatory potentials of the photoreceptors are reduced, and the implicit times are prolonged.

Pathology/Pathogenesis

The X-linked retinoschisis gene (XLRS1) has been mapped to Xp 22.2. This gene encodes retinoschisin, a photoreceptor protein secreted into the inner retina. A diffuse abnormality of the Müller cells may be the underlying cause of this condition, as suggested by ERG and histopathologic findings.

Treatment/Prognosis

Affected patients usually maintain stable visual acuity or experience a slow progression of the condition. However, if complications such as vitreous hemorrhage or retinal detachment arise, surgical management may be necessary. Hence, patients with X-linked retinoschisis should be observed.

Systemic Evaluation

No known systemic associations have been reported with this condition.

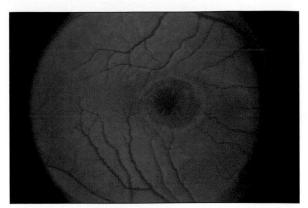

X-linked juvenile retinoschisis is characterized by cyst-like changes in the fovea. The splitting of the neurosensory retina occurs between the nerve fiber and ganglion cell layers.

Higher magnification of the macula of the patient shown in the previous figure reveals the stellate, cyst-like pattern of schisis extending from the center of the fovea.

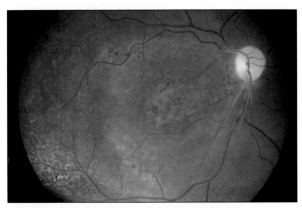

This 51-year-old man with X-linked juvenile retinoschisis had extensive macular pigmentary alterations and sheathing of the retinal vessels.

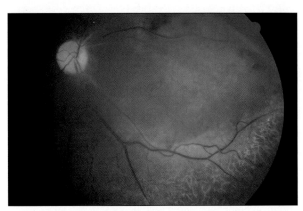

His left eye had similar findings. Note the white "fishbone" spicules that may be seen in patients with X-linked juvenile retinoschisis.

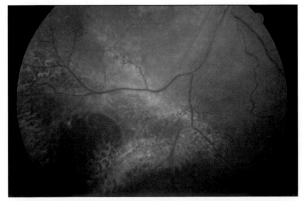

Peripheral retinoschisis may contain inner or outer retinal holes. Vitreous hemorrhage or retinal detachment may cause visual loss in patients with X-linked juvenile retinoschisis.

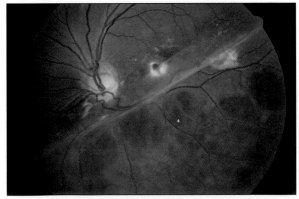

Peripheral retinoschisis may extend to the macula. This 9-year-old boy had a retinal fold extending through the macula. He also had retinal pigment epithelial alterations in the macula and peripheral retina.

SELECTED REFERENCES

Albinism

1. Biswas S, Lloyd IC. Oculocutaneous albinism. *Arch Dis Child.* 1999;80(6):565–569.

2. Gass JDM. Heredodystrophic disorders affecting the pigment epithelium and retina. In: Gass JDM, ed. *Stereoscopic Atlas of Macular Diseases: Diagnosis and Treatment.* St. Louis: Mosby-Year Book, Inc; 1997:386–388.

3. Izquierdo NJ, Townsend W, Hussels IE. Ocular findings in the Hermansky-Pudlak syndrome. *Trans Am Ophthalmol Soc.* 1995;93:191–200.

4. Lam BL, Fingert JH, Shutt BC, Singleton EM, Merin LM, Brown HH, et al. Clinical and molecular characterization of a family affected with X-linked ocular albinism (OA1). *Ophthalmic Genet.* 1997;18(4):175–184.

5. Orlow SJ. Albinism: an update. *Semin Cutan Med Surg.* 1997;16(1):24–29.

6. Shen B, Samaraweera P, Resenberg B, Orlow SJ. Ocular albinism Type 1: more than meets the eye. *Pigment Cell Res.* 2001;14(4):243–248.

Best's Disease

1. Blodi CF, Stone EM. Best's vitelliform dystrophy. *Ophthalmic Paediatr Genet.* 1990;11(1):49–59.

2. Deutman AF, Hoyng CB. Macular dystrophies. In: Schachat AP, senior ed. *Medical Retina.* Ryan SJ, ed. *Retina.* Vol 2. 3rd ed. St. Louis: Mosby, Inc; 2001:1225–1229.

3. Gass JDM. Heredodystrophic disorders affecting the pigment epithelium and retina. In: Gass JDM, ed. *Stereoscopic Atlas of Macular Diseases: Diagnosis and Treatment.* St. Louis: Mosby-Year Book, Inc; 1997:303–312.

4. Marmorstein AD, Marmorstein LY, Rayborn M, Wang X, Hollyfield JG, Petrukhin K. Bestrophin, the product of the Best vitelliform macular dystrophy gene (VMD2), localizes to the basolateral plasma membrane of the retinal pigment epithelium. *Proc Natl Acad Sci, USA.* 2000;97(23):12758–12763.

5. Marquardt A, Stohr H, Passmore LA, Kramer F, Rivera A, Weber BH. Mutations in a novel gene, VMD2, encoding a protein of unknown properties cause juvenile-onset vitelliform macular dystrophy (Best's disease). *Hum Mol Genet.* 1998;7(9):1517–1525.

6. Mohler CW, Fine SL. Long-term evaluation of patients with Best's vitelliform dystrophy. *Ophthalmology.* 1981;88(7);688–692.

7. Park DW, Arbour NC, Brown DM, Stone EM. Best's disease: molecular and clinical findings. In: Guyer DR, Yannuzzi LA, Chang S, Shields JA, Green WR, eds. *Retina-Vitreous-Macula.* Philadelphia: WB Saunders Co; 1999:989–1005.

8. Petrukhin K, Koisti MJ, Bakall B, Li W, Xie G, Marknell T, et al. Identification of the gene responsible for Best macular dystrophy. *Nat Genet.* 1998;19(3):241–247.

For more information refer to www.sph.uth.tmc.edu/RetNet/disease.htm.

Choroideremia

1. Alory C, Balch WE. Organization of the Rab-GDI/CHM superfamily: the functional basis for choroideremia disease. *Traffic.* 2001;2(8):532–543.

2. Gass JDM. Heredodystrophic disorders affecting the pigment epithelium and retina. In: Gass JDM, ed. *Stereoscopic Atlas of Macular Diseases: Diagnosis and Treatment.* St. Louis: Mosby-Year Book, Inc; 1997:366–368.

3. McCulloch C. Choroideremia: a clinical and pathologic review. *Trans Am Ophthalmol Soc.* 1969;67:142–195.

4. Noble KG. Choroidal dystrophies. In: Guyer DR, Yannuzzi LA, Chang S, Shields JA, Green WR, eds. *Retina-Vitreous-Macula.* Philadelphia: WB Saunders Co; 1999:956–960.

5. Ohba N, Isashiki Y. Clinical and genetic features of choroideremia. *Jpn J Ophthalmol.* 2000;44(3):317.

6. Rodrigues MM, Ballintine EJ, Wiggert BN, Lee L, Fletcher RT, Chader GJ. Choroideremia: a clinical, electron microscopic, and biochemical report. *Ophthalmology.* 1984;91(7):873–883.

7. Sieving PA, Niffenegger JH, Berson EL. Electroretinographic findings in selected pedigrees with choroideremia. *Am J Ophthalmol.* 1986;101(3):361–317.

8. van den Hurk JAJM, Schwartz M, van Bokhoven H, van de Pol TJ, Bogerd L, Pinckers AJ, et al. Molecular basis of choroideremia (CHM): mutations involving the Rab escort protein-1 (REP-1) gene. *Hum Mutat.* 1997;9(2):110–117.

9. Zhang K, Garabaldi DC, Carr RE, Sunness JS. Hereditary choroidal disease. In: Ogden TE, Hinton DR, senior eds. *Basic Sciences and Inherited Retinal Diseases/Tumors.* Ryan SJ, ed. *Retina.* Vol 1. 3rd ed. St. Louis: Mosby Inc; 2001:468–469.

For more information refer to www.sph.uth.tmc.edu/RetNet/disease.htm.

Cone Dystrophies/Cone-Rod Dystrophies

1. Carr RE. Abnormalities of cone and rod function. In: Ogden TE, Hinton TE, eds. *Basic Sciences and Inherited Retinal Diseases/Tumors.* Ryan SJ, ed. *Retina,* Vol 1. 3rd ed. St. Louis: Mosby Inc; 2001:471–474.

2. Carr RE. Cone dystrophies. In: Guyer DR, Yannuzzi LA, Chang S, Shields JA, Green WR, eds. *Retina-Vitreous-Macula.* Philadelphia: WB Saunders Co; 1999:942–948.

3. Deutman AF, Hoyng CB. Macular dystrophies. In: Schachat AP, senior ed. *Medical Retina.* Ryan SJ, ed. *Retina.* Vol 2. 3rd ed. St. Louis: Mosby Inc; 2001:1216–1219.

4. Downes SM, Holder GE, Fitzke FW, Payne AM, Warren MJ, Bhattacharya SS, et al. Autosomal dominant cone and cone-rod dystrophy with mutations in the guanylate cyclase activator 1A gene-encoding retinal guanylate cyclase activating protein-1. *Arch Ophthalmol.* 2001;119(1):96–105.

5. Gass JDM. Heredodystrophic disorders affecting the pigment epithelium and retina. In: Gass JDM. *Stereoscopic Atlas of Macular Diseases: Diagnosis and Treatment.* St. Louis: Mosby-Year Book, Inc; 1997:336–338, 370.

6. Mantyjarvi M, Nurmenniemi P, Partanen J, Myohanen T, Peippo M, Alitalo T. Clinical features and a follow-up study in a family with X-linked progressive cone-rod dystrophy. *Acta Ophthalmol Scand.* 2001;79(4):359–365.

7. Ripps H, Noble KG, Greenstein VC, Siegel IM, Carr RE. Progressive cone dystrophy. *Ophthalmology.* 1987;94(11):1401–1409.

8. Simunovic MP, Moore AT. The cone dystrophies. *Eye.* 1998;12(pt 3b):553–565.

For more information refer to www.sph.uth.tmc.edu/RetNet/disease.htm.

Congenital Stationary Night Blindness

1. Bech-Hansen NT, Boycott KM, Gratton KJ, Ross DA, Field LL, Pearce WG. Localization of a gene for incomplete X-linked congenital stationary night blindness to the interval between DXS6849 and DXS8023 in Xp11.2 3. *Hum Genet.* 1998;103(2):124–130.

2. Carr RE. Abnormalities of cone and rod function. In: Ogden TE, Hinton DR, senior eds. *Basic Sciences and Inherited Retinal Diseases/Tumors.* Ryan SJ, ed. *Retina.* Vol 1. 3rd ed St. Louis: Mosby Inc; 2001:474–480.

3. Dryja TP, Berson EL, Rao V, Oprian DD. Heterozygous missense mutation in the rhodopsin gene as a cause of congenital stationary night blindness. *Nat Genet.* 1993;4(3):280–283.

4. Dryja TP, Hahn LB, Reboul T, Arnaud B. Missense mutation in the gene encoding the alpha subunit of rod transducin in the Nougaret form of congenital stationary night blindness. *Nat Genet.* 1996;13(3):358–360.

5. Fuchs S, Nakazawa M, Maw M, Tamai M, Oguchi Y, Gal A. A homozygous 1-base pair deletion in the arrestin gene is a frequent cause of Oguchi disease in Japanese. *Nat Genet.* 1995;10(3):360–362.

6. Gal A, Orth U, Baehr W, Schwinger E, Rosenberg T. Heterozygous missense mutation in the rod cGMP phosphodiesterase beta-subunit gene in autosomal dominant stationary night blindness. *Nat Genet.* 1994;7(1):64–68.

7. Gass JDM. Heredodystrophic disorders affecting the pigment epithelium and retina. In: Gass JDM, ed. *Stereoscopic Atlas of Macular Diseases: Diagnosis and Treatment.* St. Louis: Mosby-Year Book, Inc; 1997:346–350.

8. Noble KG. Congenital stationary night blindness. In: Guyer DR, Yannuzzi LA, Chang S, Shields JA, Green WR, eds. *Retina-Vitreous-Macula.* Philadelphia: WB Saunders Co; 1999:934–941.

9. Pusch CM, Zeitz C, Brandau O, Pesch K, Achatz H, Feil S, et al. The complete form of X-linked congenital stationary night blindness is caused by mutations in a gene encoding a leucine-rich repeat protein. *Nat Genet.* 2000;26(3):324–327.

Dominant Drusen

1. Edwards AO, Klein ML, Berselli CB, Hejtmancik JF, Rust K, Wirtz MK, et al. Malattia leventinese: refinement of the genetic locus and phenotypic variability in autosomal dominant macular drusen. *Am J Ophthalmol.* 1998;126(3):417–424.

2. Gass JDM. Heredodystrophic disorders affecting the pigment epithelium and retina. In: Gass JDM, ed. *Stereoscopic Atlas of Macular Diseases: Diagnosis and Treatment.* St. Louis: Mosby-Year Book, Inc; 1997:110.

3. Gregory CY, Evans K, Wijesuriya SD, Kermani S, Jay MR, Plant C, et al. The gene responsible for autosomal dominant Doyne's honeycomb retinal dystrophy (DHRD) maps to chromosome 2p16. *Hum Mol Genet.* 1996;5(7):1055–1059.

4. Heon E, Piguet B, Munier F, Sneed SR, Morgan CM, Forni S, et al. Linkage of autosomal dominant radial drusen (malattia leventinese) to chromosome 2p16-21. *Arch Ophthalmol.* 1996;114(2):193–198.

5. Matsumoto M, Traboulsi EL. Dominant radial drusen and Arg345Trp EFEMP1 mutation. *Am J Ophthalmol.* 2001;131(6):810–812.

6. Pager CK, Sarin LK, Federman JL, Eagle R, Hageman G, Rosenow J, et al. Malattia leventinese presenting with subretinal neovascular membrane and hemorrhage. *Am J Ophthalmol.* 2001;131(4):517–518.

7. Song M, Small KW. Macular dystrophies. In: Regillo CD, Brown GC, Flynn HW, eds. *Vitreoretinal Disease: The Essentials.* New York: Thieme Medical Publishers, Inc; 1999:295–297.

8. Stone EM, Lotery AJ, Munier FL, Heon E, Piguet B, Guymer RH, et al. A single EFEMP1 mutation associated with both malattia leventinese and Doyne honeycomb retinal dystrophy. *Nat Genet.* 1999;22(2):199–202.

For more information refer to www.sph.uth.tmc.edu/RetNet/disease.htm.

Gyrate Atrophy

1. Gass JDM. Heredodystrophic disorders affecting the pigment epithelium and retina. In: Gass JDM, ed. *Stereoscopic Atlas of Macular Diseases: Diagnosis and Treatment.* St. Louis: Mosby-Year Book, Inc; 1997:382–384.

2. Kaiser-Kupfer MI, Caruso RC, Valle D. Gyrate atrophy of the choroid and retina: long-term reduction of ornithine slows retinal degeneration. *Arch Ophthalmol.* 1991;109(11):1539–1548.

3. Noble KG. Choroidal dystrophies. In: Guyer DR, Yannuzzi LA, Chang S, Shields JA, Green WR, eds. *Retina-Vitreous-Macula.* Philadelphia: WB Saunders Co; 1999:960–974.

4. Peltola KE, Nanto-Salonen K, Heinonen OJ, Jaaskelainen S, Heinanen K, Simell O. Ophthalmologic heterogeneity in subjects with gyrate atrophy of choroid and retina harboring the L402P mutation of ornithine aminotransferase. *Ophthalmology.* 2001;108(4):721–729.

5. Ramesh V, Gusella JF, Shih VE. Molecular pathology of gyrate atrophy of the choroid and retina due to ornithine aminotransferase deficiency. *Mol Biol Med.* 1991;8(1):81–93.

6. Weleber RG, Kennaway NG, Buist NR. Gyrate atrophy of the choroid and retina: approaches to therapy. *Int Ophthalmol.* 1981;4:23–32.

7. Wilson DJ, Weleber RG, Green WR. Ocular clinicopathologic study of gyrate atrophy. *Am J Ophthalmol.* 1991;111(1):24–33.

8. Zhang K, Garabaldi DC, Carr RE, Sunness JS. Hereditary choroidal disease. In: Ogden TE, Hinton DR, eds. *Basic Sciences and Inherited Retinal Diseases/Tumors.* Ryan SJ, ed. *Retina.* Vol 1. 3rd ed. St. Louis: Mosby Inc; 2001:468.

For more information refer to www.sph.uth.tmc.edu/RetNet/disease.htm.

Leber's Congenital Amaurosis

1. Carr RE, Noble KG. Retinitis pigmentosa and allied diseases. In: Guyer DR, Yannuzzi LA, Chang S, Shields JA, Green WR, eds. *Retina-Vitreous-Macula.* Philadelphia: WB Saunders Co; 1999:901.

2. Dharmaraj S, Li Y, Robitaille JM, Silva E, Zhu D, Mitchell TN, et al. A novel locus for Leber congenital amaurosis maps to chromosome 6q. *Am J Hum Genet.* 2000;66(1):319–326.

3. Gass JDM. Heredodystrophic disorders affecting the pigment epithelium and retina. In: Gass JDM, ed. *Stereoscopic Atlas of Macular Diseases: Diagnosis and Treatment.* St. Louis: Mosby-Year Book, Inc; 1997:362–364.

4. Hameed A, Khaliq S, Ismail M, Anwar K, Ebenezer ND, Jordan T, et al. A novel locus for Leber congenital amaurosis (LCA4) with anterior keratoconus mapping to chromosome 17p13. *Invest Ophthalmol Vis Sci.* 2000;41(3):629–633.

5. Hamel CP, Griffoin JM, Lasquellec L, Bazalgette C, Arnaud B. Retinal dystrophies caused by mutations in RPE65: assessment of visual functions. *Br J Ophthalmol.* 2001;85(4):424–427.

6. Lorenz B, Gyurus P, Preising M, Bremser D, Gu S, Andrassi M, et al. Early-onset severe rod-cone dystrophy in young children with RPE65 mutations. *Invest Ophthalmol Vis Sci.* 2000;41(9):2735–2742.

7. Lotery AJ, Namperumalsamy P, Jacobson SG, Weleber RG, Fishman GA, Murasella MA, et al. Mutation analysis of 3 genes in patients with Leber congenital amaurosis. *Arch Ophthalmol.* 2000;118 (4):538–543.

8. Perrault I, Rozet JM, Gerber S, Ghazi I, Ducroq D, Souied E, et al. Spectrum of retGC1 mutations in Leber's congenital amaurosis. *Eur J Hum Genet.* 2000;8(8):578–582.

9. Perrault I, Rozet JM, Gerber S, Ghazi I, Leowski C, Ducroq D, et al. Leber congenital amaurosis. *Mol Genet Metab.* 1999;68(2):200–208.

10. Stockton DW, Lewis RA, Abboud EB, Al-Rajhi A, Jabak M, Anderson KL, et al. A novel locus for Leber congenital amaurosis on chromosome 14q24. *Hum Genet.* 1998;103(3):328–333.

For more information refer to www.sph.uth.tmc.edu/RetNet/disease.htm.

North Carolina Macular Dystrophy

1. Gass JDM. Heredodystrophic disorders affecting the pigment epithelium and retina. In: Gass JDM, ed. *Stereoscopic Atlas of Macular Diseases: Diagnosis and Treatment.* St. Louis: Mosby-Year Book, Inc; 1997:112–114.

2. Small KW, Udar N, Yelchits S, Klein R, Garcia C, Gallardo G, et al. North Carolina macular dystrophy (MCDR1) locus: a fine resolution genetic map and haplotype analysis. *Mol Vis.* 1999;29(5):38.

3. Small KW, Weber J, Roses A, Pericak-Vance P. North Carolina macular dystrophy (MCDR1): a review and refined mapping to 6q14–q16. 2. *Ophthalmic Paediatr Genet.* 1993;14(4):143–150.

4. Song M, Small KW. Macular dystrophies. In: Regillo CD, Brown GC, Flynn HW, eds. *Vitreoretinal Disease: The Essentials.* New York: Thieme Medical Publishers, Inc; 1999:299–300.

5. Voo I, Glasgow BJ, Flannery J, Udar N, Small KW. North Carolina macular dystrophy: clinicopathologic correlation. *Am J Ophthalmol.* 2001;132(6):933–935.

For more information refer to www.sph.uth.tmc.edu/RetNet/disease.htm.

Retinitis Pigmentosa (Rod-Cone Dystrophies)

1. Berson EL. Retinitis pigmentosa: the Friedenwald lecture. *Invest Ophthalmol Vis Sci.* 1993;34:1659–1676.

2. Berson EL, Rosner B, Sandberg MA, Hayes KC, Nicholson BW, Weigel-DiFranco C, Willet W. A randomized trial of vitamin A and vitamin E supplementation for retinitis pigmentosa. *Arch Ophthalmol.* 1993;111(6):761–772.

3. Carr RE, Noble KG. Retinitis pigmentosa and allied diseases. In: Guyer DR, Yannuzzi LA, Chang S, Shields JA, Green WR, eds. *Retina-Vitreous-Macula.* Philadelphia: WB Saunders Co; 1999:891–923.

4. Gass JDM. Heredodystrophic disorders affecting the pigment epithelium and retina. In: Gass JDM, ed. *Stereoscopic Atlas of Macular Diseases: Diagnosis and Treatment.* St. Louis: Mosby-Year Book, Inc; 1997:352–360.

5. Wang Q, Chen Q, Zhao K, Wang L, Wang L, Traboulsi EI. Update on the molecular genetics of retinitis pigmentosa. *Ophthalmic Genet.* 2001;22(3):133–154.

6. Weleber RG, Gregory-Evans K. Retinitis pigmentosa and allied disorders. In: Ogden TE, Hinton DR, senior eds. *Basic Sciences and Inherited Retinal Diseases/Tumors.* Ryan SJ, ed. *Retina.* Vol 1. 3rd ed. St. Louis: Mosby Inc; 2001:362–460.

For more information refer to www.sph.uth.tmc.edu/RetNet/disease.htm.

Sorsby's Fundus Dystrophy

1. Clarke M, Mitchell KW, Goodship J, McDonnell S, Barker MD, Griffiths ID, et al. Clinical features of a novel TIMP-3 mutation causing Sorsby's fundus dystrophy: implications for disease mechanism. *Br J Ophthalmol.* 2001;85(12):1429–1431.

2. Jacobson SG, Cideciyan AV, Regunath G, Rodriguez FJ, Vandenburgh K, Sheffield VC, et al. Night blindness in Sorsby's fundus dystrophy reversed by vitamin A. *Nat Genet.* 1995;11(1):27–32.

3. Langton KP, McKie N, Curtis A, Goodship JA, Bond PM, Barker MD, et al. A novel tissue inhibitor of metalloproteinases-3 mutation reveals a common molecular phenotype in Sorsby's fundus dystrophy. *J Biol Chem.* 2000;275(35):27027–27031.

4. Noble KG. Sorsby's fundus dystrophy. In: Guyer DR, Yannuzzi LA, Chang S, Shields JA, Green WR, eds. *Retina-Vitreous-Macula.* Philadelphia: WB Saunders Co; 1999:1018–1024.

5. Song M, Small KW. Macular dystrophies. In: Regillo CD, Brown GC, Flynn HW, eds. *Vitreoretinal Disease: The Essentials.* New York: Thieme Medical Publishers, Inc; 1999:302–303.

6. Weber BH, Vogt G, Wolz W, Ives EJ, Ewing CC. Sorsby's fundus dystrophy is genetically linked to chromosome 22q13-qter. *Nat Genet.* 1994;7(2):158–161.

For more information refer to www.sph.uth.tmc.edu/RetNet/disease.htm.

Stargardt Disease

1. Armstrong JD, Meyer D, Xu S, Elfervig JL. Long-term follow-up of Stargardt's disease and fundus flavimaculatus. *Ophthalmology.* 1998;105:448–457.

2. Allikmets R, Singh N, Sun H, Shroyer NF, Hutchinson A, Chidambaram A, et al. A photoreceptor cell-specific ATP-binding transporter gene (ABCR) is mutated in recessive Stargardt macular dystrophy. *Nat Genet.* 1997;15(3):236–246.

For more information refer to www.sph.uth.tmc.edu/RetNet/disease.htm.

X-Linked Juvenile Retinoschisis

1. Deutman AF, Hoyng CB. Macular dystrophies. In: Schachat AP, senior ed. *Medical Retina.* Ryan SJ, ed. *Retina.* Vol 2. 3rd ed. St. Louis: Mosby Inc; 2001:1210–1216.

2. Edwards AO, Robertson JE. Hereditary vitreoretinal degeneration. In: Ogden TE, Hinton DR, eds. Ryan SJ, ed. *Retina,* 3rd ed. *Basic Sciences and Inherited Retinal Diseases/Tumors.* Ryan SJ, ed. *Retina.* Vol 1. 3rd ed. St. Louis: Mosby Inc; 2001:487–490.

3. Gass JDM. Heredodystrophic disorders affecting the pigment epithelium and retina. In: Gass JDM. *Stereoscopic Atlas of Macular Diseases: Diagnosis and Treatment.* St Louis: Mosby-Year Book, Inc; 1997:374–376.

4. Grayson C, Reid SN, Ellis JA, Rutherford A, Sowden JC, Yates JR, et al. Retinoschisin, the X-linked retinoschisis protein, is a secreted photoreceptor protein, and is expressed and released by Weri-Rb1 cells. *Hum Mol Genet.* 2000;9(12):1873–1879.

5. Regillo CD, Custis PH. Surgical management of retinoschisis. *Curr Opin Ophthalmol.* 1997;8(3):80–86.

6. Shinoda K, Ishida S, Oguchi Y, Mashima Y. Clinical characteristics of 14 Japanese patients with X-linked juvenile retinoschisis associated with XLRS1 mutation. *Ophthalmic Genet.* 2000;21(3):171–180.

7. Shinoda K, Ohde H, Mashima Y, Inoue R, Ishida S, Inoue M, et al. On- and off-responses of the photopic electroretinograms in X-linked juvenile retinoschisis. *Am J Ophthalmol.* 2001;131(4):489–494.

8. Tasman W. X-linked retinoschisis. In: Guyer DR, Yannuzzi LA, Chang S, Shields JA, Green WR, eds. *Retina-Vitreous-Macula.* Philadelphia: WB Saunders Co; 1999:1013–1017.

For more information refer to www.sph.uth.tmc.edu/RetNet/disease.htm.

chapter 7

Drug Toxicities

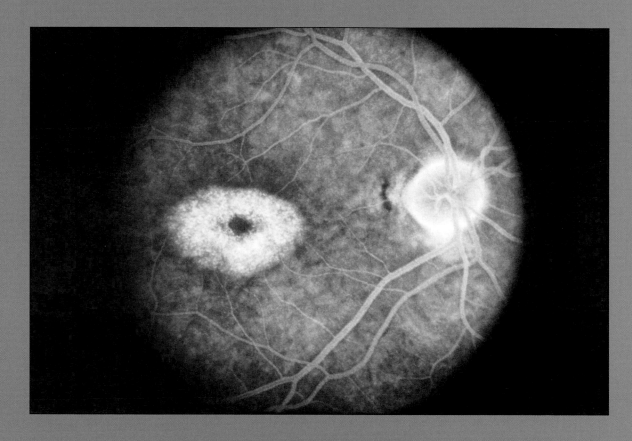

David G. Callanan, MD

AMINOGLYCOSIDE TOXICITY

The aminoglycoside antibiotics include gentamicin, amikacin, and tobramycin. These drugs are used for the treatment and prophylaxis of endophthalmitis. They are toxic to the retina when they enter the vitreous or posterior chamber in high enough concentrations. Toxicity occurs most commonly through inadvertent leakage into the eye from subconjunctival injections or direct injection into the vitreous of inappropriately diluted mixtures.

Symptoms

Aminoglycoside toxicity causes an acute and severe loss of vision.

Clinical Features

Following exposure to a toxic level of these agents, the retina exhibits significant whitening. The area of ischemic retinal whitening can have distinct borders that are irregular in contour. The involved area is typically centered near the macula. Frequently, small retinal hemorrhages are present. Findings that occur weeks to months later include optic atrophy, pigmentary irregularity, and neovascular glaucoma secondary to severe retinal ischemia.

Ancillary Testing

The fluorescein angiogram shows hypofluorescence as a result of nonperfusion of the retinal arterioles. The hypofluorescence tends to be localized to the area of retinal whitening, but can be widespread. The early- and middle-phase angiograms show hypofluorescence of the affected area. The late phases of the angiogram can demonstrate staining of the edges of the area. The electroretinogram shows a marked reduction and can become extinguished in severe cases.

Pathology/Pathogenesis

In high concentrations, the aminoglycoside drugs appear to cause a direct chemical injury to the retina and nerve fiber layer. Each of the drugs has a different dose that is toxic.

Treatment/Prognosis

Immediate pars plana vitrectomy with a washout of the posterior chamber has been suggested as treatment, if the unintended administration of the drug is recognized quickly. This may reduce the extent and severity of retinal toxicity. Other than this, there is no known treatment. The prognosis is generally poor, with loss of central visual acuity.

Systemic Evaluation

There is no systemic evaluation indicated in aminoglycoside toxicity.

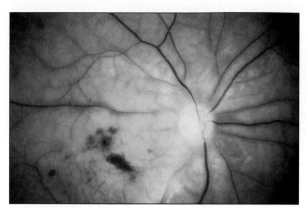

Acute gentamicin toxicity has occurred after subconjunctival injection following cataract surgery. Note the ischemic retinal whitening and intraretinal hemorrhages.

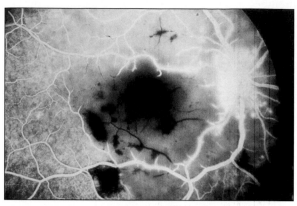

The fluorescein angiogram of the same patient reveals widespread closure of the retinal arterioles and loss of capillary perfusion.

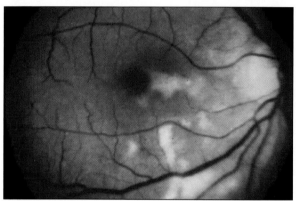

This patient developed retinal toxicity following intravitreal injection of amikacin for infectious endophthalmitis. The fundus examination revealed ischemic retinal whitening.

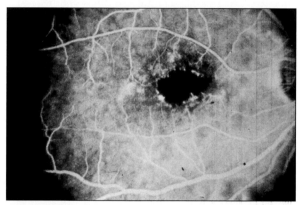

The fluorescein angiogram of the same patient revealed enlargement of the foveal avascular zone with capillary nonperfusion.

CHLOROQUINE/HYDROXYCHLOROQUINE TOXICITY

Chloroquine and hydroxychloroquine are used for the treatment of malaria and a variety of collagen vascular diseases including systemic lupus erythematosus. Irreversible retinal damage has been observed in some patients who have received long-term or high-dose therapy. Patients with collagen vascular diseases taking chloroquine or hydroxychloroquine must be monitored regularly to facilitate early detection of retinal toxicity and discontinuation of treatment.

Symptoms

Early symptoms of toxicity are paracentral scotomas. As toxicity progresses, patients report loss of acuity and nyctalopia. Dyschromatopsia can occur as well.

Clinical Features

Patients may describe paracentral scotomas and distortion on Amsler grid testing. Early in the course of retinal toxicity, no funduscopic abnormalities or mild stippling of the retinal pigment epithelium (RPE) may be visible. In the later stages, granularity of the RPE is observed in a bull's eye pattern of retinal pigment epithelial atrophy. Arteriolar narrowing, optic disc pallor, and peripheral RPE degeneration may develop as well. Poliosis, sub-epithelial corneal deposits, decreased corneal sensitivity, and even sixth cranial nerve palsies may be observed.

Ancillary Testing

How to monitor patients for the early signs of toxicity is still controversial. Central visual field testing with a red test object, Amsler grid monitoring, color vision testing, and electroretinographic studies have all been proposed. Fundus photographs may be obtained for future comparison.

Fluorescein angiography may demonstrate more prominent retinal pigment epithelial alterations than suspected by clinical examination. The classic finding is a bull's eye pattern of hypo- and hyperfluorescence related to the pigmentary alterations. The hyperfluorescence is an example of a transmission or "window" defect. The electroretinogram may be reduced or extinguished in advanced cases.

Pathology/Pathogenesis

Toxicity with chloroquine is more likely with daily doses greater than 250 mg. The drug can be found in both blood and urine up to 5 years after discontinuation of the drug, hence the reports of progressive toxicity even after the drug is stopped. Toxicity with hydroxychloroquine is unusual if the daily dose is kept below 6.5 mg/kg per day. Both of these chemicals have an affinity for melanin and cause lysosomal damage in the ganglion cell layer and degeneration of the photoreceptor outer segments.

Treatment/Prognosis

Chloroquine appears to be more toxic than hydroxy-chloroquine. Nevertheless, patients taking either medication should be monitored regularly for toxicity. The drug should be discontinued immediately if any signs or symptoms of retinal disease occur. Unfortunately, retinal toxicity may progress despite discontinuation of the medication.

Systemic Evaluation

Systemic toxicity related to chloroquine and hydroxy-chloroquine is uncommon. Systemic side effects include central nervous system reactions such as tinnitus, gastro-intestinal disturbances, blood dyscrasias, dermatologic reactions, and rare reports of neuromyotoxicity. It is important to establish and maintain good communication with the treating rheumatologist or primary physician regarding the patient's ocular status.

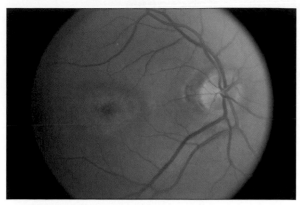

The characteristic retinal finding in chloroquine toxicity is a bull's eye maculopathy. A central region of hyperpigmentation is surrounded by a zone of hypopigmentation.

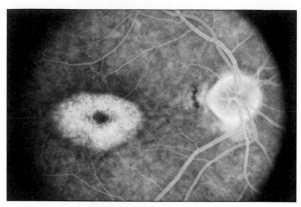

Fluorescein angiography demonstrates a transmission or "window" defect corresponding to the zone of retinal pigment epithelial atrophy.

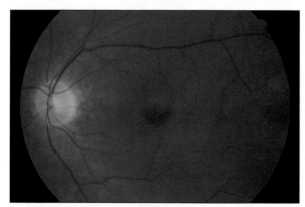

Advanced cases of chloroquine toxicity may reveal optic disc pallor, retinal vascular narrowing, and peripheral retinal pigmentary alterations in addition to the bull's eye maculopathy.

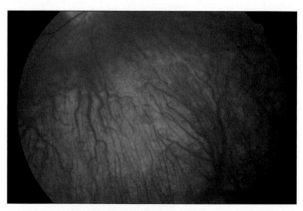

Peripheral retinal pigmentary alterations range from mild stippling of the retinal pigment epithelium to widespread retinal pigment epithelial derangement.

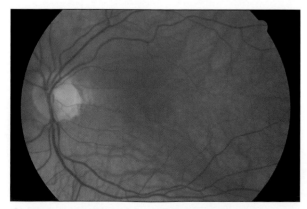

Chloroquine toxicity may progress even after cessation of the medication. This is related to the slow excretion of chloroquine from the body. This patient was found to have a bull's eye maculopathy after years of chloroquine therapy.

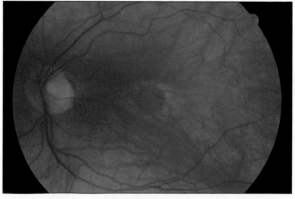

Note the progression of the bull's eye maculopathy in the same patient 1 year following discontinuation of chloroquine. The patient reported reduced vision with paracentral scotomas.

CRYSTALLINE RETINOPATHIES

Several chemicals can cause deposition of crystals in the retina. They include canthaxanthin, talc, and tamoxifen. In the majority of the cases, the patient is unaware of the presence of these crystals; they are found on a routine dilated retinal examination. Canthaxanthin has been used as an oral tanning agent, but its use seems to have diminished since the reports of deposits in the retina. Talc is typically seen in intravenous drug use, for which talc has been used as a filler in compounding the illegal drug. Tamoxifen is typically used in treating breast cancer. The number of cases with tamoxifen retinopathy has greatly declined since the daily dose was lowered to 10 to 20 mg per day.

Symptoms

Patients with either talc or canthaxanthin retinopathy are usually asymptomatic. However, talc retinopathy can be associated with arteriolar occlusions and retinal nonperfusion leading to neovascularization and even glaucoma. The original published reports of patients with tamoxifen retinopathy described mild decreases in central visual acuity.

Clinical Features

The crystals can be subtle or quite striking. Canthaxanthin can be overwhelming in the number of highly reflective crystals. Talc and tamoxifen crystals tend to be fewer and they are also less reflective. The talc crystals can be more concentrated along the major retinal vessels. The crystals tend to be located in the inner, superficial layers of the retina. Tamoxifen retinopathy may be associated with lesions at the level of the retinal pigment epithelium as well.

Ancillary Testing

It is generally not necessary to perform additional testing in these patients. A thorough history will usually guide the clinician to the diagnosis. No pathognomonic findings are found on angiographic or electrophysiologic testing.

Pathology/Pathogenesis

Canthaxanthin retinopathy is usually associated with prolonged use. The crystals do decrease slightly after cessation of its use. Talc retinopathy is commonly associated with some cardiopulmonary shunt that allows the compound to enter the arterial circulation. Tamoxifen is a cationic amphophilic drug, and the deposits have been found in the nerve fiber and inner plexiform layers. The crystals are both intra- and extracellular. Limited change is seen following discontinuation of the drug. Tamoxifen retinopathy is more likely to occur once the lifetime dose exceeds 90 g.

Treatment/Prognosis

The treatment of all the crystalline retinopathies is to stop the drug. In the case of tamoxifen, the dose could be lowered. The majority of affected patients maintain good vision in spite of the presence of the crystals. Patients with talc retinopathy can develop further problems and therefore should be followed up and strongly encouraged to discontinue the use of illicit intravenous drugs.

Systemic Evaluation

No additional systemic evaluation is necessary if a history of medication or drug use is clear. Rare metabolic disorders such as primary hyperoxaluria may be associated with a crystalline retinopathy. Bietti's crystalline retinopathy is a rare, inherited retinal disorder characterized by the presence of retinal crystals.

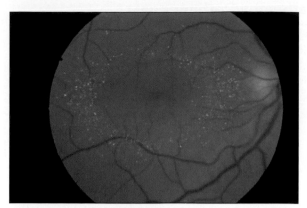

Canthaxanthin toxicity in a woman who used the drug for several months. Note the highly refractile yellowish crystals in the perifoveal region.

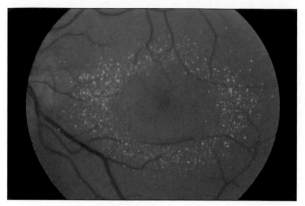

The fellow eye of the same patient reveals similar findings. The retinal crystals are located in the superficial layers of the retina.

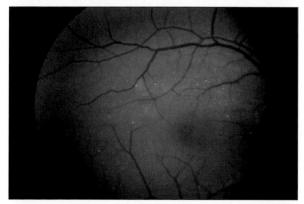

This fundus photograph reveals talc or magnesium silicate crystals in the right eye of a patient with a history of chronic intravenous drug abuse.

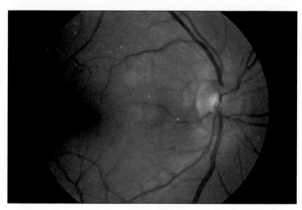

Higher-magnification photograph of talc retinopathy. Note the perivascular location of the retinal crystals.

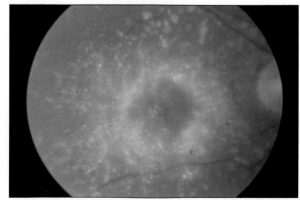

Large crystals in the right eye of a woman treated with unusually high doses of tamoxifen for several years. (Photograph reprinted with permission from Elsevier Science. [Gass JDM. Stereoscopic Atlas of Macular Diseases: Diagnosis and Treatment, 4th ed; 1997].)

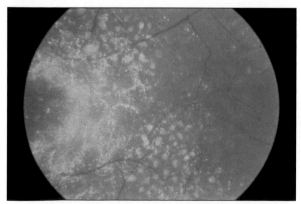

The fellow eye of the same patient had similar findings. The crystals are larger than in the other crystalline retinopathies, and retinal pigment epithelial changes are also seen. (Photograph reprinted with permission from Elsevier Science. [Gass JDM. Stereoscopic Atlas of Macular Diseases: Diagnosis and Treatment, 4th ed; 1997].)

CYSTOID MACULAR EDEMA-ASSOCIATED TOXICITIES

Several drugs may be associated with the development of cystoid macular edema (CME), including nicotinic acid (niacin), epinephrine, and latanoprost. The occurrence of CME with any of these agents is uncommon, and the causal relationship of latanoprost and CME has been questioned. Certain ocular factors may be associated with an increased risk of CME. In particular, epinephrine and latanoprost are more likely to be associated with CME in aphakic and pseudophakic eyes.

Symptoms

The usual symptoms associated with CME occur in patients with aphakia and pseudophakia. Metamorphopsia and reduced visual acuity may be found in the affected eye. These symptoms generally develop slowly over a period of weeks to months.

Clinical Features

Fundus examination reveals a cystic appearance of the fovea that is characteristic of CME. A yellowish or orange discoloration of the fovea may occur as well. In general, no evidence of ocular inflammation is noted.

Ancillary Testing

Fluorescein angiography helps confirm the diagnosis of CME except in the case of nicotinic acid. With both epinephrine and latanoprost, the typical petaloid appearance of hyperfluorescence is seen in the late phase of the angiogram. Although nicotinic acid produces a classic cystic appearance of the fovea on funduscopic examination, no evidence of hyperfluorescence is observed with fluorescein angiography.

Pathology/Pathogenesis

Each of these agents may cause CME through a different mechanism. It is unknown how nicotinic acid produces CME. It appears to be related to the dose of nicotinic acid and typically occurs when the patient is taking more than 2 g of nicotinic acid per day. Latanoprost may have a prostaglandin-like effect on the retina that contributes to the development of CME.

Treatment/Prognosis

In each case, stopping or lowering the drug dosage is the proper treatment. Epinephrine-induced CME usually resolves after discontinuing the drug. Stopping nicotinic acid or lowering the dosage will clear the CME. The CME produced by latanoprost can be quite severe, and topical steroids or nonsteroidal agents may be necessary to help alleviate the CME. An alternative pressure-lowering agent should be considered in patients with CME associated with latanoprost.

Systemic Evaluation

No systemic evaluation is necessary in patients with a history of exposure to nicotinic acid, epinephrine, or latanoprost. Other causes of CME should be excluded before CME is attributed to any of these medications.

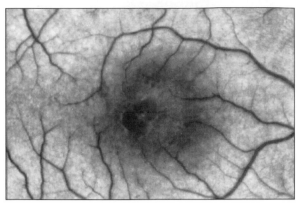

Niacin toxicity demonstrates a marked cystic appearance of the macula in this patient who took 4 g of niacin per day for 18 months.

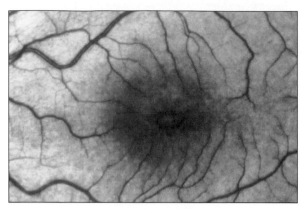

The fundus photograph of the left eye of the same patient reveals a similar cystic pattern in the fovea.

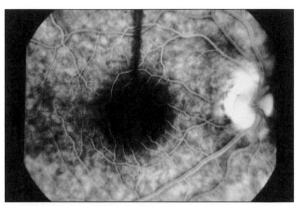

A distinguishing feature of nicotinic acid-related cystoid macular edema is the lack of hyperfluorescence on fluorescein angiography. This late-phase angiogram demonstrates normal macular hypofluorescence.

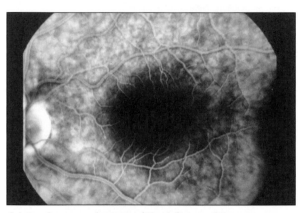

A late-phase angiogram of the left eye of the same patient is similar: the petaloid pattern of hyperfluorescence is absent.

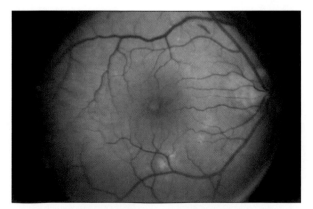

This pseudophakic patient developed cystoid macular edema while taking latanoprost for ocular hypertension. Note the yellow foveal reflex.

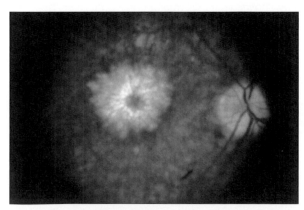

Fluorescein angiogram of the same eye of the same patient demonstrates the classic petaloid pattern of hyperfluorescence observed in patients with cystoid macular edema.

IRON TOXICITY

Iron toxicity or siderosis typically occurs following penetrating injury with a metallic foreign body. The retinal toxicity occurs gradually over time and can be completely prevented by early removal of the foreign body. It is incumbent on the physician to rule out the presence of a metallic foreign body when traumatic injury to the eye is even slightly suspected.

Symptoms

The symptoms of siderosis are insidious, and the underlying cause will not be discovered unless there is a high index of suspicion for the possibility. Loss of the peripheral visual field is gradual. Central visual acuity is affected late in the disease process.

Clinical Features

Gradual loss of the pigmentation of the retinal pigment epithelium (RPE) is the most striking finding. The optic disc may become pale and the retinal vessels attenuated (siderosis should be considered in the differential diagnosis of "unilateral retinitis pigmentosa"). The vitreous can be hazy as well. Small orange deposits in the anterior subcapsular area of the lens and darkening of the iris (iris heterochromia) may also develop in the later stages of ocular siderosis.

Ancillary Testing

The most useful test for the suspicion of iron toxicity is radiologic examination of the globe. A plain facial x-ray can most often find the foreign object. Computed tomography (CT) scan can help localize the object. The electroretinographic findings of the suspected eye can be compared to those of the other eye. The affected eye initially shows a supernormal a-wave pattern early in the disease process. As time passes a progressive decrease in the b-wave is noted, with eventual extinction of the entire electroretinographic response.

Pathology/Pathogenesis

The iron from the metallic foreign body slowly oxidizes within the eye. The iron oxide is deposited in the inner retina and RPE, which leads to atrophy of the RPE and the photoreceptors. The damage is more severe with ferrous compounds than with ferric ones.

Treatment/Prognosis

The proper treatment of siderosis is to find the foreign body and remove it from the eye. This action will halt further progression of the toxicity. The damage, however, is permanent.

Systemic Evaluation

Once a metallic foreign body is found in the eye, a complete radiologic examination of the orbit should be performed to rule out any other pathology or additional foreign objects.

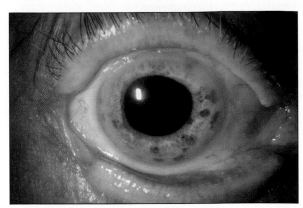

Anterior segment findings of siderosis include anterior subcapsular cataracts and iris heterochromia. The right eye has a normal blue iris.

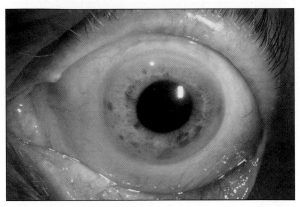

The left eye of the same patient with iron toxicity has iris heterochromia, with a greenish discoloration of the iris.

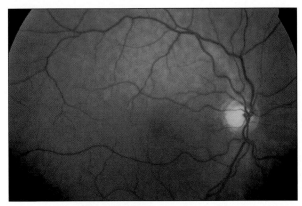

This fundus photograph shows a normal right eye in a patient with siderosis.

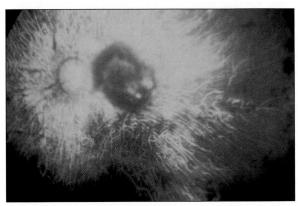

The left eye of the same patient had a metallic foreign body in the macula that was undiagnosed for 11 years. Note the optic disc pallor, retinal vascular attenuation, and extensive loss of pigmentation.

PHENOTHIAZINE TOXICITY

The phenothiazine class of compounds includes chlor-promazine and thioridazine. Both compounds are used to treat psychiatric conditions and chlorpromazine has been used to treat intractable hiccups.

Symptoms

The symptoms of toxicity include blurred vision, dyschromatopsia, and nyctalopia.

Clinical Features

Initially, the eye examination may be normal. Patients may develop brownish pigmentation of the cornea and lens. A characteristic anterior, star-shaped cataract may be observed in patients with chlorpromazine toxicity. Early in the course of the retinal toxicity, retinal pigment epithelial alterations, including retinal pigment epithelial stippling and scattered pigment clumps, are observed. Eventually, the affected patients develop geographic areas of atrophy of the retinal pigment epithelium (RPE) and retina. The optic disc and retinal vessels usually remain normal.

Ancillary Testing

The fluorescein angiogram shows irregularity of the RPE initially, with severe atrophy of the RPE and choriocapillaris in the late stages of toxicity. The electroretinogram is normal early but may be reduced or extinguished in advanced cases.

Pathology/Pathogenesis

The phenothiazines are cationic amphophilic substances that form tight bonds with the polar lipids present in lysosomes. Chlorpromazine may be less toxic, as it lacks a piperidyl side chain. The concentration in melanin granules is increased, and toxicity can progress even after the drug has been stopped. Pathology specimens show initial atrophy and disorganization of the photoreceptors followed by loss of the choriocapillaris and RPE later. A dose of greater than 800 mg/day of thioridazine is more likely to produce retinal toxicity, and the dose of chlorpromazine may be even higher (around 1 to 2 g/day).

Treatment/Prognosis

As with all toxic drugs, it is recommended that these agents be stopped immediately when signs or symptoms of toxicity appear. Discontinuation of the medication in the early stages may result in the resolution of the symptoms and retinal findings. However, because of the slow elimination of these agents, the toxicity can progress for some time after the drug is stopped.

Systemic Evaluation

No systemic evaluation is necessary. The ophthalmologist should notify the treating physician immediately when retinal toxicity is suspected.

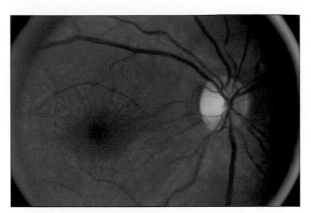

Fundus photograph of a patient with a long-standing history of thioridazine use. He had mottling of the retinal pigment epithelium that was most notable temporal to the fovea.

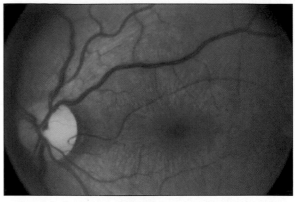

The fellow eye of the same patient had similar changes.

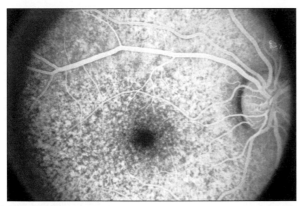

Fluorescein angiogram of the right eye of the same patient demonstrates more widespread retinal pigment epithelial alterations with a salt and pepper pattern of hyper- and hypofluorescence.

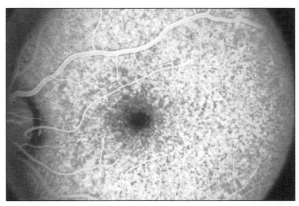

The fluorescein angiogram of the left eye of the same patient is similar to that of the right eye. Note that the retinal pigment epithelial changes are more prominent with fluorescein angiography.

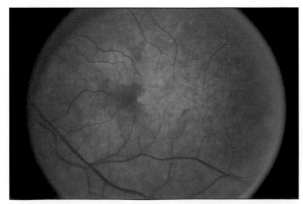

This fundus photograph shows the left eye of a patient who used thioridazine for 14 years. Large patches of geographic atrophy are present.

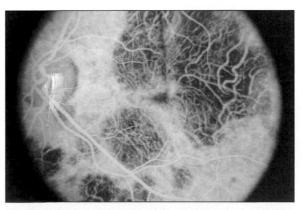

The fluorescein angiogram of the same patient reveals prominent patches of hypofluorescence corresponding to the atrophy of the retinal pigment epithelium and choriocapillaris.

SELECTED REFERENCES

Aminoglycoside Toxicity

1. Conway BP, Campochiaro PA. Macular infarction after endophthalmitis treated with vitrectomy and intravitreal gentamicin. *Arch Ophthalmol.* 1986;104:367–371.

2. Campochiaro PA, Lim JI. Aminoglycoside toxicity in the treatment of endophthalmitis: the Aminoglycoside Toxicity Study Group [see comments]. *Arch Ophthalmol.* 1994;112:48–53.

3. Chu TG, Ferreira M, Ober RR. Immediate pars plana vitrectomy in the management of inadvertent intracameral injection of gentamicin: a rabbit experimental model. *Retina.* 1994;14:59–64.

4. Talamo JH, D'Amico DJ, Hanninen LA, Kenyon KR, Shanks ET. The influence of aphakia and vitrectomy on experimental retinal toxicity of aminoglycoside antibiotics. *Am J Ophthalmol.* 1985;100:840–847.

Chloroquine/Hydroxychloroquine Toxicity

1. Easterbrook M. Chloroquine retinopathy. *Arch Ophthalmol.* 1991;109:1362.

2. Johnson MW, Vine AK. Hydroxychloroquine therapy in massive total doses without retinal toxicity. *Am J Ophthalmol.* 1987;104:139–144.

3. Levy GD, Munz SJ, Paschal J, Cohen HB, Pince KJ, Peterson T. Incidence of hydroxychloroquine retinopathy in 1,207 patients in a large multicenter outpatient practice. *Arthritis Rheum.* 1997;40:1482–1486.

4. Weiner A, Sandberg MA, Gaudio AR, Kini NM, Berson EL. Hydroxychloroquine retinopathy. *Am J Ophthalmol.* 1991;112:528–534.

5. Moorthy RS, Valluri S. Ocular toxicity associated with systemic drug therapy. *Curr Opin Ophthalmol.* 1999;10:438–446.

Crystalline Retinopathies

1. Cortin P, Corriveau LA, Rosseau AP, Tardif Y, Malenfant M, Boudreault G. Maculopathie en paillettes d'or. *Can J Ophthalmol.* 1982;17:103–106.

2. Gorin MB, Day R, Costantino JP, Fisher B, Redmond CK, Wickerham L, et al. Long-term tamoxifen citrate use and potential ocular toxicity [published erratum appears in *Am J Ophthalmol.* 1998;126:338]. *Am J Ophthalmol.* 1998;125:493–501.

3. Harnois C, Samson J, Malenfant M, Rousseau A. Canthaxanthin retinopathy: anatomic and functional reversibility. *Arch Ophthalmol.* 1989;107:538–540.

4. Heier JS, Dragoo RA, Enzenauer RW, Waterhouse WJ. Screening for ocular toxicity in asymptomatic patients treated with tamoxifen. *Am J Ophthalmol.* 1994;117:772–775.

5. Jampol LM, Setogawa T, Rednam KRV, Tso MOM. Talc retinopathy in primates: a model of ischemic retinopathy, I: clinical studies. *Arch Ophthalmol.* 1981;99:1273–1280.

6. McLane NJ, Carroll DM. Ocular manifestations of drug abuse. *Surv Ophthalmol.* 1986;30:298–313.

Cystoid Macular Edema-Associated Toxicities

1. Callanan D, Fellman RL, Savage JA. Latanoprost-associated cystoid macular edema. *Am J Ophthalmol.* 1998;126:134–135.

2. Schumer RA, Camras CB, Mandahl AK. Latanoprost and cystoid macular edema: is there a causal relation? *Curr Opin Ophthalmol.* 2000;11:94–100.

3. Callanan D, Blodi BA, Martin DF. Macular edema associated with nicotinic acid (niacin) [letter]. *JAMA.* 1998;279:1702.

4. Gass JDM. Nicotinic acid maculopathy. *Am J Ophthalmol.* 1973;76:500–510.

5. Kolker AE, Becker B. Epinephrine maculopathy. *Arch Ophthalmol.* 1968;79:552–562.

Iron Toxicity

1. Knave B. Electroretinography in eyes with retained intraocular metallic foreign bodies: a clinical study. *Acta Ophthalmol.* 1969;100:1–63.

2. Masciulli L, Anderson DR, Charles S. Experimental ocular siderosis in the squirrel monkey. *Am J Ophthalmol.* 1972;74:638–661.

3. Stokes WH. Retained intraocular foreign bodies: a clinical study with a review of 300 cases. *Arch Ophthalmol.* 1938;19:205–216.

Phenothiazine Toxicity

1. Connell MM, Poley BJ, McFarlane JR. Chorioretinopathy associated with thioridazine therapy. *Arch Ophthalmol.* 1964;71:816–821.

2. Meredith TA, Aaberg TM, Willerson WD. Progressive chorioretinopathy after receiving thioridazine. *Arch Ophthalmol.* 1978;96:1172–1176.

3. Miller FS III, Bunt-Millam AH, Kalina RE. Clinical-ultrastructural study of thioridazine retinopathy. *Ophthalmology.* 1982;89:1478–1488.

4. Siddall JR. The ocular toxic findings with prolonged and high dosage chlopromazine intake. *Arch Ophthalmol.* 1965;74:460–464.

chapter | 8

Intraocular Tumors

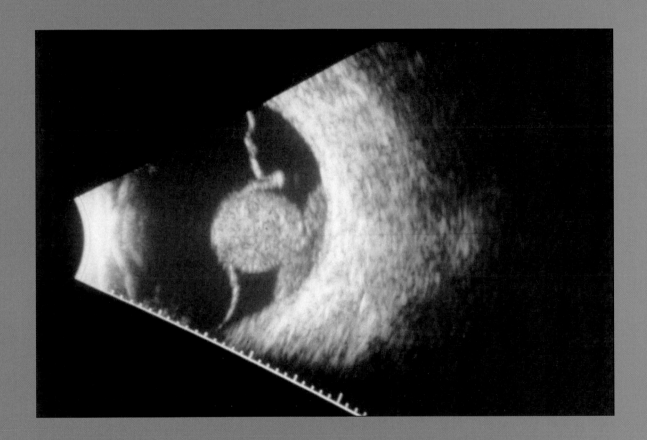

J. William Harbour, MD

Dean J. Bonsall, MD, FACS

CHOROIDAL HEMANGIOMA

Choroidal hemangiomas are benign vascular tumors with no malignant potential. Circumscribed choroidal hemangiomas are usually isolated lesions, whereas diffuse hemangiomas are most often found in patients with Sturge-Weber syndrome. (See "Phakomatoses: Sturge-Weber Syndrome" later in this chapter.) Circumscribed hemangiomas can usually be distinguished from melanomas and metastatic lesions on the basis of their clinical appearance, angiographic features, and ultrasonographic characteristics.

Symptoms

Patients with circumscribed choroidal hemangiomas may be asymptomatic or report reduced visual acuity, visual field defect, metamorphopsia, or photopsias due to leakage of subretinal fluid into the macula. Occasionally, a large exudative retinal detachment can cause profound loss of vision.

Clinical Features

Choroidal hemangiomas are usually moderately elevated, dome shaped, and orange (often difficult to distinguish from the surrounding choroid). They often have pigment clumping or fibrous retinal pigment epithelial metaplasia over the surface. Subretinal fluid is often found overlying the tumor, tracking into the macula, or, less commonly, producing a large exudative retinal detachment. Diffuse choroidal hemangiomas may be seen in patients with Sturge-Weber syndrome. The fundus is described as having a "tomato catsup" appearance. The lesions may be difficult to identify with ophthalmoscopy unless the choroidal color is compared to the other, uninvolved eye.

Ancillary Testing

Ultrasonography is extremely useful in distinguishing choroidal hemangiomas from melanomas and metastatic lesions. On A-scan ultrasonography, hemangiomas typically demonstrate high internal reflectivity with relatively regular spikes. Fluorescein angiography is helpful but not diagnostic, and classically shows lobular early filling with late diffuse staining. Indocyanine green angiography may reveal a distinctive pattern of late hypofluorescence with "washout" of the dye.

Pathology/Pathogenesis

These tumors appear histopathologically as cavernous hemangiomas that replace the normal choroid. Most circumscribed choroidal hemangiomas arise spontaneously with no hereditary pattern or other systemic associations. The pathogenesis is unknown.

Treatment/Prognosis

Since choroidal hemangiomas are benign, they are usually observed without treatment unless they are affecting vision. Depending on the degree of subretinal fluid, treatment can include laser photocoagulation, transpupillary thermotherapy, photodynamic therapy, plaque radiotherapy, or external beam radiation. Patients may suffer visual loss in spite of successful control of associated subretinal fluid.

Systemic Evaluation

Circumscribed choroidal hemangiomas are usually isolated lesions and do not require systemic evaluation. Diffuse choroidal hemangiomas may be associated with Sturge-Weber syndrome.

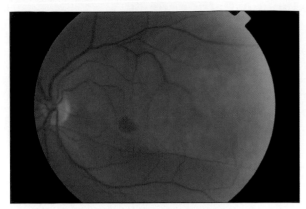

Fundus photograph of a choroidal hemangioma occupying most of the temporal macula. Note that the tumor color is virtually indistinguishable from the surrounding choroid.

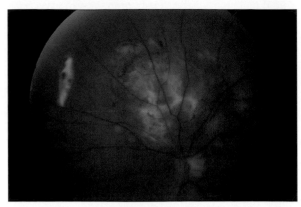

Choroidal hemangioma with extensive fibrous metaplasia over the surface and surrounding pigmentary alterations consistent with a long-standing choroidal hemangioma.

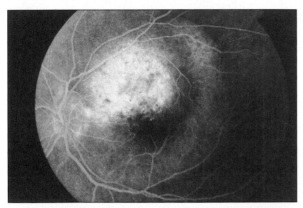

Late-phase fluorescein angiogram of a juxtapapillary choroidal hemangioma, demonstrating a diffuse, lobular pattern of hyperfluorescence.

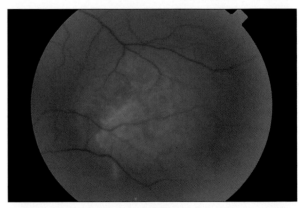

Subtle choroidal hemangioma is difficult to distinguish from the surrounding choroid except for an area of gray fibrous metaplasia in the lower left region of the tumor.

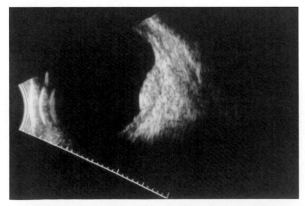

B-scan ultrasonography of a choroidal hemangioma demonstrates a bright dome-shaped lesion with no choroidal excavation.

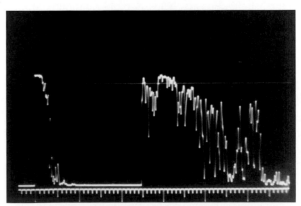

A-scan ultrasonography of a choroidal hemangioma demonstrates medium to high internal reflectivity and relatively uniform spikes.

CHOROIDAL MELANOMA

Choroidal melanoma is the most common primary intraocular cancer. The incidence in the United States is about five to eight cases per million per year. Risk factors include light skin pigmentation, blue irides, and increasing age. Although choroidal melanoma can be diagnosed at any age, most patients are in their sixth or seventh decade at diagnosis.

Symptoms

Patients may be asymptomatic or they may experience metamorphopsia, photopsia, peripheral field changes, floaters, or decreased visual acuity from direct obstruction of the visual axis, exudative retinal detachment, or vitreous hemorrhage. Pain is not a typical symptom except in neglected cases.

Clinical Features

Most melanomas are pigmented, although 20% to 30% are amelanotic. Most are dome shaped or mushroom shaped (indicating a rupture through Bruch's membrane). Melanomas are thicker than nevi, ranging from around 2 mm to more than 15 mm in thickness. Findings may include orange lipofuscin pigment over the tumor surface, exudative retinal detachment, and subretinal or vitreous hemorrhage in larger tumors. Ciliary body melanomas can be associated with sentinel episcleral vessels, extrascleral extension, and induced lenticular astigmatism.

Ancillary Testing

Ultrasonography is the most important ancillary test. Choroidal melanomas typically display low to medium internal reflectivity on A-scan, which distinguishes them from metastatic deposits, hemangiomas, and other simulating lesions. Fluorescein angiography classically demonstrates intrinsic tumor vessels or the "double circulation," and it can help to rule out a hemorrhagic process that would block fluorescence. Magnetic resonance imaging typically shows hyperintensity on T1 weighting.

Pathology/Pathogenesis

The modified Callander system is usually used to classify choroidal melanomas into spindle, mixed, and epithelioid cell types, in order of worsening prognosis. Unlike cutaneous melanoma, no strong link exists between choroidal melanoma and sunlight exposure, and the vast majority of these tumors are sporadic, with no familial pattern.

Treatment/Prognosis

Treatment options include observation, transpupillary thermotherapy, plaque radiotherapy, charged particle therapy, stereotactic radiotherapy, local resection, or enucleation, depending on the size and location of the tumor, the overall health of the patient, and other factors. The Collaborative Ocular Melanoma Study demonstrated that the mortality rates following iodine 125 brachytherapy did not differ from mortality rates following enucleation for up to 12 years after treatment. Clinical risk factors for metastasis include larger tumors, anterior location, and greater age.

Systemic Evaluation

A metastatic workup should be performed before treatment. Choroidal melanoma has a propensity to metastasize to the liver and less commonly to the lung and other sites. A metastatic evaluation should minimally include liver function studies, chest x-ray, and physical examination. Abnormalities should be followed up with further imaging studies.

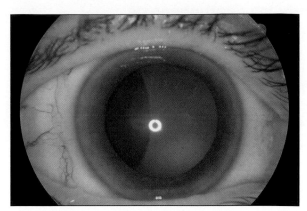

Slit lamp photograph demonstrates large temporal ciliochoroidal melanoma blocking the red reflex of the fundus.

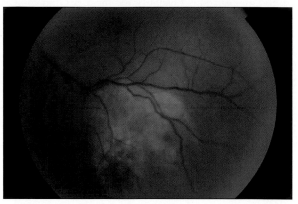

Fundus photograph of a choroidal melanoma. The elevated, pigmented tumor had orange lipofuscin pigment over the tumor surface and subretinal fluid consistent with a choroidal melanoma.

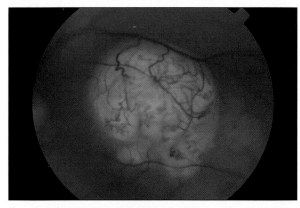

Amelanotic choroidal melanoma with prominent intrinsic vessels.

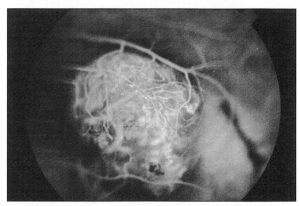

Fluorescein angiogram of the same lesion in the previous figure shows irregular, intrinsic tumor vessels, the so-called double circulation, which can be distinguished from the overlying retinal vessels.

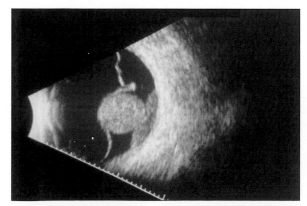

B-scan ultrasonography of a choroidal melanoma, demonstrating choroidal excavation and the classic mushroom shape that is seen in some tumors due to a break through Bruch's membrane.

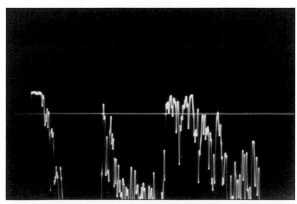

A-scan ultrasonography of a choroidal melanoma, demonstrating low to medium internal reflectivity and a tendency for spike height to decrease from left to right.

CHOROIDAL METASTASIS

Choroidal metastasis is probably the most common intraocular malignancy, but it often goes undiagnosed, depending on the overall condition of the patient. These tumors often have a characteristic clinical appearance, and can often be treated to optimize the visual function and quality of life of the cancer patient. Depending on the type of primary cancer, many of these patients will already have a diagnosis of primary cancer elsewhere, which can aid in reaching the correct diagnosis. The most common etiologies of choroidal metastasis are breast carcinoma in women and lung carcinoma in men.

Symptoms

Metamorphopsia, peripheral field changes, and decreased visual acuity may result from direct tumor involvement of the macula or exudative retinal detachment.

Clinical Features

These tumors may be solitary or multiple, unilateral or bilateral, and they usually appear creamy-yellow, often with pigment mottling over the surface. They have a tendency to produce subretinal fluid and can cause a significant exudative retinal detachment. Most tumors are located in the posterior pole with a plaque or domed shape.

Ancillary Testing

Ultrasonography is helpful in distinguishing a choroidal metastasis from a melanoma. Whereas melanomas have low, regular internal reflectivity on A-scan ultrasonography, choroidal metastases usually have medium to high, irregular internal reflectivity due to the irregular arrangement of nests and chords of tumor cells within the choroid. By magnetic resonance imaging, these tumors are usually less hyperintense on T1 weighting than melanomas. In the absence of a known primary cancer, fine-needle aspiration biopsy may be required to reach the correct diagnosis.

Pathology/Pathogenesis

Histopathologically, choroidal metastasis appears with chords and nests of cancer cells (usually carcinoma) infiltrating the choroid. Choroidal metastases have been reported from virtually every site in the body.

Treatment/Prognosis

Observation may be appropriate in asymptomatic patients. Most tumors will respond to systemic chemotherapy or external beam radiation.

Systemic Evaluation

In patients suspected of having choroidal metastasis but with no known primary cancer, a thorough systemic workup for cancer of unknown etiology should be coordinated with a medical oncologist.

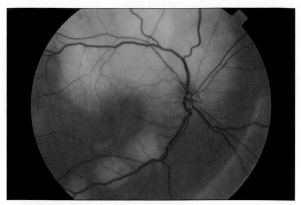

Multifocal, creamy choroidal deposits from metastatic breast carcinoma. Breast carcinoma is the most common cause of choroidal metastasis in women.

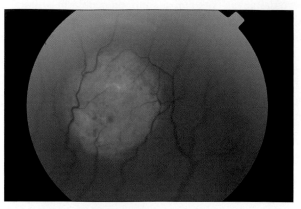

Solitary, vascularized choroidal metastasis from alveolar cell sarcoma in a 14-year-old.

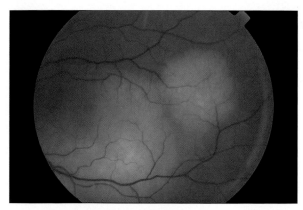

Multilobular amelanotic choroidal tumor in a patient with no history of systemic malignancy.

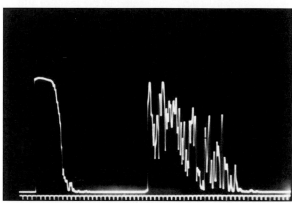

A-scan ultrasonogram of the lesion in the previous figure. Note that the tumor has irregular, medium to high internal reflectivity consistent with a metastatic lesion.

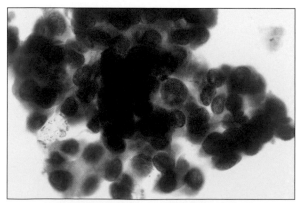

Fine-needle aspiration biopsy of the choroidal tumor depicted in the previous two figures, demonstrating adenocarcinoma with formation of glandular structures.

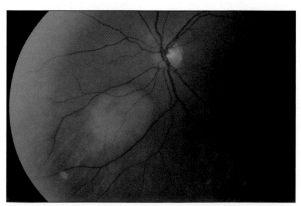

Solitary, choroidal metastasis from breast cancer. Note that the tumor is relatively flat and yet produced a large, inferior exudative retinal detachment.

CHOROIDAL NEVUS

Choroidal nevus is the most common neoplasm of the uveal tract. This benign tumor usually arises early in life. It may grow slightly during puberty, but the vast majority remain benign throughout life. However, a few of these lesions will undergo malignant degeneration into a choroidal melanoma, and an important diagnostic challenge is to distinguish a large choroidal nevus from a small choroidal melanoma.

Symptoms

Patients often have no symptoms, but metamorphopsia and blurred vision can result from subretinal fluid extending into the macula.

Clinical Features

Choroidal nevi are typically pigmented but can occasionally be amelanotic. They are located at the level of the choroid and usually have feathery, indistinct borders. They are usually flat or minimally elevated. Long-standing lesions often have drusen over the surface, which is a negative predictor of future growth. Features associated with a higher risk of growth include greater tumor thickness, posterior tumor margin touching the optic disc, subretinal fluid, and orange pigmentation on the tumor surface. Documentation of significant growth must be viewed as a probable sign of malignant degeneration.

Ancillary Testing

Ultrasonography can occasionally be helpful in distinguishing a choroidal nevus from a nonmelanocytic lesion. Choroidal nevi that are more than 1.5 mm thick usually demonstrate low internal reflectivity on A-scan ultrasonography. Fluorescein angiographic features are not diagnostic but can support the diagnosis. Pigmented nevi are usually hypofluorescent in the early frames, with patchy hyperfluorescence as the study progresses. Pinpoint hotspots often coincide with clinical evidence of subretinal fluid, and are a risk factor for growth.

Pathology/Pathogenesis

Choroidal nevi arise from melanocytes in the uveal tract and appear histopathologically as low-grade spindle cell melanocytic tumors that replace the normal choroidal architecture. The pathogenesis is unknown. A strong family history of melanocytic tumors is uncommonly elicited, and there is no known relationship to sunlight exposure.

Treatment/Prognosis

Treatment is not usually necessary unless subretinal fluid affects vision, in which case treatment options include scatter laser photocoagulation, transpupillary thermotherapy, and plaque radiotherapy. If substantial growth is documented, the lesion is treated as a choroidal melanoma.

Systemic Evaluation

Systemic screening for metastasis is not necessary for a choroidal nevus unless the lesion degenerates into a melanoma. Examination of the skin for cutaneous nevi may rarely reveal evidence of multiple melanocytic lesions.

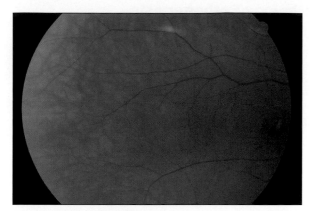

Fundus photograph of a typical choroidal nevus demonstrating a flat, pigmented lesion with feathery, indistinct borders.

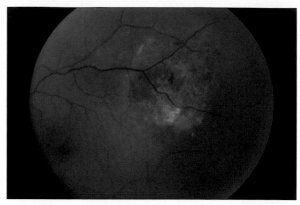

Relatively flat, pigmented choroidal nevus with drusen and fibrous metaplasia over the surface, indicative of chronicity.

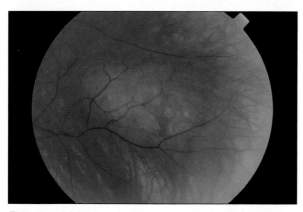

This choroidal nevus is slightly elevated with feathery margins. Greater tumor thickness is associated with an increased risk of growth.

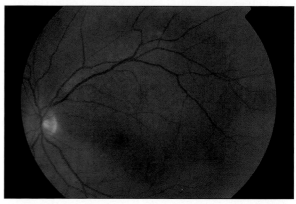

Fundus photograph of a large, suspicious choroidal nevus with risk factors for growth such as orange lipofuscin pigmentation, a thin layer of subretinal fluid over the tumor surface, and posterior tumor margin touching the optic disc.

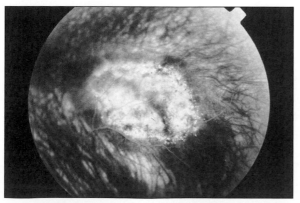

Fluorescein angiogram of a choroidal nevus, demonstrating late diffuse staining, leakage, and pinpoint hotspots, which are a risk factor for growth.

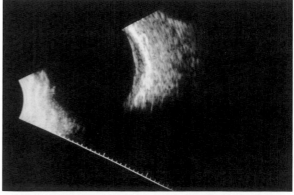

B-scan ultrasonography of a choroidal nevus. Note that the lesion is relatively thin.

CHOROIDAL OSTEOMA

Choroidal osteoma is a benign, ossifying tumor of the choroid, with a distinct clinical and histopathologic appearance. These tumors are found most commonly in young women but can also be seen in other patients. Choroidal osteomas are frequently unilateral, but can also be bilateral. No family history is found in most patients.

Symptoms

Metamorphopsia, scotoma, and blurred vision may be due to direct tumor involvement of the macula, or more commonly to choroidal neovascularization.

Clinical Features

Ophthalmoscopic examination usually reveals a relatively thin, plaque-like, yellow-tan lesion with sharp, scalloped borders. The tumors usually arise adjacent to the optic nerve and may increase slightly in size on serial examination. However, they have no malignant potential. The most common cause of visual loss is choroidal neovascularization, which often occurs on the temporal margin of the tumor and may produce subretinal fluid, lipid, or hemorrhage into fixation.

Ancillary Testing

B-scan ultrasonography shows a highly reflective, plaque-like structure at the level of the choroid that persists as a strong signal when the gain is reduced to a level where other ocular structures can no longer be seen. Similarly, computed tomography shows a strong signal indicating calcium within the lesion. Fluorescein angiography reveals early hyperfluorescence with late staining of the osteoma. Fluorescein angiography also can be helpful in demonstrating choroidal neovascularization.

Pathology/Pathogenesis

The pathogenesis of choroidal osteomas is unknown. Choroidal osteomas are composed of mature bone elements within the choroid, including osteoblasts, osteoclasts, osteocytes, and a calcium-containing matrix.

Treatment/Prognosis

Laser photocoagulation may be indicated for treatment of choroidal neovascularization. The role of photodynamic therapy for choroidal neovascularization in patients with choroidal osteomas is unclear.

Systemic Evaluation

No consistent systemic abnormalities have been associated with choroidal osteoma, although a simulating lesion, sclerochoroidal calcification, can be associated with hyperparathyroidism, chronic renal failure, and other abnormalities in calcium and phosphorus metabolism.

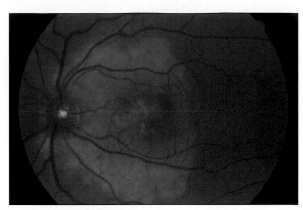

Fundus photograph of a thin, plaque-like, peripapillary tumor with scalloped borders consistent with a choroidal osteoma.

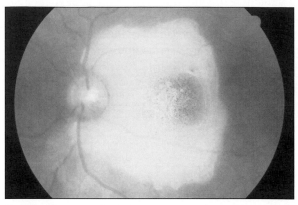

Fundus photograph of the same eye taken with a red filter demonstrates the refractile nature of the choroidal osteoma.

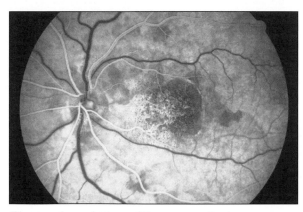

Fluorescein angiogram of the same patient demonstrates irregular hyperfluorescence as a result of retinal pigment epithelial atrophy.

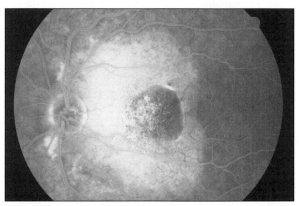

Late-phase angiogram of the same patient reveals mild staining of the choroidal osteoma. There is no evidence of choroidal neovascularization.

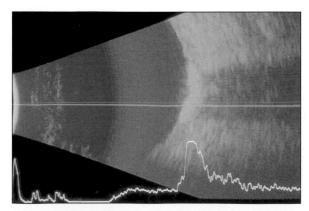

B-scan ultrasonogram of a choroidal osteoma shows a highly reflective, plaque-like structure and an acoustically empty region behind the tumor.

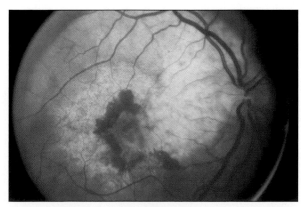

Visual loss in patients with choroidal osteomas may be related to the development of a choroidal neovascular membrane. Note the subretinal hemorrhage in this patient with a large choroidal osteoma.

CONGENITAL HYPERTROPHY OF THE RETINAL PIGMENT EPITHELIUM

Congenital hypertrophy of the retinal pigment epithelium (CHRPE) is a benign condition that has been mistaken for melanoma and can be confused with a similar abnormality that is associated with familial colon cancer.

Symptoms

Patients with CHRPE are asymptomatic.

Clinical Features

Congenital hypertrophy of the retinal pigment epithelium is a solitary, flat, circumscribed, pigmented lesion that is usually found in the fundus midperiphery. It is often surrounded by a depigmented halo, and it may contain depigmented "lacunae" within the body of the lesion. Congenital hypertrophy of the retinal pigment epithelium (RPE) can become depigmented in older individuals. By indirect ophthalmoscopy, the lesion may appear to be elevated, but with careful slit lamp biomicroscopy, the lesion is seen to be flat. These lesions are not true tumors and do not grow or produce subretinal fluid. Lesions similar to CHRPE can be found in clustered groups in a sectorial distribution that resembles "bear tracks."

Ancillary Testing

Ultrasonography will confirm that the lesion is flat. Fluorescein angiography will show a blocking defect in pigmented areas and a transmission defect in depigmented portions. No intrinsic vessels or dye flush are seen, as with a true tumor.

Pathology/Pathogenesis

Congenital hypertrophy of the RPE is composed of elongated RPE cells that have unusually dense cytoplasmic pigmentation.

Treatment/Prognosis

No treatment is required and the visual prognosis is excellent. Although it is extremely rare, malignant degeneration of CHRPE into an adenocarcinoma has been described; therefore, CHRPE lesions must be followed up regularly.

Systemic Evaluation

Pigmented lesions similar to grouped CHRPE can be seen in familial adenomatous polyposis, which is associated with a high risk of colon cancer. Unlike typical CHRPE, these lesions are usually bilateral, multifocal, asymmetrically distributed, and irregularly shaped. If there is any suggestion of this lesion or a strong family history of colon cancer, the patient should be referred for colonoscopy and further evaluation.

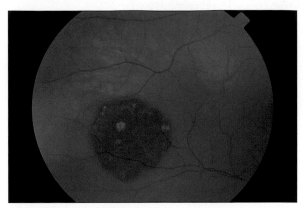

Congenital hypertrophy of the retinal pigment epithelium in a young patient. The lesion is darkly pigmented and flat, with well-defined borders. Note the small, depigmented lacunae.

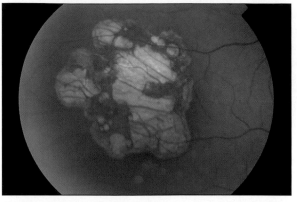

Fundus photograph of a solitary congenital hypertrophy of the retinal pigment epithelium (CHRPE) lesion. Note the multiple lacunae that reveal the underlying large choroidal vessels and sclera characteristic of an older CHRPE lesion.

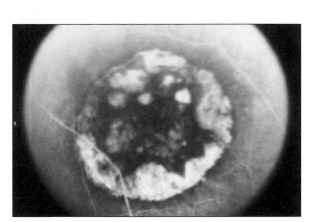

Fluorescein angiogram of a congenital hypertrophy of the retinal pigment epithelium demonstrating a central blocking defect corresponding to the pigmented portion and surrounding transmission defects corresponding to depigmented areas.

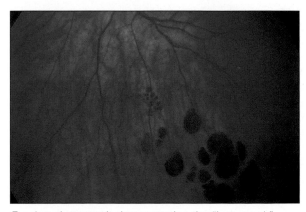

Fundus photograph demonstrating the "bear track" pattern of relatively uniform lesions grouped in a sectorial fashion.

INTRAOCULAR LYMPHOMA

Intraocular lymphoma can be part of a primary, multicentric central nervous system-ocular lymphoma or it can occur as a metastatic uveal deposit associated with visceral lymphoma. In the older ophthalmic literature, primary ocular lymphoma has been called "reticulum cell sarcoma." Intraocular lymphoma is more common in older and immunocompromised individuals. Diagnosis may be difficult to establish and is often delayed. Primary intraocular lymphoma is considered one of the "masquerade syndromes" because the clinical presentation can mimic those of other ocular conditions. Intraocular lymphoma should be considered in older patients with uveitis that is refractory to medical therapy.

Symptoms

Blurred vision and floaters may occur as a result of lymphomatous infiltration of the vitreous and other intraocular structures.

Clinical Features

Central nervous system-ocular lymphoma typically presents with a cellular vitreous infiltration with or without the presence of creamy deposits involving the retina, subretinal space, and retinal pigment epithelium (RPE). When present, the RPE detachments are the hallmark of ocular lymphoma. Intraocular lymphoma may mimic multifocal choroiditis with vitreous cells and multiple yellowish white RPE infiltrates. Uveal metastasis from a visceral lymphoma usually appears as an elevated, amelanotic choroidal mass. Most of these patients will have a previous diagnosis of systemic lymphoma. In some patients, there is overlap between these two presentations.

Ancillary Testing

Ultrasonography of the uveal mass can be helpful in ruling out melanoma. In the absence of known systemic lymphoma, definitive diagnosis usually requires a tissue biopsy. When vitreous cells are present, a core vitrectomy is often sufficient to obtain a specimen that can be diagnosed by cytopathology, immunohistochemistry, and flow cytometry. Occasionally, a retinal or choroidal biopsy is required.

Pathology/Pathogenesis

Most intraocular lymphomas are large cell lymphomas of B-cell lineage. These cells may infiltrate the vitreous, retina, subretinal space, sub-RPE space, and choroid. Rarely, T-cell lymphomas can involve the eye, and these cells are usually more aggressive.

Treatment/Prognosis

Central nervous system-ocular lymphoma is usually treated with external beam radiotherapy. Controversy exists as to whether the brain should be irradiated prophylactically or only if intracranial disease is present. Some centers also use adjunctival intrathecal chemotherapy. Uveal metastatic lymphoma can also be treated with external beam radiation if it does not respond to systemic therapy for the primary tumor. Prognosis is generally poor.

Systemic Evaluation

Systemic workup should include tests such as cranial magnetic resonance imaging, chest and abdominal computed tomography, bone marrow biopsy, and lumbar puncture to evaluate other potential sites of lymphoma. Lymphoma can be associated with immune deficiency, such as acquired immunodeficiency syndrome and immunosuppression following organ transplantation.

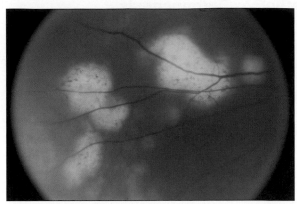

Fundus photograph of a 78-year-old woman with subretinal infiltrates. She was diagnosed with intraocular lymphoma.

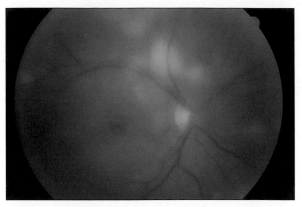

Fundus photograph of a patient with intraocular lymphoma. Prominent vitreous cells reduce the quality of the photograph. Subretinal infiltrates were found in the peripapillary and superior fundus.

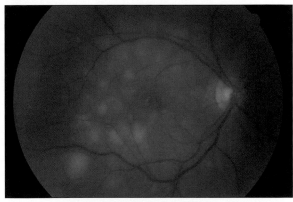

This 58-year-old man had abrupt onset of floaters and blurred vision. He was originally diagnosed with multifocal choroiditis but diagnostic vitrectomy revealed lymphoma cells.

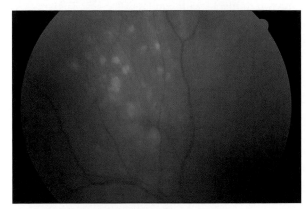

Midperipheral photograph of the same patient demonstrates the multifocal lesions at the level of the retinal pigment epithelium mimicking multifocal choroiditis.

MELANOCYTOMA

Melanocytoma is a special form of benign melanocytic uveal neoplasm that has a distinctive clinical and pathologic appearance. It can present in all age groups and races.

Symptoms

Melanocytoma is usually asymptomatic. Occasionally, a scotoma is noted due to nerve fiber layer damage.

Clinical Features

Melanocytomas commonly occur adjacent to or within the optic nerve, but they can arise anywhere in the uveal tract. Juxtapapillary tumors can cause nerve fiber layer defects or an afferent pupillary defect. Central retinal vascular obstruction has been described with melanocytoma of the optic nerve. Melanocytomas are a distinctive dark brown to black, with feathery margins. They are usually slightly elevated. Orange lipofuscin pigment and subretinal fluid are not often found. The vast majority of these tumors remain stable or grow only slightly over time, but there have been case reports of malignant degeneration.

Ancillary Testing

Baseline fundus photography is important for future monitoring. Visual field testing may identify visual field defects.

Pathology/Pathogenesis

Melanocytomas are composed of large, plump magnocellular nevus cells that are heavily pigmented. Bleaching of the specimen to remove the pigment reveals bland, regular, small nuclei consistent with a benign tumor.

Treatment/Prognosis

No treatment is usually recommended except in the rare instances of malignant degeneration, in which case the tumor is treated as a choroidal melanoma. The prognosis for survival is excellent except when malignant degeneration occurs. Vision may be affected by nerve fiber layer defects but usually remains stable.

Systemic Evaluation

No systemic evaluation is necessary.

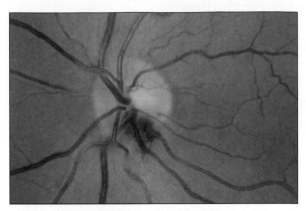

Fundus photograph of a small melanocytoma. Melanocytomas usually occur adjacent to or within the optic disc.

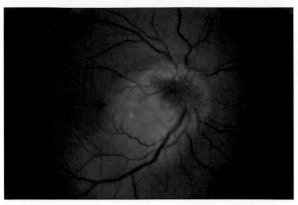

Juxtapapillary choroidal melanoma with optic nerve invasion. Note that this tumor has orange lipofuscin pigment over its surface, more consistent with melanoma than melanocytoma.

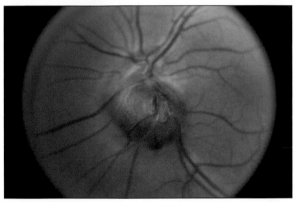

Fundus photograph of a melanocytoma of the optic disc. Note the dark pigmentation. Importantly, there is no optic disc edema or hemorrhages that may indicate optic nerve invasion by a malignant tumor.

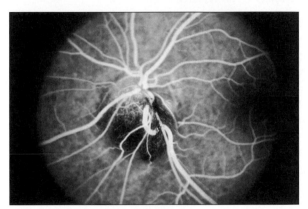

Fluorescein angiogram of a melanocytoma demonstrates hypofluorescence as a result of the darkly pigmented tumor.

PHAKOMATOSES: NEUROFIBROMATOSIS

Neurofibromatosis is a disease that primarily affects nerves of sensation, Schwann cells, and melanocytes. Two genetically distinct forms of neurofibromatosis have been described: type 1 or peripheral (NF1) and type 2 or central (NF2). NF1 is the most common form and can present at any age.

Symptoms

In NF1, vision loss can occur secondary to optic nerve glioma, menigiomas, glaucoma, or glial hamartomas of the retina. Learning disabilities occur frequently.

For patients with NF2, vision loss can occur secondary to juvenile posterior subcapsular cataracts or meningiomas. Hearing loss and vestibular problems commonly occur in the second to third decade of life.

Clinical Features

Diagnosis of NF1 requires that the patient have two or more of the following: six or more café-au-lait patches (larger than 5 mm in prepubescent patients and larger than 15 mm in postpubescent patients), two or more neurofibromas, one plexiform neurofibroma (s-shaped lid), axillary or inguinal freckling, optic nerve glioma (proptosis), two or more Lisch nodules, sphenoid wing dysplasia (pulsating exophthalmos), and a first-degree relative with NF1.

Posterior segment manifestations described in NF1 include hamartomas of the optic disc, retina, and choroid; retinal hemangioma; congenital hypertrophy of the retinal pigment epithelium; and myelinated nerve fibers. The finding of astrocytic hamartoma is less common in neurofibromatosis compared to tuberous sclerosis.

Diagnosis of NF2 requires that the patient meet the following criteria: bilateral eighth nerve masses; or a first-degree relative with NF2 and either unilateral eighth nerve mass or two of the following: neurofibroma, menigioma, schwannoma, and juvenile posterior subcapsular cataracts. Combined hamartomas of the retinal pigment epithelium and neurosensory retina have been described in patients with NF2.

Ancillary Testing

Magnetic resonance imaging (MRI) and computed tomography (CT) scans are necessary to assess central nervous system disease.

Pathology/Pathogenesis

NF1 is inherited as an autosomal dominant trait with an incidence of one in 3000 live births. The gene for NF1 has been located on chromosome 17q11.2.

NF2 is inherited as an autosomal dominant trait with an incidence of one in 50 000 live births. The gene for NF2 has been located on chromosome 22q11.2-q13.1.

Treatment/Prognosis

Most of the intraocular lesions of NF1 are benign and only warrant observation. However, patients with optic nerve gliomas need regular MRIs and visual fields and neuro-ophthalmological follow-up. In patients with NF2, cataract extraction may be necessary to restore visual function in patients with visually significant cataracts.

Systemic Evaluation

Baseline CT/MRI studies are necessary to detect subclinical visual pathway gliomas. Patients should have a cardiac echocardiogram to rule out a cardiac rhabdomyoma. A chest x-ray to rule out cystic lung lesions should be obtained. Patients should also be screened for leukemia, seizures, pheochromocytoma, and other endocrinological abnormalities. Patients with NF1 should also have a baseline neurological evaluation. These screening examinations can be coordinated through the patient's primary care provider. Patients with NF2 may require otolaryngology consultation for evaluation of hearing loss or abnormal vestibular function.

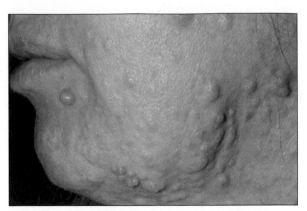

This patient with neurofibromatosis type 1 demonstrates numerous subcutaneous neurofibromas on her face and neck.

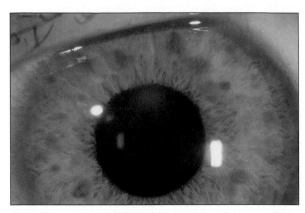

The slit lamp examination of the same patient revealed multiple Lisch nodules on the iris surface of each eye.

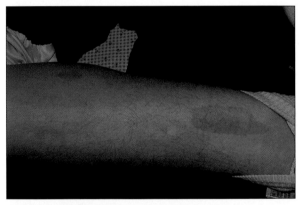

Other common cutaneous manifestations of neurofibromatosis include café-au-lait spots, as seen on the arm of this 13-year-old boy.

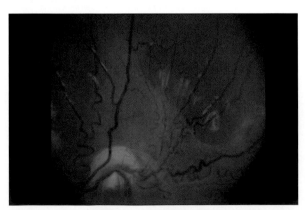

Fundus photograph of a juxtapapillary combined hamartoma of the retinal pigment epithelium and retina in a patient with neurofibromatosis type 2. The three characteristic findings in this lesion are epiretinal membrane, tortuous retinal vessels, and underlying thickened and/or pigmented retinal pigment epithelium.

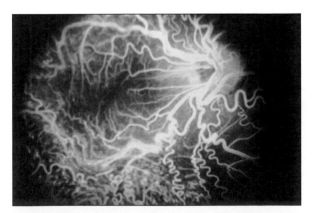

Fluorescein angiogram of the combined hamartoma of the retinal pigment epithelium and retina demonstrates markedly tortuous vessels.

PHAKOMATOSES: STURGE-WEBER SYNDROME

Sturge-Weber syndrome consists of a facial cutaneous angioma with an ipsilateral leptomeningeal vascular malformation. The classic findings include cerebral calcifications, seizures, focal neurological defects, and mental deficiency.

Symptoms

Vision loss can occur secondary to glaucoma, amblyopia, cystoid macular degeneration, exudative retinal detachment, or vascular abnormalities of the occipital lobe.

Clinical Features

Sturge-Weber syndrome is a spectrum. Most patients have a forme fruste rather than the full syndrome. The full syndrome consists of facial hemangioma, ipsilateral intracranial hemangioma, ipsilateral choroidal hemangioma, and congenital glaucoma. Developmental delay occurs in up to 50% of patients with leptomeningeal angiomatosis.

Ophthalmic findings in Sturge-Weber syndrome include eyelid hemangiomatosis, prominent conjunctival/episcleral vascular plexi, diffuse choroidal hemangioma with "tomato-catsup fundus," tortuous retinal vessels, cystoid macular degeneration, exudative retinal detachment, heterochromia iridis, glaucoma, and hyperopic amblyopia.

Systemic findings in Sturge-Weber syndrome include railroad track calcifications of the leptomeninges in the occipital/parietal area, seizures, developmental delay, hypertrophy of the face, hemangiomatosis involvement of airway, and cutaneous hemangiomas.

Ancillary Testing

Glaucoma is a significant cause of vision loss in patients with Sturge-Weber syndrome; therefore, intraocular pressure measurements and visual field testing are essential. Fluorescein angiography in patients with diffuse choroidal hemangioma may show diffuse leakage. Ultrasonography demonstrates a thickened choroid with medium to high internal reflectivity, and exudative retinal detachments may be detected.

Pathology/Pathogenesis

Sturge-Weber syndrome is not inherited and occurs in one in 50 000 live births. There is no race or sex predilection. The lesions in Sturge-Weber syndrome are anomalies of neuroectoderm. Sturge-Weber syndrome is believed to be caused by an abnormality in the early fetal development of the neural crest. The choroidal hemangioma is classified as a mixed hemangioma.

Treatment/Prognosis

If the V1 distribution is not involved there is a low chance of intracranial involvement. Glaucoma in Sturge-Weber syndrome is typically poorly responsive to medications and requires surgical management. Intraoperative complications such as expulsive ocular hemorrhage are common. Hyperopic amblyopia can occur in children with unilateral choroidal hemangioma hence, these patients need careful refraction and amblyopia therapy if warranted. External radiation therapy may be necessary to resolve exudative retinal detachment. Cutaneous hemangiomas can be treated with laser to lessen their appearance and improve cosmesis.

Systemic Evaluation

Patients with Sturge-Weber syndrome should have neurological evaluation. Evaluation of the airway must be performed before performing any surgical intervention.

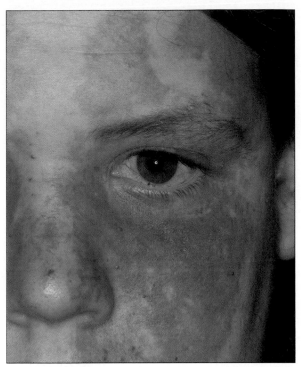

A 15-year-old boy with Sturge-Weber syndrome demonstrates the "port wine" facial hemangioma.

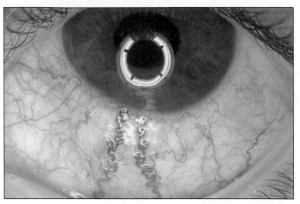

He had glaucoma refractory to medical management and required surgery. Note the prominently dilated conjunctival and episcleral vessels of his right eye.

PHAKOMATOSES: TUBEROUS SCLEROSIS

The classic triad of tuberous sclerosis includes seizures, mental retardation, and facial angiofibromas (adenoma sebaceum).

Symptoms

Vision loss can occur secondary to cortical tubers, astrocytic hamartomas of the retina, optic nerve gliomas, and optic atrophy (secondary to hydrocephalus).

Clinical Features

Ophthalmic findings in tuberous sclerosis include astrocytic hamartomas of the retina, leaf-shaped retinal pigment epithelium defects, sectoral iris hypopigmentation, optic nerve glioma, angiofibromas of the eyelids, and retinal detachment. Astrocytic hamartomas are typically elevated, nodular, calcific, mulberry-like lesions.

Systemic findings in tuberous sclerosis include ash-leaf spots, café-au-lait spots, shagreen patches, subungual fibromas, cortical tubers of basal ganglia, lateral ventricles and third ventricle, obstructive hydrocephalus, subependymal nodules, subependymal giant cell astrocytoma, and tumors or cysts of the bone, lung, heart, liver, and kidney.

Diagnosis of tuberous sclerosis requires that the patient have one of the following: cortical tuber, subependymal glial nodules, subependymal-intraventricular giant cell astrocytoma, retinal hamartoma, facial angiofibromas (70% by 4 years of age), periungual/subungual fibromas, forehead/scalp fibrous plaques, and multiple renal angiomyolipomas.

Presumptive diagnosis of tuberous sclerosis can be made if the patient has two of the following: infantile spasms, seizures (90%), areas of increased attenuation in cerebral cortex, calcified lesion in cortex/subcortex, ash-leaf spots, peripapillary retinal hamartoma, gingival fibromas, dental enamel pits, and multiple renal tumors, multiple renal cysts, cardiac rhabdomyoma, pulmonary lymphangiomyomatosis, radiographic honeycomb lungs, and an immediate relative with tuberous sclerosis.

Ancillary Testing

Astrocytic hamartomas may be autofluorescent depending on the extent of calcification. In the arterial phase of the fluorescein angiogram, the astrocytic hamartoma is hypofluorescent and tortuous vessels are seen around the tumor. In the venous phase, the fine vessels on the tumor surface begin to leak and lead to homogeneous staining of the mass. Ultrasonography is of use in the larger calcified astrocytic hamartomas. The lesion is acoustically solid, well demarcated, and lacks choroidal excavation. The tumors have high internal reflectivity with attenuation of orbital echoes posterior to the tumor.

Pathology/Pathogenesis

Tuberous sclerosis is inherited as an autosomal dominant trait with an incidence of one in 15 000 live births. The genes for tuberous sclerosis have been located on chromosomes 9q and 11q. There is no race or sex predilection. The retinal astrocytic hamartoma arises from the nerve fiber layer. It contains elongated fibrous astrocytes that are well differentiated. Mitotic figures are rare. Sometimes calcified bodies are present within the tumor.

Treatment/Prognosis

Patients with tuberous sclerosis have a normal life expectancy. The seizures typically present in infancy as infantile spasms and progress to grand mal seizures later in life. Patients may need a shunt procedure for obstructive hydrocephalus. The retinal astrocytic hamartomas usually remain stable over time and have no effect on visual function.

Systemic Evaluation

Patients should have a multidisciplinary evaluation including dermatology, ophthalmology, neurology, cardiology, urology, and pulmonology. These examinations can be coordinated through the patient's primary care provider.

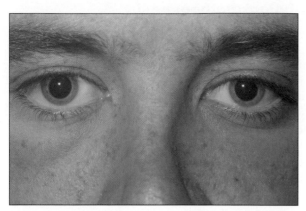

This photograph demonstrates the facial angiofibromas (adenoma sebaceum) seen with tuberous sclerosis.

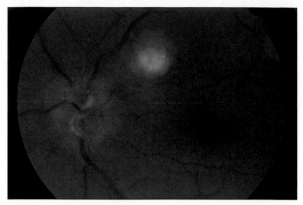

Fundus photograph of the same patient reveals a calcific astrocytic hamartoma in the superior macula of the left eye. The tumor has mulberry-like deposits and fine vascularization. Note the associated disc edema.

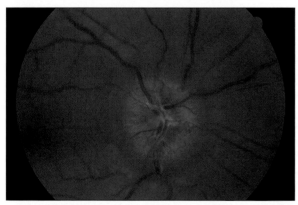

Fundus photograph of the same patient's right eye reveals prominent optic disc edema. He was diagnosed with papilledema and sent for an immediate neuroimaging study.

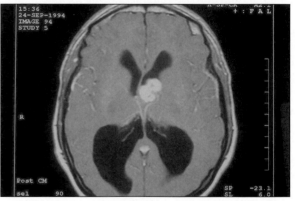

The computed tomography scan revealed a prominent subependymal astrocytoma with dilated ventricles consistent with obstructive hydrocephalus.

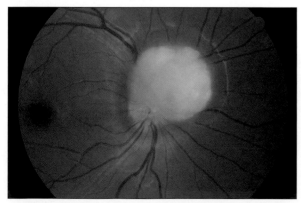

Astrocytic hamartomas may arise from the optic disc and retina. This child had a calcific tumor extending from the optic disc.

PHAKOMATOSES: VON HIPPEL-LINDAU DISEASE

Von Hippel-Lindau disease is a disorder characterized by vascular tumors of the retina and central nervous system. In addition, patients are predisposed to developing additional tumors including renal cell carcinoma, pheochromocytoma, and renal, pancreatic, and epididymal cysts. Most patients present in the third to fourth decade of life, but manifestations of von Hippel-Lindau disease can be observed at birth.

Symptoms

Vision loss can occur from the retinal hemangioma or cerebellar/cerebral hemangioblastoma.

Clinical Features

Diagnosis of von Hippel-Lindau disease requires one of the following: cerebellar, spinal, medullary, or cerebral hemangioblastoma; retinal capillary hemangioma; multiple renal cysts; or renal cell carcinoma; pancreatic cysts; cystadenocarcinoma; islet cell tumor; pheochromocytoma; and epididymal cystadenoma (male infertility); plus a relative who has a central nervous system or eye lesion, renal cysts, or adenocarcinoma.

The retinal capillary hemangiomas are often multifocal and bilateral. The classic presentation is a vascularized tumor mass with prominent feeder and draining vessels. Retinal capillary hemangiomas may be associated with exudation of fluid and lipid. Severe cases are characterized by an exudative retinal detachment, which may lead to retinal ischemia, iris neovascularization, and neovascular glaucoma.

Ancillary Testing

Fluorescein angiography will typically demonstrate in the early arterial phase a dilated feeder arteriole. A few seconds later, the tumor will rapidly fill with fluorescein. In the venous phase, the dilated draining vein will appear. In the late phase, the tumor will demonstrate leakage. Ultrasonography demonstrates high internal reflectivity within the acoustically solid mass. Retinal detachment and subretinal fluid can also be seen on ultrasound.

Pathology/Pathogenesis

Von Hippel-Lindau disease is inherited as an autosomal dominant trait with an incidence of one in 36 000 live births. The lesions in this disease are primarily of mesodermal origin. The gene for von Hippel-Lindau disease is located on chromosome 3p25. There is no race or sex predilection. The retinal hemangioma is a mass of fenestrated capillaries that locally replaces retinal architecture. The tumors consist of endothelial cells, pericytes, and lipid-laden foam cells. They are classified as endophytic or exophytic depending on their direction of growth.

Treatment/Prognosis

Von Hippel-Lindau disease is a potentially lethal condition. The most common cause of death is the cerebellar hemangioblastoma or renal cell carcinoma. Patients with confirmed von Hippel-Lindau disease have a median survival of 49 years. Visual prognosis is variable. Treatment of the retinal capillary hemangiomas depends on size, location, and clarity of the media. Small tumors (less than 5 mm) can usually be treated with laser photocoagulation or cyrotherapy. Treatment of large tumors (greater than 5 mm) is more difficult and may require cryotherapy or plaque radiotherapy and retinal detachment surgery. Patients may experience a marked increase in exudation immediately following treatment, particularly with larger tumors. Enucleation may be necessary for uncontrolled hemangiomas causing advanced glaucoma.

Systemic Evaluation

Patients should have periodic evaluations, including a physical, an eye exam, a urine analysis, a urine 24-hour collection for VMA, and a renal ultrasound. Every three years they should have a brain magnetic resonance imaging (MRI) and computed tomography (CT) scan and a CT scan of the kidneys. At-risk relatives need a yearly eye examination and physical. They also need a yearly urine analysis, urine 24-hour collection for VMA, and renal ultrasound. Every three years at risk relatives also need a brain MRI or CT scan starting at age 15 years. They also need a CT scan of the kidneys every three years starting at age 20. Genetic testing is available but the benefits must be weighed in each case.

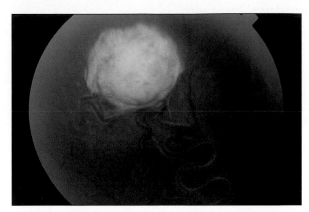

Fundus photograph of a retinal capillary hemangioma in a patient with von Hippel-Lindau disease. Note the dilated feeder vessel and the vascularized tumor mass. There was dependent lipid exudation into the macula.

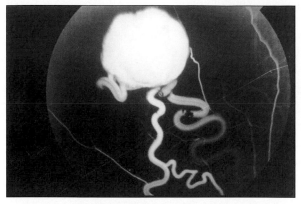

Fluorescein angiogram of the same patient demonstrates rapid filling of the arterial feeder vessel and marked hyperfluorescence of the retinal capillary hemangioma.

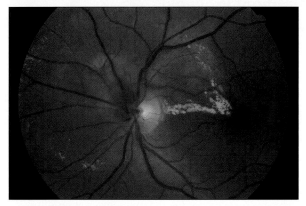

Exophytic tumors arise from the outer layers of the retina and tend to be found in the peripapillary distribution. This 36-year-old man had a peripapillary lesion associated with fluid and lipid exudation into the fovea.

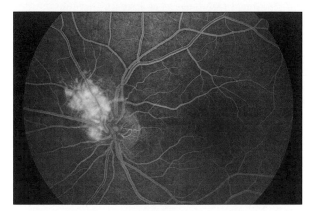

The fluorescein angiogram of the same patient revealed hyperfluorescence in the superior nasal peripapillary region with late leakage. The lesion was located in the outer retinal layers. The differential diagnosis for exophytic tumors includes peripapillary choroidal neovascularization.

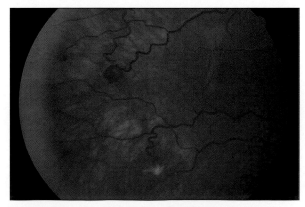

This 21-year-old woman was diagnosed with von Hippel-Lindau disease after resection of a large cerebellar hemangioblastoma. Her retina examination revealed bilateral, multifocal retinal capillary hemangiomas. This fundus photograph shows a characteristic endophytic lesion with dilated feeder and draining vessels. Inferiorly, there is a less common sessile exophytic hemangioma.

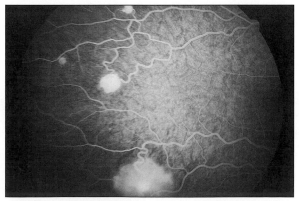

Fluorescein angiography of the same patient demonstrates three hyperfluorescent spots superiorly and a larger hyperfluorescent lesion inferiorly corresponding to the tumors.

PHAKOMATOSES: WYBURN-MASON SYNDROME

The coexistence of arteriovenous malformations between the retina and the midbrain has been referred to as the Wyburn-Mason syndrome. The ocular manifestations are usually unilateral.

Symptoms

The vision in patients with Wyburn-Mason syndrome ranges from normal to severely impaired. Vision loss can occur secondary to abnormal vessels in the macula, vitreous hemorrhage, retinal hemorrhage, microvascular decompensation or compressive nerve fiber layer loss, macular hole formation, retinal vein occlusion, neovascular glaucoma, or strabismus.

Clinical Features

Ocular findings in Wyburn-Mason syndrome may include unilateral widely dilated and tortuous retinal vessels, orbital arteriovenous malformation with proptosis, cranial nerve III, IV, VI palsies, and visual field defects. The appearance of the arteriovenous malformation may vary from a localized abnormality between an artery and a vein to marked dilation and tortuosity of the retinal vessels.

Systemic findings include ipsilateral intracranial vascular malformation (thalamus, midbrain, orbit), headaches, seizures, subarachnoid hemorrhage, hydrocephalus, trigeminal distribution nevi, hemiparesis, epistaxis, gingival hemorrhages secondary to arteriovenous malformations in the maxilla/mandible, and mental retardation.

Ancillary Testing

Fluorescein angiography shows rapid filling of the arteriovenous malformation without leakage. Patients usually have visual field abnormalities related to either retinal or intracranial abnormalities.

Pathology/Pathogenesis

Wyburn-Mason syndrome is not inherited. There is no race or sex predilection. This syndrome is thought to arise secondary to an embryonic insult to the primitive anterior vascular plexus during cerebral angiogenesis, which produces an anomalous anastomosis between the arterial and venous circulation of the retina and brain.

Treatment/Prognosis

The retinal vascular lesions are typically not treated. The role of laser photocoagulation in cases of retinal edema is unclear. Patients may require strabismus surgery for diplopia secondary to cranial neuropathies.

Systemic Evaluation

Patients with arteriovenous malformations should have a comprehensive neurological evaluation. Magnetic resonance imaging or computed tomography scans should be performed to evaluate for central nervous system vascular malformations. Dental extractions should be approached with extreme caution.

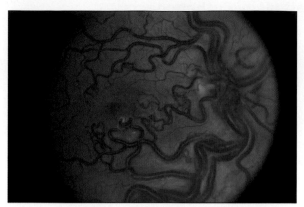

Fundus photograph of a patient with Wyburn-Mason syndrome demonstrating marked dilation and tortuosity of the retinal vessels as a result of the arteriovenous malformation.

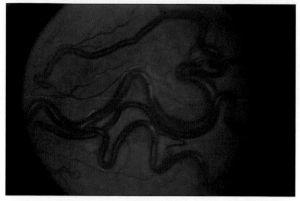

Fundus photograph of the nasal retina of the same patient reveals significant arterial and venous dilation. It is difficult to distinguish between the arteries and the veins.

RETINOBLASTOMA

Retinoblastoma is the most common childhood intraocular malignancy. The majority of cases of retinoblastoma manifest before age 3 years. It is hereditary in about 40% of all cases and sporadic in the other 60%. Patients with the hereditary trait transmit the disease in an autosomal dominant fashion and are at high risk of other primary cancers throughout life. These patients also have the potential for multifocal unilateral tumors, bilateral tumors, and the possibility of transmitting the defect to offspring.

Symptoms

Because it usually occurs in small children, retinoblastoma is often asymptomatic. The most common presenting signs are leukokoria and strabismus.

Clinical Features

Nonhereditary retinoblastoma commonly presents between ages 1 and 3 years, with a large, unilateral tumor. Hereditary retinoblastoma presents somewhat earlier, often with bilateral, multifocal tumors. Exophytic tumors appear as white, vascularized masses in the subretinal space with associated retinal detachment. Endophytic tumors grow into the vitreous cavity and usually produce vitreous seeding. Tumors arise within the retina but can secondarily involve the iris, anterior chamber, and orbit.

Ancillary Testing

In children less than 5 years old, the presence of calcium in a suspected intraocular tumor is highly consistent with retinoblastoma. Computed tomography (CT) establishes the presence of calcium, and also can detect optic nerve invasion and midline intracranial tumors. Ultrasonography can also demonstrate calcium if CT is not available. Magnetic resonance imaging (MRI) may also be useful on initial or subsequent examinations to rule out optic nerve involvement or intracranial tumors.

Pathology/Pathogenesis

Retinoblastoma results from the mutational loss of both copies of the retinoblastoma gene (RB) in a developing retinoblast. The RB gene is located in chromosome 13q14. Both alleles of chromosome 13 must be affected for the neoplasm to develop (Knudsen's "two hit" hypothesis). Mutations of the retinoblastoma gene result in deregulation of DNA synthesis; as a result, cells proliferate unchecked, leading to tumor development and growth. These tumors arise from immature neuronal elements of the retina and may demonstrate varying degrees of retinal differentiation. Tumor invasion of the optic nerve and choroid are risk factors for metastasis.

Treatment/Prognosis

Treatment options include laser photocoagulation, transpupillary thermotherapy, cryotherapy, plaque radiotherapy, external beam radiotherapy, systemic or local chemotherapy, and enucleation, depending on the clinical circumstances. More than 95% of patients survive retinoblastoma in developed countries, but hereditary patients often succumb to second primary cancers such as midline intracranial primitive neuroectodermal tumors, osteosarcomas, soft tissue sarcomas, and melanomas. Visual prognosis depends on the location and number of tumors.

Systemic Evaluation

Patients with hereditary retinoblastoma must be monitored with MRI until age 5 to 6 years for midline intracranial tumors. Metastatic workup (eg, lumbar puncture, chest and abdominal CT, bone marrow biopsy) should be performed if optic nerve invasion or extraocular extension is suspected.

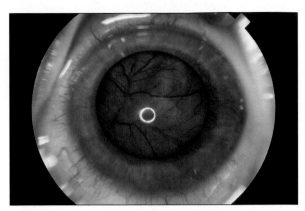

Slit lamp photograph of an eye with exophytic retinoblastoma. Note the total retinal detachment and white subretinal masses. Retinoblastoma is in the differential diagnosis for leukokoria.

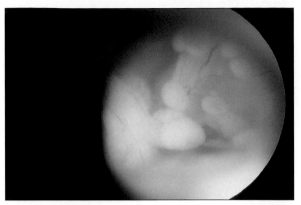

External view of an eye with endophytic retinoblastoma. Note the multiple vascularized fingerlike tumor projections and globular vitreous seeds.

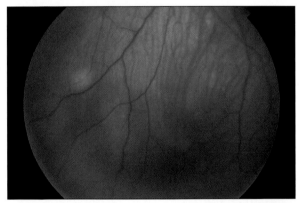

New tumor in a hereditary retinoblastoma patient with multiple bilateral tumors. Children at risk for hereditary retinoblastoma should be examined regularly for new tumors.

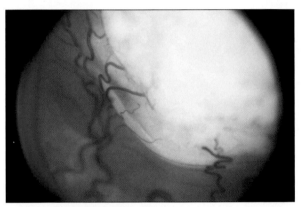

Fundus photograph of a large retinoblastoma. Note that the retinal vessels dive into the tumor substance. Areas of the tumor are chalk white, indicating the presence of calcium.

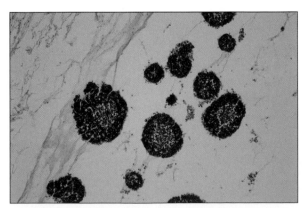

Vitreous seeding from retinoblastoma can be extremely difficult to treat with chemotherapy, laser photocoagulation, and cryotherapy. Radiotherapy and enucleation are often required.

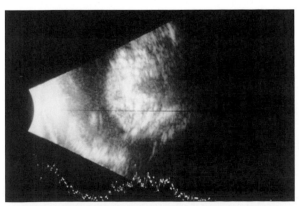

B-scan ultrasonography of a large retinoblastoma. Intratumoral calcium is indicated by the multiple, highly reflective areas within the tumor and the marked orbital shadowing.

SELECTED REFERENCES

Choroidal Hemangioma

1. Garcia-Arumi J, Ramsay LS, Guraya BC. Transpupillary thermotherapy for circumscribed choroidal hemangiomas. *Ophthalmology*. 2000;107:351–356.

2. Madreperla SA. Choroidal hemangioma treated with photodynamic therapy using verteporfin. *Arch Ophthalmol*. 2001;119:1606–1610.

3. Schalenbourg A, Piguet B, Zografos L. Indocyanine green angiographic findings in choroidal hemangiomas: a study of 75 cases. *Ophthalmologica*. 2000;214:246–252.

4. Shields CL, Honavar SG, Shields JA, Carter J, Demirci H. Circumscribed choroidal hemangioma: clinical manifestations and factors predictive of visual outcome in 200 consecutive cases. *Ophthalmology*. 2001;108:2237–2248.

5. Verbeek AM, Koutentakis P, Deutman AF. Circumscribed choroidal hemangioma diagnosed by ultrasonography: a retrospective analysis of 40 cases. *Int Ophthalmol*. 1995;19:185–189.

Choroidal Melanoma

1. Char DH, Quivey JM, Castro JR, Kroll S, Phillips T. Helium ions versus iodine 125 brachytherapy in the management of uveal melanoma: a prospective, randomized, dynamically balanced trial. *Ophthalmology*. 1993;100:1547–1554.

2. Diener-West M, Earle JD, Fine SL, Hawkins BS, Moy CS, Reynolds SM, et al. The COMS randomized trial of iodine 125 brachytherapy for choroidal melanoma, III: initial mortality findings. COMS Report No. 18. *Arch Ophthalmol*. 2001;119(7):969–982.

3. Garretson BR, Robertson DM, Earle JD. Choroidal melanoma treatment with iodine 125 brachytherapy. *Arch Ophthalmol*. 1987;105:1394–1397.

4. Kivela T, Eskelin S, Makitie T, Summanen P. Exudative retinal detachment from malignant uveal melanoma: predictors and prognostic significance. *Invest Ophthalmol Vis Sci*. 2001;42:2085–2093.

5. Oosterhuis JA, Journee-de Korver HG, Keunen JE. Transpupillary thermotherapy: results in 50 patients with choroidal melanoma. *Arch Ophthalmol*. 1998;116:157–162.

Choroidal Metastasis

1. Albert DM, Zimmermann AW Jr, Zeidman I. Tumor metastasis to the eye: the fate of circulating tumor cells to the eye. *Am J Ophthalmol*. 1967;63(4):733–738.

2. Augsburger JJ. Fine needle aspiration biopsy of suspected metastatic cancers to the posterior uvea. *Trans Am Ophthalmol Soc*. 1988;86:499–560.

3. Sobottka B, Kreissig I. Ultrasonography of metastases and melanomas of the choroid. *Curr Opin Ophthalmol*. 1999;10(3):164–167.

Choroidal Nevus

1. Augsburger JJ, Schroeder RP, Territo C, Gamel JW, Shields JA. Clinical parameters predictive of enlargement of melanocytic choroidal lesions. *Br J Ophthalmol*. 1989;73:911–917.

2. Butler P, Char DH, Zarbin M, Kroll S. Natural history of indeterminate pigmented choroidal tumors. *Ophthalmology*. 1994;101:710–716.

3. Shields GL, Shields JA, Kiratli H, DePotter P, Carter JR. Risk factors for growth and metastasis of small choroidal melanocytic lesions. *Ophthalmology*. 1995;102:1351–1361.

4. Sumich P, Mitchell P, Wang JJ. Choroidal nevi in a white population: the Blue Mountains Eye Study. *Arch Ophthalmol*. 1998;116:645–650.

Choroidal Osteoma

1. Aylward GW, Chang TS, Pautler SE, Gass JD. A long-term follow-up of choroidal osteoma. *Arch Ophthalmol*. 1998;116:1337–1341.

2. Gass JD, Guerry RK, Jack RL, Harris G. Choroidal osteoma. *Arch Ophthalmol*. 1978;96:428–435.

3. Ide T, Ohguro N, Hayashi A, Yamamoto S, Nakagawa Y, Nagae Y, et al. Optical coherence tomography patterns of choroidal osteoma. *Am J Ophthalmol*. 2000;130(1):131–134.

4. Kadrmas EF, Weter JJ. Choroidal osteoma. *Int Ophthalmol Clin*. 1997;37:171–182.

Congenital Hypertrophy of the Retinal Pigment Epithelium

1. Lloyd WC, Eagle RC Jr, Shields JA, Kwa DM, Arbizo VV. Congenital hypertrophy of the retinal pigment epithelium: electron microscopic and morphometric observations. *Ophthalmology*. 1990;97:1052–1060.

2. Shields JA, Shields CL, Shah PG, Pastore DJ, Imperiale SM Jr. Lack of association among typical congenital hypertrophy of the retinal pigment epithelium, adenomatous polyposis, and Gardner syndrome. *Ophthalmology*. 1992;99:1709–1713.

3. Shields JA, Shields CL, Eagle RC Jr, Singh AD. Adenocarcinoma arising from congenital hypertrophy of the retinal pigment epithelium. *Arch Ophthalmol*. 2001;119:597–602.

4. Tiret A, Parc C. Fundus lesions of adenomatous polyposis. *Curr Opin Ophthalmol*. 1999;10:168–172.

5. Ziskind A, Kitze MJ, Grobbelaar JJ. The relationship between congenital hypertrophy of the retinal pigment epithelium (CHRPE) and germline mutations in the adenomatous polyposis coli (APC) gene. *Ophthalmic Genet*. 1999;20:53–56.

Intraocular Lymphoma

1. Akpek EK, Ahmed I, Hochberg FH, Soheilian M, Dryja TP, Jakobiec FA, et al. Intraocular-central nervous system lymphoma: clinical features, diagnosis, and outcomes. *Ophthalmology.* 1999;106:1805–1810.
2. Char DH, Ljung BM, Miller T, Phillips T. Primary intraocular lymphoma (ocular reticulum cell sarcoma) diagnosis and management. *Ophthalmology.* 1988;95:625–630.
3. Gill MK, Jampol LM. Variations in the presentation of primary intraocular lymphoma: case reports and a review. *Surv Ophthalmol.* 2001;45:463–471.
4. Margolis L, Fraser R, Lichter A, Char DH. The role of radiation therapy in the management of ocular reticulum cell sarcoma. *Cancer.* 1980;45:688–692.

Melanocytoma

1. Antcliff RJ, Ffytche TJ, Shilling JS, Marshall J. Optical coherence tomography of melanocytoma. *Am J Ophthalmol.* 2000;130:845–847.
2. Joffe L, Shields JA, Osher RH, Gass JD. Clinical and follow-up studies of melanocytomas of the optic disc. *Ophthalmology.* 1979;86:1067–1083.
3. LoRusso FJ, Boniuk M, Font RL. Melanocytoma (magnocellular nevus) of the ciliary body: report of 10 cases and review of the literature. *Ophthalmology.* 2000;107:795–800.
4. Reidy JJ, Apple DJ, Steinmetz RL, Craythorn JM, Loftfield K, Gieser SC, et al. Melanocytoma: nomenclature, pathogenesis, natural history and treatment. *Surv Ophthalmol.* 1985;29:319–327.
5. Shields JA, Shields CL, Eagle RC Jr, Singh AD, Berrocal MH, Berrocal JA. Central retinal vascular obstruction secondary to melanocytoma of the optic disc. *Arch Ophthalmol.* 2001;119(1):129–133.

Phakomatoses: Neurofibromatosis

1. Barker D, Wright E, Nguyen K, Cannon L, Fain P, Goldgar D, et al. Gene for von Recklinghausen neurofibromatosis is in the pericentromeric region of chromosome 17. *Science.* 1987;236:1100–1102.
2. Greenwald MJ, Weiss A. Ocular manifestations of the neurocutaneous syndromes. *Pediatr Dermatol.* 1984;2:98–117.
3. Harbour JW. Tumor suppressor genes in ophthalmology. *Surv Ophthalmol.* 1999;44:235–246.
4. National Institutes of Health Consensus Development Conference Statement on Neurofibromatosis. *Arch Neurol.* 1988;45:575.
5. Ragge NK, Baser ME, Riccardi VM, Falk RE. The ocular presentation of neurofibromatosis 2. *Eye.* 1997;11:12–8.

6. Ragge NK, Traboulsi EI. The phakomatoses. In: Traboulsi EI, ed. *Genetic Diseases of the Eye.* New York: Oxford University Press; 1998:733–775.
7. Rouleau GA, Wertelecki W, Haines JL, Hobbs WJ, Trofatter JA, Seizinger BR, et al. Genetic linkage of bilateral acoustic neurofibromatosis to a DNA marker on chromosome 22. *Nature.* 1987;329:246–248.
8. Sippel KC. Ocular findings in neurofibromatosis type 1. *Int Ophthalmol Clin.* 2001;41:25–40.
9. von Recklinghausen FD. *Ueber die multiplen Fibrome der Haut und ihre Beziehung zu den multiplen Neuromen Festschrift zur Feier des funfundzwanzigjahrigen Bestehens des pathologischen Instituts zu Berlin.* Berlin, Germany: Hirschwald; 1882.
10. Wertelecki W, Rouleau GA, Superneau DW, Forehand LW, Williams JP, Haines JL, et al. Neurofibromatosis 2: clinical and DNA linkage studies of a large kindred. *N Engl J Med.* 1988;319(5):278–283.

Phakomatoses: Sturge-Weber Syndrome

1. Celebi S, Alagoz G, Aykan U. Ocular findings in Sturge-Weber syndrome. *Eur J Ophthalmol.* 2000;10:239–243.
2. Enjolras O, Riche MC, Merland JJ. Facial port-wine stains and Sturge-Weber syndrome. *Pediatrics.* 1985;76:48.
3. Shields JA, Shields CL. Vascular tumors of the uvea. In: Shields JA, Shields CL, eds. *Intraocular Tumors: A Text and Atlas.* Philadelphia: WB Saunders; 1992:239.
4. Susac JO, Smith JL, Scelfo RJ. The "tomato-catsup" fundus in Sturge-Weber syndrome. *Arch Ophthalmol.* 1974;92:69.
5. Tan OT, Gilchrest BA. Laser therapy for selected cutaneous vascular lesions in the pediatric population: a review. *Pediatrics.* 1988;82:652.

Phakomatoses: Tuberous Sclerosis

1. Bourneville DM. Sclerose tubereuse des circonvolutions cerebrales: Idiote et epilepsie hemiplegique. *Arch Neurol.* 1880;1:81.
2. Fryer AE, Chalmers A, Connor JM, Fraser I, Povey S, Yates AD, et al. Evidence that the gene for tuberous sclerosis is on chromosome 9. *Lancet.* 1987;1:659–661.
3. Nyboer JH, Robertson DM, Gomez MR. Retinal lesions in tuberous sclerosis. *Arch Ophthalmol.* 1976;94:1277.
4. Ragge NK, Traboulsi EI. The phakomatoses. In: Traboulsi EI, ed. *Genetic Diseases of the Eye.* New York: Oxford University Press; 1998:733–775.
5. Shields JA, Shields CL. Glial tumors of the retina and optic disc. In: Shields JA, Shields CL, eds. *Intraocular Tumors: A Text and Atlas.* Philadelphia: WB Saunders; 1992:421.

6. Shields JA, Shields CL. The systemic hamartomatoses. In: Shields JA, Shields CL, eds. *Intraocular Tumors: A Text and Atlas.* Philadelphia: WB Saunders; 1992:519.

Phakomatoses: von Hippel-Lindau Disease

1. De Potter P, Shields CL, Shields JA. Disorders of the orbit: tumors and pseudotumors of the retina. In: De Potter P, Shields JA, Shields CL, eds. *MRI of the Eye and Orbit.* Philadelphia: JB Lippincott; 1995:93.

2. Maher ER, Yates JRW, Harries R, Benjamin C, Harris R, Moore AT, et al: Clinical features and natural history of von Hippel-Lindau disease. *Q J Med.* 1990;77:1151–1163.

3. Neumann HPH, Wiestler OD. Clustering of features of von Hippel-Lindau syndrome: evidence of a complex gene locus. *Lancet.* 1991;337:1052.

4. Ragge NK, Traboulsi EI. The phakomatoses. In: Traboulsi EI, ed. *Genetic Diseases of the Eye.* New York: Oxford University Press; 1998:733–775.

5. Seizinger BR, Rouleau GA, Ozelius LJ, Lane AH, Farmer GE, Lamiell JM, et al. von Hippel-Lindau disease maps to the region of chromosome 3 associated with renal cell carcinoma. *Nature.* 1988;332:268–269.

Phakomatoses: Wyburn-Mason Syndrome

1. Archer DB, Deutman A, Ernest JT, Krill AE. Arteriovenous communication of the retina. *Am J Ophthalmol.* 1973;75:224.

2. Magnus H. Aneurysma arterioso-venosum retinale. *Virchows Arch Pathol Anat Physiol.* 1874;60:38.

3. Wyburn-Mason R. Arteriovenous aneurysm of mid-brain and retina, facial naevi, and mental changes. *Brain.* 1943;66:163.

Retinoblastoma

1. Eng C, Li FP, Abramson DH, Ellsworth RM, Wong FL, Goldman MB, et al. Mortality from second tumors among long-term survivors of retinoblastoma. *J Natl Cancer Inst.* 1993;85:1121–1128.

2. Murphree AL, Villablanca JG, Deegan WR, Sato JK, Malogolowkin M, Fisher A, et al. Chemotherapy plus local treatment in the management of intraocular retinoblastoma. *Arch Ophthalmol.* 1996;114:1348–1356.

3. Scott IU, Murray TG, Feuer WJ, Van Quill K, Markoe AM, Ling S, et al. External beam radiotherapy in retinoblastoma: tumor control and comparison of 2 techniques. *Arch Ophthalmol.* 1999;117:766–770.

chapter 9

Inflammatory Diseases

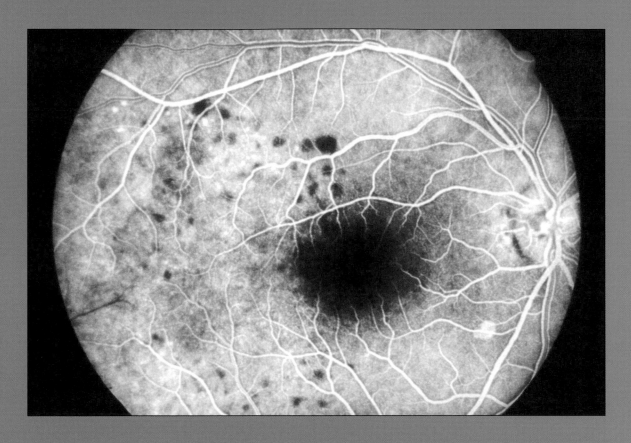

Justin L. Gottlieb, MD

Nancy M. Holekamp, MD

Robert E. Parnes, MD

ACUTE POSTERIOR MULTIFOCAL PLACOID PIGMENT EPITHELIOPATHY

Acute posterior multifocal placoid pigment epitheliopathy (APMPPE) is one of the inflammatory white dot syndromes. It is characterized by acute, bilateral loss of vision in young healthy men or women between the ages of 20 and 50 years. Approximately one third of individuals report an antecedent viral illness.

Symptoms

Symptoms of APMPPE include a rapid onset of blurred vision often associated with central and paracentral scotomas. Visual loss is usually bilateral but may be asymmetric. Individuals may complain of photopsia, a symptom reported by persons with other inflammatory white dot disorders as well.

Clinical Features

In APMPPE, the anterior segment usually appears normal, although episcleritis, iritis, and bilateral perilimbal anterior stromal corneal infiltrates have been reported. Mild vitreous cells usually are present. The ophthalmoscopic examination is characterized by bilateral, multifocal yellowish white placoid lesions located primarily in the posterior pole at the level of the retinal pigment epithelium (RPE). The lesions fade over the course of 1 to 2 weeks. The acute lesions are replaced by varying degrees of RPE abnormalities including atrophy and hyperpigmentation. Atypical findings include papillitis, periphlebitis, central retinal vein occlusion, disc neovascularization, and subhyaloid hemorrhage.

Ancillary Testing

Intravenous fluorescein angiography (IVFA) reveals a characteristic "block early, stain late" pattern. In the early phase of the angiogram, the acute lesions are hypofluorescent. The hypofluorescence is related to both the gray-white opacification of the RPE and choroidal nonperfusion. The lesions become hyperfluorescent in the late phase of the study. In the quiescent stage of APMPPE, varying degrees of hypofluorescence and hyperfluorescence are revealed by IVFA, depending on the extent of the RPE derangement.

Indocyanine green (ICG) angiography reveals hypofluorescence of the active and healed lesions, highlighting the role of choroidal nonperfusion in APMPPE. Electrophysiologic testing may demonstrate an abnormal electro-oculogram.

Pathology/Pathogenesis

The etiology of APMPPE is not well understood. An abnormal immune response to an inciting agent—possibly viral—has been postulated. The early hypofluorescence of the acute lesions demonstrated by IVFA and ICG angiography suggests that nonperfusion or infarction of the choroid, perhaps secondary to vasculitis, may be the primary disorder; the multifocal placoid lesions may be related to RPE ischemia or infarction.

Acute posterior multifocal placoid pigment epitheliopathy has been described in association with mumps, Wegener's granulomatosis, ulcerative colitis, group A streptococcal infection, tuberculosis, previous hepatitis B vaccination, and Lyme disease; however, the nature of these associations is unclear. Associations with HLA-B7 and HLA-DR2 also have been reported.

Treatment/Prognosis

In general, no treatment is required for APMPPE. Most individuals have an excellent prognosis, with spontaneous recovery of visual acuity to 20/40 or better within 3 to 6 weeks. Recurrences are rare. Long-term loss of vision may be related to extensive RPE alterations, choroidal neovascularization, or the atypical features described herein.

Systemic corticosteroid treatment has been suggested in cases with foveal involvement and/or associated central nervous system (CNS) vasculitis. Although extremely rare, there are reports of death associated with CNS vasculitis that developed within several weeks after the onset of APMPPE.

Systemic Evaluation

No systemic investigation is necessary for typical APMPPE. A neurology workup including magnetic resonance imaging is indicated in individuals with evidence of CNS vasculitis, including severe headache or other neurological signs or symptoms.

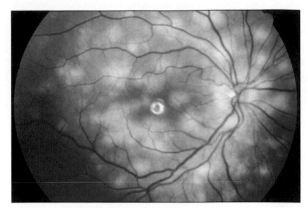

Acute posterior multifocal placoid pigment epitheliopathy is characterized by sudden onset of multifocal yellowish white placoid lesions located at the level of the retinal pigment epithelium.

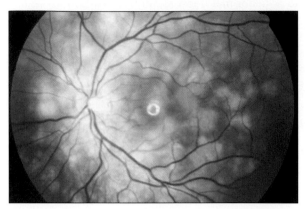

The fellow eye of the same patient demonstrates the bilateral, symmetric nature of acute posterior multifocal placoid pigment epitheliopathy.

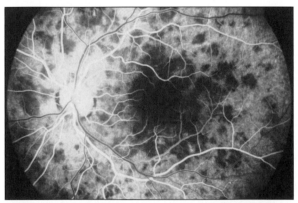

Fluorescein angiography is important in the diagnosis of acute posterior multifocal placoid pigment epitheliopathy. It is characterized by a "block early, stain late" pattern. The lesions are hypofluorescent in the early phase of the angiogram.

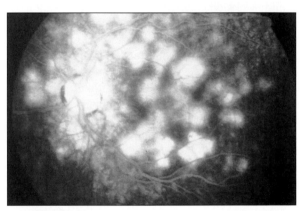

In the late phase of the angiogram, the lesions become hyperfluorescent.

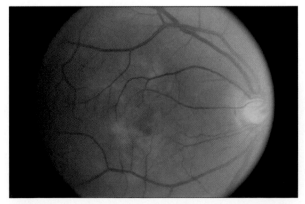

Another example of acute posterior multifocal placoid pigment epitheliopathy shows that the macular lesions are beginning to fade.

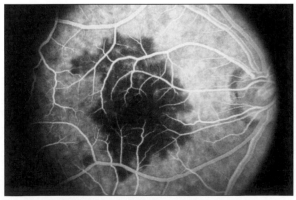

The fluorescein angiogram of the same patient reveals prominent hypofluorescence corresponding to the lesions observed clinically. The hypofluorescence is believed to result from choroidal nonperfusion.

ACUTE RETINAL NECROSIS

Acute retinal necrosis (ARN) is a syndrome of rapidly spreading retinal necrosis, occlusive arteriolar vasculitis, and vitritis that affects both healthy and immunocompromised individuals. In immunocompromised patients ARN is particularly virulent and is designated progressive outer retinal necrosis.

Symptoms

Acute retinal necrosis may present with mild ocular discomfort due to inflammation. Vitritis usually causes floaters or decreased vision due to vitreous haze. A rapid deterioration of vision may occur due to spread of necrosis, optic neuropathy, or retinal vascular occlusion.

Clinical Features

Patients with ARN may present with conjunctival injection, mild to moderate anterior chamber inflammation with keratic precipitates, and normal to elevated intraocular pressure. Vitritis is usually substantial, with dense cellular and protein exudation. Acute retinal necrosis is characterized by peripheral multifocal areas of retinal whitening that rapidly become confluent with full-thickness retinal necrosis. Retinal opacification usually spreads posteriorly and may spare the macula. The whitened retina is replaced with thinned retina and pigmentary scarring. The retinal arterioles often demonstrate perivascular infiltrate, which may cause occlusion and retinal hemorrhage. Optic neuropathy may be a cause of significant visual loss. Retinal detachment is a frequent outcome due to the development of large irregular holes in necrotic retina and severe proliferative vitreoretinopathy. Less common findings are optic neuritis, retinal vascular occlusion, and ocular neovascularization.

Ancillary Testing

Fluorescein angiography demonstrates decreased perfusion to areas of retinal necrosis. Arterial occlusion may be demonstrated posterior to necrotic retina. Inflammation and breakdown of the blood-retinal barrier cause fluorescein leakage from retinal capillaries. Laboratory testing may rule out other causes of retinal whitening.

Pathology/Pathogenesis

Reports have linked ARN with varicella-zoster virus, herpes simplex virus, cytomegalovirus, and toxoplasmosis. Polymerase chain reaction demonstration of herpesvirus family DNA in the vitreous of patients with ARN as well as the positive response to intravenous acyclovir suggests that herpesvirus family is the cause of ARN.

Histopathologic examination shows sharply defined zones of full-thickness necrotizing retinitis associated with replicating herpesvirus along with occlusive vasculitis of the choroid and retina.

Treatment/Prognosis

Early studies indicate that the natural course of untreated eyes is poor, with less than 28% of eyes obtaining a final visual acuity better than 20/200 because of retinal detachment. Antiviral therapy and advanced vitreoretinal techniques have decreased this degree of visual loss to less than 30% of cases. The percentage of bilateral disease has also been decreased by the early recognition of disease and immediate use of intravenous acyclovir. Anticoagulation with aspirin as well as corticosteroids has been recommended to prevent severe visual loss due to ischemic optic neuropathy. Corticosteroids may also serve to decrease the chorioretinal and vitreous inflammation.

Prophylactic confluent laser photocoagulation applied posterior to the areas of retinitis has been used to reduce the risk of retinal detachment. Surgery for retinal detachment following ARN invariably uses silicone oil because of the atrophic nature of the retina.

Systemic Evaluation

It is important to assess the patient's level of systemic immunocompetence, as this may influence the treatment regimen. Intravitreal antiviral medications have been suggested for immunocompromised patients.

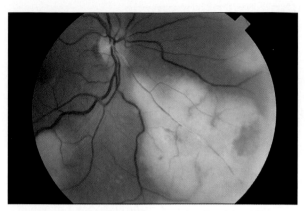

Acute retinal necrosis with areas of yellowish white, full-thickness retinitis with perivascular sheathing of the inferonasal retinal arteriole.

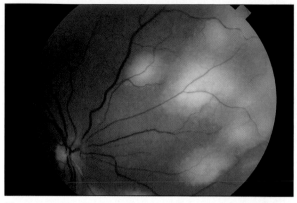

The areas of retinal necrosis may become confluent. This finding is most notable in the peripheral retina.

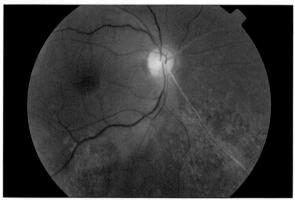

Fundus photograph of the same patient following treatment with acyclovir. Necrosis is replaced with retinal atrophy and retinal pigmentary alterations. The arteriole is sclerotic.

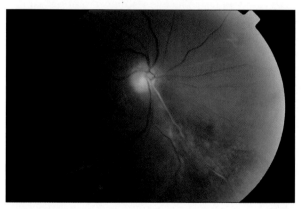

Retinal detachment is a common cause of visual loss in patients with acute retinal necrosis. The retina becomes atrophic, with multiple holes leading to retinal detachment.

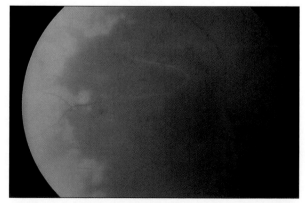

Fundus photograph of an otherwise healthy man who developed acute retinal necrosis is characterized by widespread peripheral retinal necrosis and arteritis.

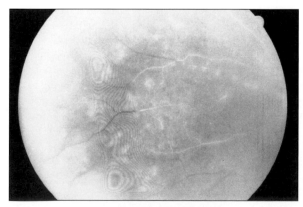

Fluorescein angiogram of the same patient demonstrates multifocal branch retinal artery occlusions as a result of arteritis.

BEHÇET'S DISEASE

Behçet's disease is an immune complex disease with occlusive vasculitis as the main pathologic feature. The disease is found worldwide but predominantly in the Middle and Far East.

Symptoms

The symptoms of Behçet's disease are primarily those of iridocyclitis—periorbital pain, erythema, photophobia, and blurred vision. The vitritis, vaculitis, and retinal infiltrates of posterior disease may lead to visual loss.

Clinical Features

The diagnosis of Behçet's disease is based on the presence of various clinical features. The diagnosis requires recurrent oral ulcerations plus two of the following: recurrent genital ulcerations, eye lesions, skin lesions, and a positive pathergy test. The eye findings are observed in most patients, usually occurring 3 to 4 years after buccal and genital lesions. There may be asymmetric and non-concurrent disease, but it is nearly always bilateral.

The anterior segment disease is classically iridocyclitis with hypopyon. The anterior uveitis may have a rapid, "explosive" onset. Without treatment, the iridocyclitis may resolve in 3 to 4 weeks, but usually recurs.

The characteristic posterior segment lesion is retinal vasculitis, which may involve both the arteries and veins, with arterial occlusion and retinal necrosis. Perivascular sheathing and retinal exudation are observed. Vitritis is always present acutely. Papillitis is present acutely in 25% of cases.

Recurrences are the rule, and visual loss is associated with iris atrophy and posterior synechiae; cataract; vitreous cells; narrowed, occluded retinal vessels; and optic atrophy. Retinal neovascularization may be seen in late disease due to ischemic retinopathy.

Ancillary Testing

Fluorescein angiography shows leakage from retinal vessels before sheathing may be seen clinically. Macular cystic leakage may be found. Decreased fluorescein leakage may serve as a marker of response to therapy.

Pathology/Pathogenesis

The cause of Behçet's disease remains unknown. It has a strong association with HLA-B5 phenotype and subtype HLA-Bw51, suggesting genetic susceptibility. Behçet's disease is likely due to a dysregulation of the immune response, resulting in immune complex formation and vasculitis.

Treatment/Prognosis

Immunosuppressive agents are required for effective treatment. These agents suppress inflammation, reduce the frequency and severity of recurrences, and may halt retinal involvement. Along with the acute use of corticosteroids, other immunosuppressive agents include chlorambucil, colchicine, and dapsone. Sustained intraocular drug delivery systems for patients with chronic uveitis are being studied.

The natural course of Behçet's disease is poor. Most patients will lose most vision within 5 years without treatment. Even with aggressive treatment many patients may experience visual loss.

Systemic Evaluation

The ophthalmologist must follow up patients along with the dermatologist, neurologist, rheumatologist, and others. The greatest mortality arises from central nervous system involvement—untreated neurologic disease is associated with 50% mortality.

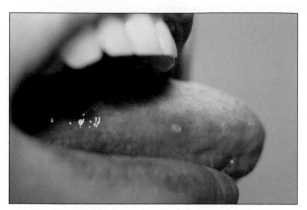

Systemic findings in Behçet's disease include oral aphthous ulcers, recurrent genital ulcerations, and skin lesions.

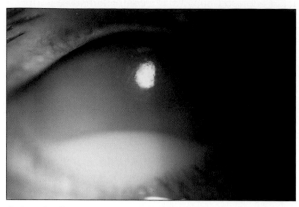

Behçet's disease may present with iridocyclitis and hypopyon, as seen in this patient.

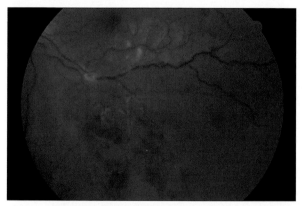

Retinal findings in patients with Behçet's disease include retinal vasculitis, retinal vascular occlusions, and focal areas of retinitis. This woman had vasculitis with a branch retinal vein occlusion.

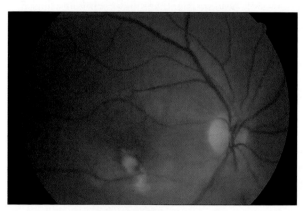

Fundus photograph of a 40-year-old woman with Behçet's disease. She had a focal retinal infiltrate, intraretinal hemorrhage, and an epiretinal membrane.

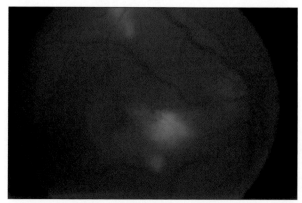

This patient had areas of retinal whitening, with the most notable lesion in the macula. Also present are intraretinal hemorrhage and mild disc edema.

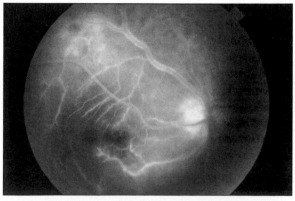

Fluorescein angiogram of the same patient reveals ischemia corresponding to the area of retinal whitening.

BIRDSHOT CHORIORETINOPATHY

Birdshot chorioretinopathy is a rare, bilateral posterior uveitis and chorioretinitis with distinctive fundus lesions and a strong HLA-A29 association. It is a chronic disorder characterized by intermittent exacerbations and remissions. Birdshot chorioretinopathy typically affects healthy individuals in the fifth through seventh decades; women are affected more than men.

Symptoms

Symptoms of birdshot chorioretinopathy include blurred vision, floaters, photopsia, nyctolopia, and dyschromatopsia. Visual loss is insidious, and exacerbations and remissions are common.

Clinical Features

The anterior segment of affected patients is usually normal, although mild iritis and keratic precipitates may be seen. Vitreous cells are prominent. Characteristic fundus lesions are bilateral, cream-colored, oval spots located at the level of the retinal pigment epithelium and choroid. The lesions vary from one-fourth to three-fourths disc diameter in size and are distributed in the postequatorial fundus (usually, they are most notable nasal to the optic disc). Sequelae include cystoid macular edema (CME), optic disc edema or pallor, epiretinal membrane formation, and choroidal neovascularization. Retinal vascular abnormalities include arteriolar narrowing, vascular tortuosity, and intraretinal hemorrhages.

Ancillary Testing

Intravenous fluorescein angiography demonstrates hypofluorescence of the lesions in the early phase, with or without hyperfluorescence in the late phase. Vascular leakage and CME are common.

Indocyanine green angiography is interesting in that it often reveals more lesions than detected by ophthalmoscopy or fluorescein angiography. Lesions are usually hypofluorescent in the early and mid-phases of the study. They may become isofluorescent or remain hypofluorescent in the late phase.

Electrophysiologic testing may demonstrate an abnormal electroretinogram and a subnormal electro-oculogram.

Pathology/Pathogenesis

The etiology of birdshot chorioretinitis is unclear. Because of the strong HLA-A29 association and cell-mediated responses to retinal S antigen (approximately 50%), an unspecified immune mechanism is postulated.

Treatment/Prognosis

Treatment for birdshot chorioretinitis is directed mainly at the vitritis and CME. The mainstay of treatment is immunosuppressive agents such as topical, periocular, and systemic corticosteroids and low-dose cyclosporine (2.5 to 5.0 mg/kg/day).

Systemic Evaluation

Birdshot chorioretinitis may be associated with vitiligo and hearing loss. HLA-A29 blood testing is helpful in distinguishing birdshot chorioretinitis from the other inflammatory white dot syndromes.

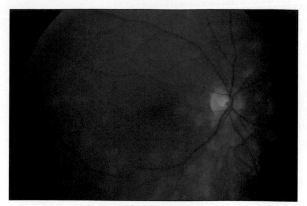

Birdshot choroidopathy is characterized by bilateral, symmetric, cream-colored, oval spots at the level of the retinal pigment epithelium.

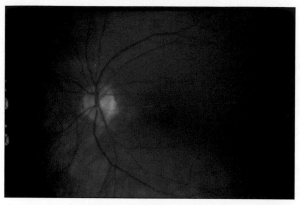

Common associations include vitritis, retinal vascular narrowing, disc pallor, and cystoid macular edema.

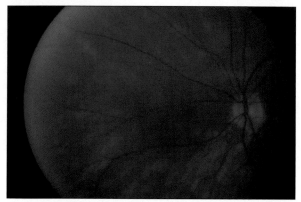

The inflammatory white dots are most notable in the posterior fundus nasal to the optic disc.

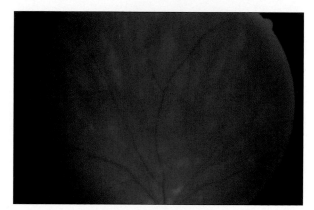

The inflammatory white dots are usually one-fourth to three-fourths disc diameter in size. They often assume a radiating pattern from the optic disc.

CYTOMEGALOVIRUS RETINITIS

Cytomegalovirus (CMV) retinochoroiditis occurs primarily in the unborn infant and the immunocompromised adult. This once uncommon disease became common with the advent of acquired immunodeficiency syndrome (AIDS). In the early years of the US AIDS epidemic, 30% of human immunodeficiency virus (HIV)-positive patients developed CMV retinitis. Since the introduction of antiretroviral therapy in 1996, the prevalence of this disease has decreased dramatically.

Symptoms

Symptoms of CMV are present in up to 75% of infected eyes. Peripheral CMV retinitis typically produces floaters and visual field cuts. Posterior pole disease is more frequently accompanied by blurred vision or blind spots. Isolated macular disease or CMV optic neuritis is uncommon but can cause profound and sudden loss of vision.

Clinical Features

Cytomegalovirus retinitis has two clinical presentations: fulminant and indolent. Fulminant CMV retinitis is classically described as a "pizza" fundus; it causes a necrotizing retinitis that produces confluent retinal whitening associated with retinal hemorrhages and vascular sheathing. Vitreous and anterior chamber cells are invariably present. Indolent or granular CMV retinitis has less edema and a faint, gray opacification with little hemorrhage or vascular sheathing. In both types, the leading edge of infection will display an advancing, irregular, granular border often with small, isolated satellite lesions. Healed, old infection is characterized by fibroglial retinal scarring and mottling of the underlying retinal pigment epithelium.

Frosted branch angiitis is a rare association. Immune recovery uveitis may be seen in patients following successful anti-HIV therapy.

Ancillary Testing

Fluorescein angiography is not necessary for the diagnosis or management of CMV retinitis. Serial fundus photography is integral to the management of this disease.

Pathology/Pathogenesis

Cytomegalovirus is a DNA virus and a member of the herpesvirus family. It has been identified in all layers of the retina. Infection spreads by cell-to-cell transmission of the virus. Histopathologically, CMV retinitis destroys retinal architecture; many enlarged cells containing Cowdry type A intranuclear eosinophilic inclusions with surrounding clear zones give the cells an "owl's eye" appearance.

Treatment/Prognosis

Immune reconstitution in transplant patients or AIDS patients can induce resolution of CMV retinitis. The first three drugs approved for treatment of CMV retinitis are ganciclovir, foscarnet, and cidofovir. Although the choice of agent and route of therapy is complex, in general, patients are started on induction therapy followed by maintenance therapy. Approximately 85% of treated patients will respond, but reactivation is the rule, prompting reinduction or switching to a new agent. Intravitreal gancyclovir implants are an alternative to systemic antiviral therapy. Retinal detachment is a particularly severe complication that may occur in 15% to 40% of eyes.

Systemic Evaluation

All patients suspected of having CMV retinitis should undergo HIV testing. If positive, CD4+ and viral load counts should be performed. Cytomegalovirus retinitis is most commonly observed in patients with CD4+ counts less than 50 µL. Most HIV-positive patients are CMV seropositive, so attempts to isolate virus from nonocular body fluids are non-diagnostic. Polymerase chain reaction (PCR)-based analysis of vitreous fluid offers highly diagnostic sensitivity and specificity and can be used in atypical or unresponsive cases.

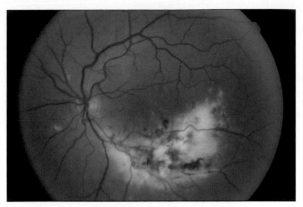

Cytomegalovirus retinitis is characterized by full-thickness retinitis associated with retinal hemorrhage. It commonly affects the posterior fundus in a perivascular distribution.

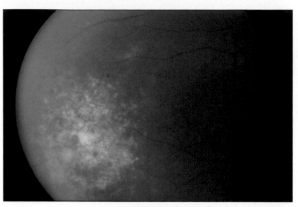

Peripheral cytomegalovirus retinitis often has a granular pattern with less intraretinal hemorrhage. Small satellite lesions extending from the main area of retinitis are common.

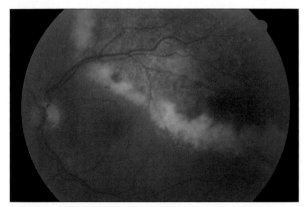

Cytomegalovirus retinitis may demonstrate a leading edge of active retinitis and a wake of atrophy of the retina and retinal pigment epithelium reminiscent of a brush fire.

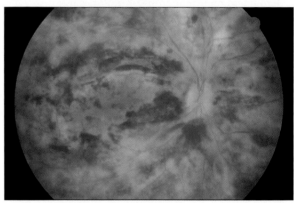

Untreated cytomegalovirus retinitis may result in a diffuse retinitis associated with intraretinal hemorrhage resembling a "pizza" fundus.

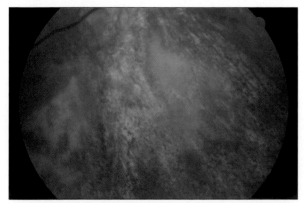

Old cytomegalovirus infection is characterized by fibroglial retinal scarring and mottling of the underlying retinal pigment epithelium.

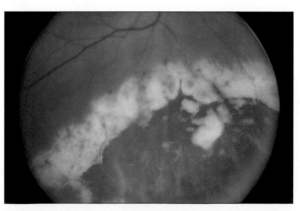

A late complication of cytomegalovirus retinitis is retinal detachment, as seen inferiorly below the active retinitis in this figure. Retinal detachment results from multiple holes in the thin, atrophic retina in areas of previous infection.

DIFFUSE UNILATERAL SUBACUTE NEURORETINITIS

Diffuse unilateral subacute neuroretinitis (DUSN) is an infectious disease caused by a nematode that may be found in the vitreous or subretinal space. It may cause profound loss of vision in one eye, usually in children or young adults. There is one case report of bilateral DUSN.

Symptoms

Patients can present with acute visual loss ranging from 20/30 to 20/200. Floaters and ocular discomfort are less common symptoms. In approximately 50% of patients, particularly children, visual loss is insidious, and the patient comes to medical attention only late in the course of disease. By that time severe visual loss is permanent.

Clinical Features

Findings in early DUSN include mild vitritis, mild optic disc edema, and recurrent crops of multifocal, gray-white outer retinal lesions. The round, white nematode may be found adjacent to these active lesions. Findings in late DUSN include optic atrophy, narrowed retinal arterioles, and striking degenerative changes in the retinal pigment epithelium (RPE) and retina ("unilateral wipe-out syndrome"). A relative afferent pupillary defect is usually present.

Ancillary Testing

Fluorescein angiography in early DUSN shows that the gray-white areas of retinitis are hypofluorescent early but stain late. There is optic nerve hyperfluorescence. Angiography is not helpful in locating the nematode. Fluorescein angiography in late DUSN shows widespread hyperfluorescence caused by window defects resulting from the damaged RPE. The electroretinographic findings range from subnormal to extinguished in the affected eye (and normal in the fellow eye).

Pathology/Pathogenesis

Diffuse unilateral subacute neuroretinitis is caused by at least two different nematodes, neither of which has been definitively identified. The smaller of the two measures 400 μm to 1000 μm in length and is thought to possibly be *Ancylosytoma caninum*. The larger measures 1500 μm to 2000 μm in length and is thought to possibly be *Baylisascaris procyonis*. The pathogenesis of DUSN appears to be mediated by worm waste products acting as toxins damaging both the inner and outer retina. Thus, visual loss is thought to be caused by physiologic retinal damage by worm end products rather than by anatomic retinal damage by the migrating worm itself.

Treatment/Prognosis

Photocoagulation of the nematode is the treatment of choice. It effectively kills the worm, causes little or no inflammation, and inactivates the disease process. Visual prognosis is good only if the worm is killed shortly after the onset of visual loss. In eyes in which the nematode cannot be located and destroyed, oral thiabendazole or ivermectin have been tried to arrest the disease.

Systemic Evaluation

Patients with DUSN do not manifest systemic disease. Stool samples do not show ova or parasites. Eosinophilia is rare. Serologic studies are prone to error in interpretation. Thus, a systemic evaluation is of little help in making the diagnosis of DUSN.

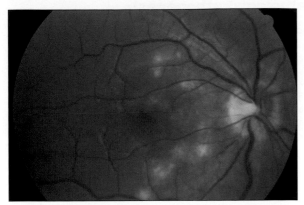

Diffuse unilateral subacute neuroretinitis is considered one of the inflammatory white dot syndromes. Clusters of small white dots are visible in the vicinity of the nematode.

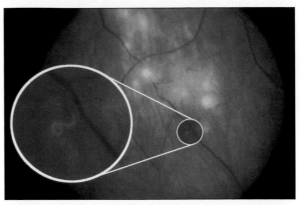

Diffuse unilateral subacute neuroretinitis is caused by a mobile, small, white nematode located in the potential space between the neurosensory retina and the retinal pigment epithelium. (Photograph courtesy Ditte Hess, CRA, and Rick Stratton.)

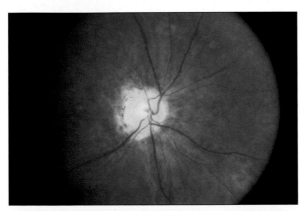

End-stage diffuse unilateral subacute neuroretinitis is characterized by optic disc pallor, retinal vascular narrowing, and diffuse mottling of the retinal pigment epithelium.

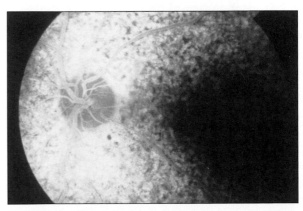

This fluorescein angiogram reveals a "salt and pepper" pattern of hyperfluorescence as a result of the retinal pigment mottling.

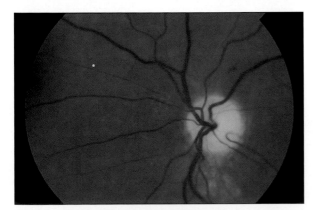

Fundus photograph in a patient with diffuse unilateral subacute neuroretinitis reveals a small nematode located nasal to the optic disc.

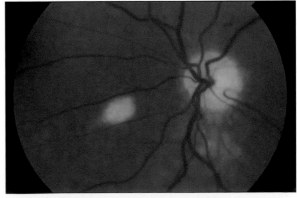

Fundus photograph of the same patient following laser photocoagulation of the nematode. Laser photocoagulation is effective when the nematode is detected early in the disease course.

ENDOPHTHALMITIS

Endophthalmitis refers to inflammation that may ulti-mately involve all tissues of the eye. Exogenous endoph-thalmitis occurs when trauma or surgery allows microorganisms access into the eye. Endogenous endophthalmitis occurs when microorganisms spread to the eye from another source in the body, usually via the bloodstream. Endophthalmitis is an infrequent clinical entity but has the potential to cause severe visual loss.

Symptoms

In postoperative and posttraumatic endophthalmitis, patients will notice increasing redness and decreasing vision within 1 to 7 days. Pain is usually but not neces-sarily present. The upper eyelid may become edematous and difficult to open. Discharge may be seen in the con-junctival cul-de-sac. In endogenous endophthalmitis, susceptible patients (eg, septic, immunocompromised, users of intravenous drugs) will notice progressively blurred vision or floaters. A chronic bacterial endoph-thalmitis following cataract surgery may masquerade as a chronic uveitis that occurs months to years following intraocular surgery.

Clinical Features

In exogenous endophthalmitis, ophthalmologic examina-tion shows conjunctival injection and chemosis, variable degrees of corneal edema, anterior chamber cells, flare, fibrin, hypopyon, and heavy cellular debris in the vitre-ous. In endogenous endophthalmitis, examination shows vitreous cells and debris with either retinal involvement or a reduced red reflex. In chronic bacterial endoph-thalmitis caused by *Propionibacterium acnes,* a creamy-white plaque may be visible within the peripheral lens capsule.

Ancillary Testing

The clinical diagnosis is confirmed by obtaining aqueous and vitreous for culture on blood agar, chocolate agar, Sabouraud's media or broth, and thioglycolate broth. Material is also placed on two glass slides for Gram and Giemsa stains. In post-traumatic endophthalmitis an orbital computed tomography scan is necessary to rule out an intraocular foreign body.

Pathology/Pathogenesis

Bacteria, fungi, protozoa, parasites, and viruses are all capable of producing endophthalmitis. The most com-mon organisms causing acute bacterial endophthalmitis after cataract surgery are *Staphylococcus aureus* and *S epidermidis. Streptococcus pneumoniae* and *Haemophilus influenzae* are common causes of bacterial endophthalmitis following glaucoma filtering surgeries. In traumatic endophthalmitis, *Bacillus* species are fre-quent pathogens. *Propionibacterium acnes* is the most commonly recognized organism causing chronic bacter-ial endophthalmitis following cataract surgery.

Treatment/Prognosis

Intravitreal injection of antibiotics, with or without victrectomy, is the standard of care in endophthalmitis. Antibiotics can also be administered via systemic, peri-ocular, and topical routes. The role of corticosteroids remains controversial. Regarding visual outcome, the most important prognostic indicator is the virulence of the infecting organism. Although the use of prophylactic antibiotics to reduce the occurrence of post-cataract sur-gery endophthalmitis is controversial, most surgeons rec-ommend using preoperative povidone-iodine antisepsis.

Systemic Evaluation

Systemic evaluation is generally not necessary for exogenous endophthalmitis. For endogenous endoph-thalmitis, an aggressive search for the systemic source of infection is indicated, including cultures of the blood, urine, indwelling catheters, and intravenous lines. Involvement of an infectious disease specialist or internist is essential.

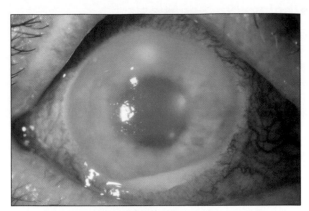

Acute bacterial endophthalmitis following cataract surgery is characterized by conjunctival injection and chemosis, corneal edema, anterior chamber cell and flare, and hypopyon. The degree of pain is variable.

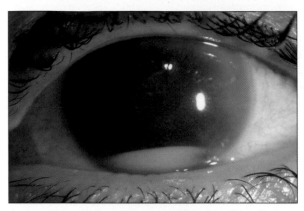

Some patients with acute bacterial endophthalmitis have fibrin in the pupil in addition to the hypopyon. Common organisms include Staphylococcus aureus and S epidermidis.

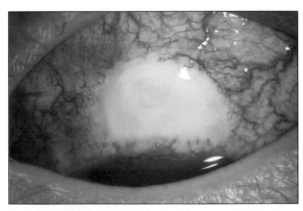

Endophthalmitis may develop in patients following glaucoma filtering surgery, with or without the use of topical antimetabolites. Common bacteria include Streptococcus pneumoniae and Haemophilus influenzae.

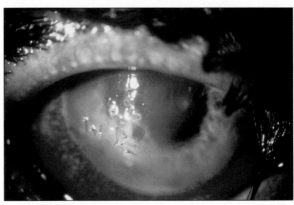

This patient developed endophthalmitis following a penetrating corneal injury. Bacillus species are common causes of traumatic endophthalmitis.

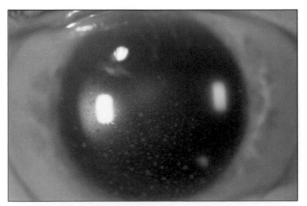

Propionibacterium acnes is the most commonly recognized organism causing chronic bacterial endophthalmitis following cataract surgery. P acnes endophthalmitis may mimic chronic uveitis.

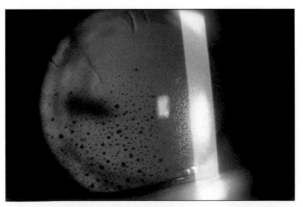

Retroillumination of the same eye reveals the shadow of a capsular plaque in the 9 o'clock position. The patient responded well to pars plana vitrectomy and intraocular vancomycin.

HUMAN IMMUNODEFICIENCY VIRUS RETINOPATHY

Human immunodeficiency virus (HIV) is a retrovirus implicated in the development of acquired immunodeficiency syndrome (AIDS). Infection of helper T cells results in a profound disruption of the cell-mediated immune system. Immunodeficiency leads to susceptibility to blinding infections.

Symptoms

Noninfectious retinopathy is generally asymptomatic. Symptomatic disease is most often secondary to infectious disease occurring with the development of AIDS.

Clinical Features

The most common finding is a noninfectious retinopathy characterized by cotton wool spots, retinal hemorrhages, and microvascular disease. The noninfectious retinopathy does not correlate with the clinical severity of HIV disease. Chorioretinal infectious disease associated with AIDS includes cytomegalovirus retinitis, toxoplasmosis, *Mycobacterium avium-intracellulare* choroiditis, cryptococcus choroiditis, and *Pneumocystis carinii* choroiditis.

Ancillary Testing

Human immunodeficiency virus retinopathy does not require other testing.

Pathology/Pathogenesis

Cotton wool spots result from microinfarction of the nerve fiber layer. Arteriolar deposition of immunoglobulin in the microvasculature around the cotton wool spots suggests an immune complex disease. Attempts to isolate organisms from cotton wool spots have been unsuccessful.

Treatment/Prognosis

Noninfectious HIV retinopathy does not require treatment. While some investigators have speculated that cotton wool spots may represent *P carinii* infection or early cytomegalovirus retinopathy, patients with noninfectious HIV retinopathy should not be subjected to toxic medications. Infectious retinopathy must be aggressively treated.

Systemic Evaluation

The diagnosis of HIV must be considered in patients with unexplained cotton wool spots or intraretinal hemorrhages. Patients with HIV disease or AIDS must be followed up closely by internists or infectious disease specialists for the many systemic diseases associated with immunodeficiency.

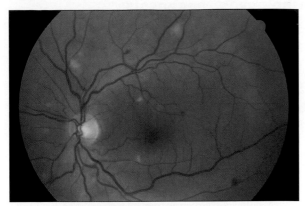

Fundus photograph of a 39-year-old man with human immunodeficiency virus (HIV) disease reveals numerous cotton wool spots and intraretinal hemorrhages characteristic of HIV retinopathy.

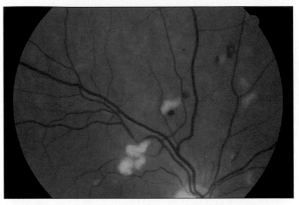

Higher-magnification view of same patient reveals cotton wool spots and intraretinal hemorrhages. A few of the intraretinal hemorrhages have white centers.

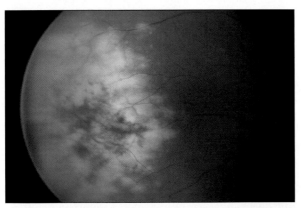

Cytomegalovirus retinitis is the most common opportunistic ocular infection in patients with acquired immunodeficiency syndrome. Cytomegalovirus retinitis is characterized by full-thickness retinitis and intraretinal hemorrhage.

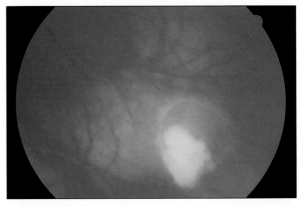

Patients with acquired immunodeficiency syndrome may develop toxoplasmosis retinochoroiditis. The extent of vitritis is low because of the immunodeficiency. Patients may develop diffuse infection with acute retinal necrosis.

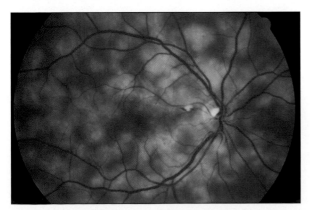

Pneumocystis carinii choroiditis was seen in patients with acquired immunodeficiency syndrome before the use of systemic therapy. Patients were usually asymptomatic in spite of the dramatic appearance of the choroidal lesions.

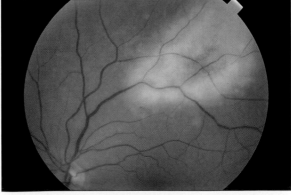

Progressive outer retinal necrosis is a form of acute retinal necrosis seen in patients with acquired immunodeficiency syndrome. It is characterized by full-thickness retinitis without evidence of intraocular inflammation or vasculitis.

INTERMEDIATE UVEITIS

Intermediate uveitis is an idiopathic syndrome of intraocular inflammation centered around the peripheral retina and pars plana. The average age at onset is during the third decade of life, but intermediate uveitis is a common cause of uveitis in children. It represents between 4% and 16% of cases in a uveitis referral practice and 16% to 33% of all uveitis cases in children.

Symptoms

Most commonly, a patient with intermediate uveitis presents with unilateral, painless blurring of vision with floaters. A more dramatic loss of vision may occur in patients with cystoid macular edema (CME), vitreous hemorrhage, or even retinal detachment. Anterior segment symptoms of inflammation are mild and rare but may include pain, redness, and photophobia. While initial symptoms are often unilateral, the disease is ultimately bilateral in 80% of cases.

Clinical Features

Intermediate uveitis is defined by fibrocellular exudative aggregates in the anterior vitreous base over the pars plana and anterior retina. These aggregates may coalesce to form a distinctive "snowbank." Chronic cases may develop neovascularization within or bridging the snowbank as well as vitreous hemorrhage. The intraocular inflammation often leads to CME, the most common cause of visual loss. The vitreous cells often lead to development of epiretinal membrane formation. Acute inflammation may be associated with focal areas of phlebitis and venous dilation. Resultant ischemia may lead to neovascularization and serous and rhegmatogenous retinal detachment. Often, optic nerve edema is present, and neovascularization of the disc may occur.

Ancillary Testing

Fluorescein angiography is important in the evaluation of CME and may be helpful in monitoring response to therapy. Fluorescein angiography is useful in the investigation of cases with phlebitis and/or retinal ischemia.

Pathology/Pathogenesis

The cause of intermediate uveitis is unknown but is presumed to be autoimmune.

Treatment/Prognosis

The majority of patients with intermediate uveitis do well. The final visual outcome depends mostly on macular involvement. Chronic CME, epiretinal membrane formation, and retinal detachment are associated with poorer visual outcome. The most common complications include visually significant cataract, chronic CME, retinal neovascularization, epiretinal membrane, and retinal detachment.

Corticosteroids are very effective in the treatment of the inflammation associated with intermediate uveitis. Systemic and periocular administration is usually required. Neovascularization of the vitreous base requires cryotherapy or panretinal laser photocoagulation. Antimetabolite and immunosuppressive therapy may be required for recalcitrant disease.

Systemic Evaluation

No diagnostic test is available for intermediate uveitis. Diagnostic testing is undertaken primarily to rule out other causes of posterior uveitis.

Intermediate uveitis may be associated with the development of multiple sclerosis. There is a reported 20% chance of developing multiple sclerosis or optic neuritis during a 5-year period after diagnosis with intermediate uveitis. Testing for HLA-DR2 and magnetic resonance imaging of the brain may be indicated in patients with unexplained weakness or optic neuritis.

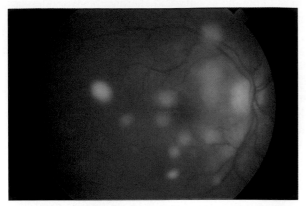

Visual loss in patients with intermediate uveitis is caused by vitreous floaters and cystoid macular edema. The fundus details in this photograph are poor because of vitreous inflammation.

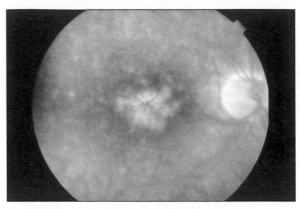

Fluorescein angiography reveals cystoid macular edema in a patient with intermediate uveitis.

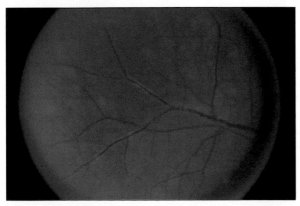

Perivascular sheathing may be seen in patients with intermediate uveitis. The inflammation usually produces a periphlebitis. Peripheral retinal ischemia and retinal neovascularization may develop.

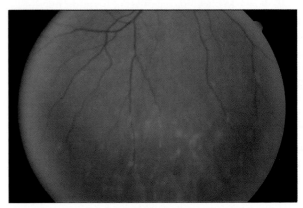

Aggregation of vitreous cells may result in the formation of vitreous "snowballs." This patient had numerous opacities in the inferior vitreous.

MULTIFOCAL CHOROIDITIS AND PANUVEITIS

Multifocal choroiditis and panuveitis (MCP) is a syndrome simulating presumed ocular histoplasmosis syndrome but includes vitreous inflammation, anterior uveitis, and active choroidal lesions. Punctate inner choroiditis (PIC) is a similar syndrome characterized by myopia, photopsia, and scotomas in women, with the choroidal lesions largely confined to the posterior pole. Punctate inner choroiditis has no associated vitritis. These two syndromes likely represent a continuum of severity of one syndrome. Some patients with MCP or PIC may go on to develop localized or widespread subretinal fibrosis.

Symptoms

Patients may present with decreased vision due to floaters and vitritis. Acute choroidal lesions beneath the macula center, cystoid macular edema (CME), or exudation secondary to choroidal neovascularization may cause decreased vision. Retinal pigment epithelial metaplasia and the formation of fibrotic scars in the macula may also cause loss of vision. Some patients may develop peripheral visual field loss not corresponding to focal areas of choroiditis.

Clinical Findings

Punched-out chorioretinal scars with pigmented borders within the posterior pole and periphery similar to those found in presumed ocular histoplasmosis syndrome are typically found in patients with MCP. These lesions are usually 50 µm to 100 µm in diameter. Acute lesions are yellow-white and primarily involve the choroid and outer retina. There is the frequent development of macular and juxtapapillary choroidal neovascularization, which is the most frequent cause of severe visual loss. The presence of vitritis and/or iritis is an important requirement for the definition of MCP, excluding a diagnosis of presumed ocular histoplasmosis syndrome. Some patients initially classified as having PIC may go on to develop vitritis.

The disease is usually bilateral but may be asymmetric, with delayed development of disease in the second eye. There is a predilection for women, and most are affected within their third decade of life.

Ancillary Testing

Fluorescein angiography may demonstrate lesions within the macula that are not visible by ophthalmoscopy. Acute lesions demonstrate early hypofluoresence with late hyperfluorescent staining. Such lesions may develop in the course of observation of a patient. The fluorescein angiogram may demonstrate CME, leakage from acute lesions within the macula, and choroidal neovascularization arising from juxtapapillary or macular scars.

Visual field testing may demonstrate peripheral visual field loss not corresponding to acute choroiditis. Enlarged blind spots have also been reported.

Electrophysiologic study has yielded variable results. Some patients with MCP may have severely reduced electroretinograms, while others may have normal findings. Multifocal electroretinography may demonstrate decreased function within the macula.

Pathology/Pathogenesis

The cause of this disorder is unknown. It has been hypothesized that an exogenous pathogen stimulates an immune response. Subsequent exacerbations may occur without an inciting pathogen.

Treatment/Prognosis

Multifocal choroiditis and panuveitis tends to be a chronic disorder lasting months to years. Visual prognosis is guarded. Severe visual loss may occur due to disciform macular scarring, macular fibrotic scarring, atrophy, or chronic CME.

The use of systemic or periocular steroids may be effective in controlling MCP. Some authors have reported success in the treatment of choroidal neovascularization with corticosteroids, although this may be the natural course of regression of some lesions. Corticosteroids are recommended for treatment of acute infiltrative choroidal lesions within the macula causing visual loss or for the treatment of CME.

Systemic Evaluation

No systemic association has been found. A generalized systemic evaluation for infectious and autoimmune causes of uveitis should be performed.

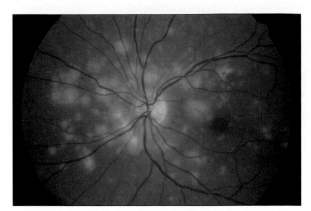

Multiple acute areas of deep chorioretinal infiltration appear yellow-white. A moderate vitritis is present.

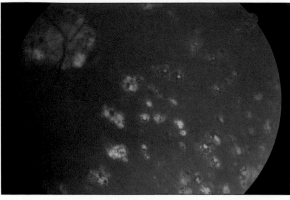

Inactive lesions of multifocal choroiditis are difficult to distinguish from presumed ocular histoplasmosis syndrome. The chorioretinal scars may become more pigmented over time, and subretinal fibrosis is common.

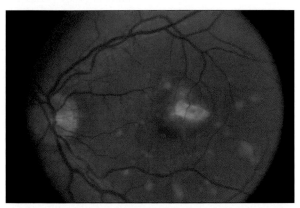

The most common cause of vision loss in patients with multifocal choroiditis and panuveitis is choroidal neovascularization. Note the subretinal blood and fluid in the fovea.

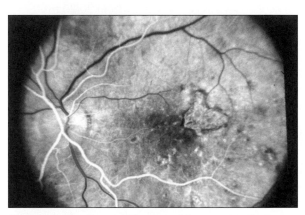

Early venous-phase angiogram of the same patient reveals a classic choroidal neovascular membrane.

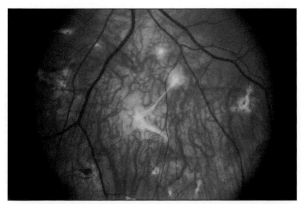

The finding of subretinal fibrotic bands is suggestive of multifocal choroiditis rather than presumed ocular histoplasmosis syndrome.

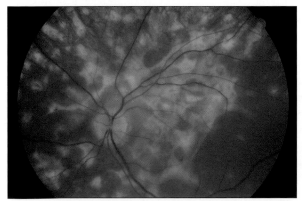

Diffuse subretinal fibrosis syndrome is believed to be an advanced form of multifocal choroiditis with panuveitis.

MULTIPLE EVANESCENT WHITE DOT SYNDROME

Multiple evanescent white dot syndrome (MEWDS) primarily affects young adults between the ages of 20 and 45 years. There is a strong female predilection. Although typically unilateral, bilateral cases of MEWDS have been described. Spontaneous recovery usually occurs within several weeks or months. There are no known racial or hereditary associations.

Symptoms

Patients with MEWDS usually present with sudden visual alterations in one eye. Symptoms include blurred vision, temporal or paracentral scotomas, photopsia, and dyschromatopsia. A preceding viral illness is reported in approximately one third of cases.

Clinical Features

Visual acuity is variable and ranges from 20/20 to 20/400. A small degree of myopia is common. A relative afferent pupillary defect may be present. The anterior segment appears normal, without signs of inflammation. Vitreous cells are mild. The optic disc may be hyperemic or edematous. The characteristic lesions are multiple small, ill-defined white dots located at the level of the outer retina or retinal pigment epithelium (RPE). The lesions may be subtle and usually fade within the first few weeks of the disease. The fovea may have an unusual orange-yellow granularity; this granularity may persist after resolution of the white dot lesions. Atypical findings include circumpapillary patches with or without paramacular involvement and choroidal neovascularization.

Ancillary Testing

Visual field testing often reveals enlargement of the blind spot. Other temporal and paracentral scotomas may be detected.

Fluorescein angiography demonstrates early and late hyperfluorescence of the white dots at the level of the outer retina/RPE. The optic disc may appear hyperfluorescent in the late phase of the study. Indocyanine green (ICG) angiography reveals multiple small, round hypofluorescent spots in the posterior and midperipheral fundus. The number of spots seen on ICG angiography may be more numerous than those seen clinically or with fluorescein angiography.

Electrophysiologic testing may demonstrate a reduced a-wave on the electroretinogram (ERG). The electro-oculogram (EOG) also may be abnormal. The ERG and EOG abnormalities usually normalize with resolution of symptoms.

Pathology/Pathogenesis

The cause of MEWDS is unknown. A viral etiology has been suggested. Fluorescein angiographic and electrophysiologic studies have demonstrated the involvement of the RPE and photoreceptors in MEWDS. The findings with ICG angiography suggest that MEWDS affects the choroidal circulation as well. Multiple evanescent white dot syndrome has been associated with other inflammatory conditions including acute macular neuroretinopathy and multifocal choroiditis and panuveitis.

Treatment/Prognosis

Multiple evanescent white dot syndrome resolves spontaneously without need for treatment. The prognosis is excellent, with most patients achieving normal vision and visual fields within several weeks to months. Visual field loss, photopsia, and dyschromatopsia may persist. Recurrence is unusual but has been reported. Bilateral cases with asymmetric involvement or progressive bilateral involvement have occurred, but are rare. Multiple evanescent white dot syndrome should be considered in the differential diagnosis of acute idiopathic blind spot enlargement syndrome (AIBSES). Controversy exists as to whether AIBSES is the same condition as MEWDS following resolution of the white dots.

Systemic Evaluation

No systemic evaluation is required. Multiple evanescent white dot syndrome has been described following hepatitis B vaccination, but the importance of this association is unclear.

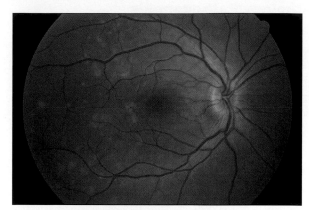

Multiple evanescent white dot syndrome is characterized by the presence of subtle white inflammatory lesions located at the level of the retinal pigment epithelium.

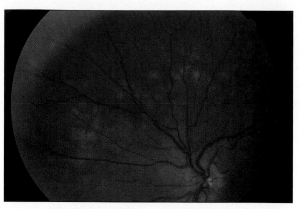

The white dots are located in the posterior fundus. They occasionally assume a "wreath-like pattern" around the optic disc.

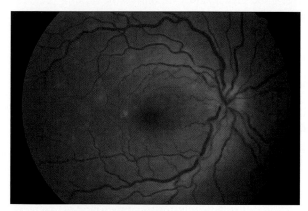

Optic disc edema is common in patients with multiple evanescent white dot syndrome. If present, vitreous inflammation is usually mild.

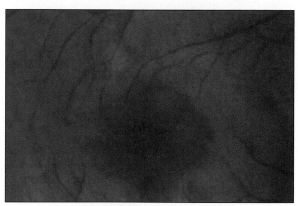

A peculiar orange granularity of the fovea is seen in some patients with multiple evanescent white dot syndrome. The orange granularity usually develops during the resolution phase of the condition.

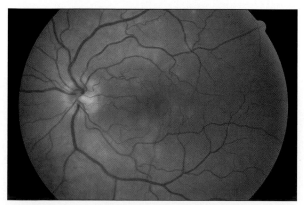

This 31-year-old woman presented with photopsia and temporal visual field loss in her left eye. Ophthalmoscopic examination reveals acute multiple evanescent white dot syndrome.

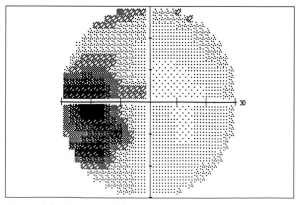

A visual field study of the same patient demonstrates marked enlargement of the blind spot. This blind spot enlargement may persist for several months.

NEURORETINITIS

Neuroretinitis is more appropriately termed optic neuritis with secondary retinal involvement. A number of known disease entities can produce the clinical syndrome of unilateral visual loss, optic disc swelling, and macular star with spontaneous resolution. The term Leber's idiopathic stellate neuroretinitis is reserved for those cases in which no specific etiologic agent has been identified.

Symptoms

The presenting symptom is blurred vision, usually in one eye. Color vision is often affected out of proportion to changes in visual acuity. Rarely, patients will complain of retrobulbar pain with eye movement. A viral prodrome has been reported in approximately 50% of cases.

Clinical Features

Visual acuity is generally between 20/40 and 20/200. Due to optic nerve involvement, an afferent pupillary defect in unilateral disease can usually be elicited. Early in the disease, optic disc edema may be mild to severe, and produces a shallow exudative detachment of the macula. As the optic nerve involvement resolves, lipid deposition occurs in the macula, producing a characteristic macular star. Focal retinochoroiditis and areas of retinal vasculitis may be seen. Vascular occlusions are less common findings.

Ancillary Testing

Fluorescein angiography demonstrates intense hyperfluorescence of the optic nerve. No leakage from the retinal vessels is seen in the macula. Visual field testing will usually be abnormal, demonstrating a cecocentral scotoma or, less commonly, a central scotoma or arcuate defect. Color vision testing will be subnormal.

Pathology/Pathogenesis

Stellate maculopathy can be caused by any disease that affects capillary permeability in the optic nerve. An exudate rich in protein and lipid leaks from deep optic nerve capillaries into the peripapillary retina and macula. With resorption of the serous component, the lipid and protein precipitate in the outer plexiform layer are engulfed by macrophages, creating the characteristic macular star.

Treatment/Prognosis

If all treatable causes of neuroretinitis have been ruled out, no treatment is indicated for Leber's idiopathic stellate neuroretinitis. The optic nerve findings resolve spontaneously in 6 to 12 weeks, and the macular star resolves in 6 to 12 months. In some cases, optic nerve pallor or macular pigmentary changes remain. Most patients recover good visual acuity. In one study, 66% of patients regained 20/20 visual acuity.

Systemic Evaluation

Cat scratch disease is a frequent cause of neuroretinitis. All patients should undergo blood testing for IgG and IgM titers to *Bartonella henselae* and *B quintana*. Syphilis and Lyme disease should be excluded with Venereal Disease Research Laboratories (VDRL) test, fluorescent treponemal antibody absorption (FTA-ABS) test, and Lyme titers. Other conditions that may produce these clinical findings, including systemic hypertension, diabetes mellitus, and anterior ischemic optic neuropathy, should be evaluated with a complete physical examination.

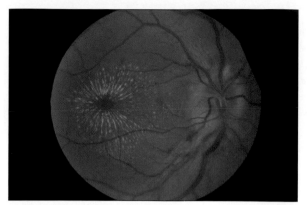

Neuroretinitis related to cat scratch disease is characterized by optic disc edema with a macular star in one eye.

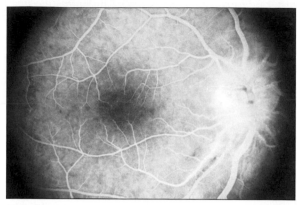

Fluorescein angiography reveals optic disc hyperfluorescence related to optic disc edema. The retinal blood vessels appear normal.

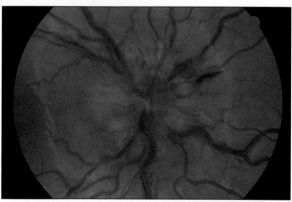

Early in the disease course, optic disc edema may be present without the macular star.

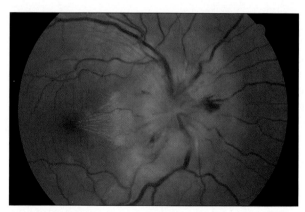

The macular star is most prominent nasal to the fovea in the papillomacular bundle. The macular star results from protein and lipid deposition in the outer plexiform layer.

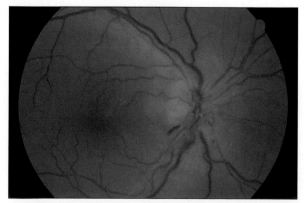

This pair of photographs demonstrates the natural course of cat scratch neuroretinitis. Leakage of fluid from the optic disc causes fluid extension into the fovea.

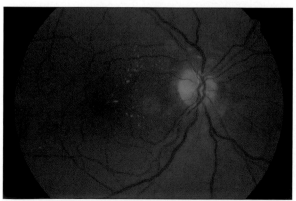

As the fluid resorbs, the macular star becomes more prominent. The star may persist for several months.

POSTERIOR SCLERITIS

Posterior scleritis is defined as scleral inflammation that occurs primarily posterior to the equator. It is the rarest form of scleritis. Posterior scleritis is typically unilateral, more common in women, and most likely to present in middle age. Up to 50% of patients will have an underlying disease. As many as 40% of patients will have recurrences.

Symptoms

The most common symptoms are decreased vision, pain, and redness. The extent of visual loss depends on the extent of macular involvement. The pain may be severe, and is frequently described as deep, boring pain behind the globe. The degree of redness is highly variable, and some cases of posterior scleritis may appear white and quiet.

Clinical Features

Visual acuity may range from normal to no light perception. The globe may be tender to touch. The anterior segment may be quiet or show iridocyclitis or anterior scleritis. The posterior segment may show vitreous cells, optic nerve edema, retinovascular occlusion, choroidal folds, focal choroidal mass, or exudative retinal detachment. Orbital involvement may produce ptosis, proptosis, or restricted motility.

Ancillary Testing

Ultrasonography is an important test. It is diagnostic if thickening of the sclera and uvea are associated with edema within Tenon's space, producing the classic "T" sign. A computed tomographic scan with contrast will show diffuse scleral thickening. It may also aid in finding any adjacent orbital disease. Fluorescein angiography is non-diagnostic but may show multiple small leaks at the level of the retinal pigment epithelium that then fill a neurosensory detachment. Optic nerve leakage, vasculitis, and chorioretinal folds can also be seen.

Pathology/Pathogenesis

While vasculitis has been implicated in the pathogenesis, histopathologic examination shows the posterior sclera to be thickened with granulomatous inflammation. A predominance of T lymphocytes was identified in one case. Lymphoid follicles can also be seen in the choroid and episclera.

Treatment/Prognosis

Oral nonsteroidal agents may be tried initially. Refractory cases require oral corticosteroids. In rare cases, immunosuppressive agents such as cyclophosphamide, cyclosporine, or azathioprine have been tried alone or with corticosteroids. Duration of treatment depends on response to treatment, and the majority of cases will respond well. Recurrences are common. Visual prognosis is associated with extent of optic nerve or macular involvement.

Systemic Evaluation

Associated systemic diseases include rheumatoid arthritis, systemic lupus erythematosus, Wegener's granulomatosis, inflammatory bowel disease, sarcoidosis, and syphilis. A complete blood cell count, erythrocyte sedimentation rate, antinuclear antibodies, antineutrophil cytoplasmic antibodies, angiotensin-converting enzyme, and chest x-ray are recommended.

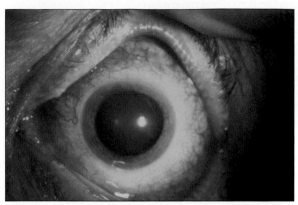

Slit lamp photograph of a patient with posterior scleritis reveals scleral injection in the equatorial region of the globe. The eye remains injected following instillation of tropicamide and phenylephrine for dilation.

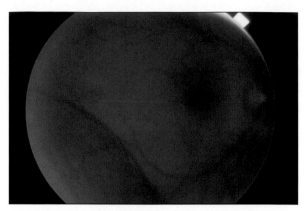

Ophthalmoscopic findings in posterior scleritis may simulate a focal choroidal mass, as seen in this patient.

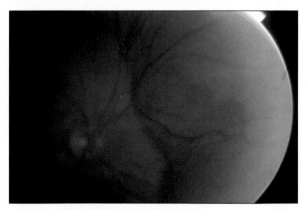

Patients may develop peripheral choroidal effusions and exudative retinal detachment. Chorioretinal folds are common.

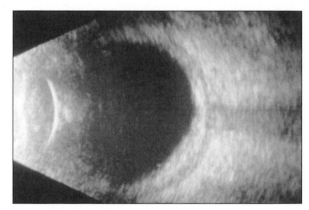

B-scan ultrasonography demonstrates the "T" sign that results from edema within Tenon's space. The sclera and choroid are thickened.

PRESUMED OCULAR HISTOPLASMOSIS SYNDROME

Presumed ocular histoplasmosis syndrome is the clinical triad of peripheral atrophic chorioretinal scars, peripapillary atrophy, and hemorrhagic macular disciform scarring, presumably due to previous exposure to *Histoplasmosis capsulatum* through inhalation of the fungal spores.

Symptoms

Most individuals with clinical signs of ocular histoplasmosis are asymptomatic. Symptoms of metamorphopsia, scotoma, or visual loss may occur with the development of exudative choroidal neovascularization within the macula.

Clinical Findings

The chorioretinal scars of ocular histoplasmosis are multiple, discrete, atrophic lesions that have hypertrophic pigmented borders. The lesions may form linear streaks peripherally. Peripheral scarring is bilateral in more than 60% of individuals. Ocular histoplasmosis is also characterized by peripapillary atrophic scarring. Choroidal neovascularization may arise from macular scars or peripapillary scarring. The chorioretinal findings are not associated with aqueous or vitreous inflammation.

Ancillary Testing

Fluorescein angiography may be used to investigate choroidal neovascularization. Chorioretinal scarring will only show window defects by angiography.

Pathology/Pathogenesis

Evidence that ocular histoplasmosis syndrome is caused by *H capsulatum* includes the following: (1) most cases occur in endemic areas of the United States, (2) almost all patients with ocular histoplasmosis have lived at least some of their lives in endemic regions, (3) positive reactions to histoplasmin skin testing are more common among patients with disciform lesions of ocular histoplasmosis than among controls, and (4) activation of inactive lesions of ocular histoplasmosis after skin testing has been reported. Gass and Wilkinson proposed that the scars result from a single prior systemic infection, in which *H capsulatum* is disseminated hematogenously from the lungs to the choroid, forming choroidal granulomas that heal into focal scars with resolution of the granulomas.

Treatment/Prognosis

Peripheral scars require no treatment. As most choroidal neovascularization arises from macular scars, patients with high-risk lesions should be instructed on self-monitoring with an Amsler grid. The Macular Photocoagulation Study demonstrated the beneficial effect of laser photocoagulation for extra- and juxtafoveal choroidal neovascularization. Photodynamic therapy should be considered in patients with classic subfoveal choroidal neovascularization. The results of surgical excision of subfoveal choroidal neovascularization are encouraging, but frequent recurrences have been reported.

Systemic Evaluation

Histoplasmin skin testing is helpful in indicating previous exposure to *H capsulatum*. Skin testing has been reported to cause reactivation of inactive scars. Chest x-ray may demonstrate calcified lung lesions.

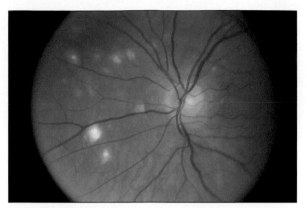

The classic triad of presumed ocular histoplasmosis syndrome includes punched-out chorioretinal scars, peripapillary pigmentary changes, and macular abnormalities such as choroidal neovascularization.

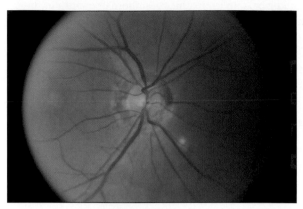

This fundus photograph demonstrates characteristic peripapillary findings. Also, a small chorioretinal scar is seen inferonasal to the optic disc.

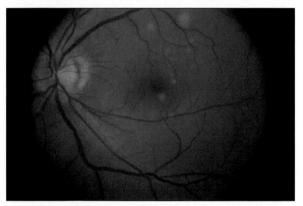

This pair of fundus photographs demonstrates the major complication of presumed ocular histoplasmosis syndrome—choroidal neovascularization. This woman was found to have chorioretinal scars in her left macula during a routine eye examination.

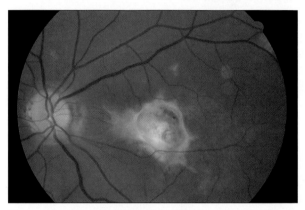

The same patient subsequently developed choroidal neovascularization followed by fibrovascular scarring.

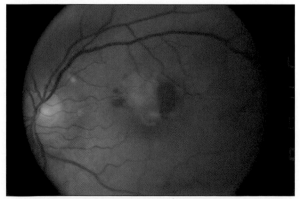

Choroidal neovascularization arises from chorioretinal scars. Breaks in the Bruch's membrane-retinal pigment epithelial complex allow choroidal new vessels to proliferate under the retina.

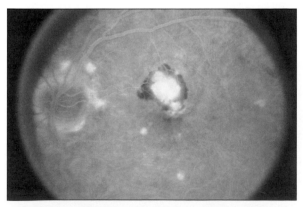

Fluorescein angiogram of the same patient reveals hyperfluorescence of the choroidal new vessels. The hypofluorescence corresponds to blood.

SARCOIDOSIS

Sarcoidosis is an idiopathic, granulomatous inflammation that may affect nearly any part of the body. Ocular involvement may be present in up to 50% of patients with histologically proven sarcoidosis. Often sarcoidosis is not a known diagnosis in a patient presenting with uveitis.

Symptoms

Posterior segment involvement is often associated with decreased vision due to floaters and vitritis. Symptoms of anterior uveitis including photophobia, conjunctival injection, and eye pain may be presenting signs of sarcoid uveitis. Decreased vision may be due to posterior uveitis from chronic macular edema, epiretinal membrane formation, and retinal ischemia due to vasculitis.

Clinical Features

Retinal lesions occur in approximately 25% of patients with sarcoid-associated uveitis. Vitritis is a major manifestation of posterior segment involvement with sarcoidosis. Retinal vasculitis is the most common retinal abnormality associated with sarcoidosis. The vasculitis primarily affects the venules and may be associated with focal perivascular exudates ("candlewax drippings"). The vasculitis may lead to vascular occlusion, retinal ischemia, and retinal neovascularization. The chorioretinitis of sarcoidosis is nonspecific, although focal choroidal granulomas have been reported. These granulomas are associated with overlying neurosensory detachment. Optic nerve granulomas may occur. Posterior uveitis may lead to the development of cystoid macular edema (CME) and epiretinal membrane formation.

Ancillary Testing

Fluorescein angiography is important in the diagnosis and monitoring of CME. In cases with severe vitritis, fluorescein angiography may help identify vasculitis and retinal lesions. Choroidal granulomas demonstrate early hypofluorescence and late hyperfluorescent staining.

Pathology/Pathogenesis

Sarcoid nodules consist of noncaseating epithelioid granulomatous disease.

Treatment/Prognosis

Sarcoid uveitis usually responds well to corticosteroid therapy. Treatment of eye disease is commonly part of treatment of the systemic disease. The nature of the disease and process usually requires prolonged therapy. Nonsteroidal anti-inflammatory medications may supplement systemic therapy or even periocular steroid treatment. Cystoid macular edema requires the use of systemic or periocular corticosteroids. Neovascularization may respond to control of ocular inflammation but may require peripheral scatter laser photocoagulation if there is extensive nonperfusion.

Systemic Evaluation

The ultimate diagnosis of sarcoidosis depends on histologic confirmation of sarcoid granulomas. Less invasive testing to support clinical suspicion of disease include the demonstration of hilar adenopathy on chest x-ray, gallium scan demonstration of inflammatory cell infiltration, and elevated angiotensin-converting enzyme levels.

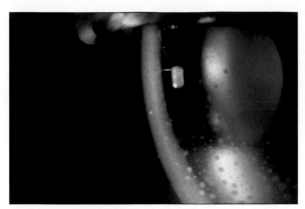

Sarcoidosis commonly involves the eye. Anterior segment manifestations include iritis and iridocyclitis. This woman presented with pain, redness, and photophobia. She had prominent keratic precipitates.

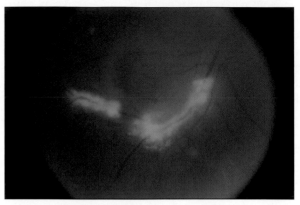

The characteristic retinal finding in patients with sarcoidosis is a periphlebitis described as "candlewax drippings."

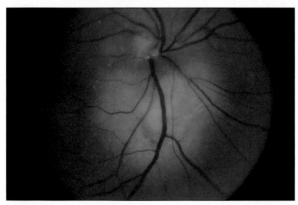

Focal choroidal granulomas may be observed. These usually are associated with overlying subretinal fluid.

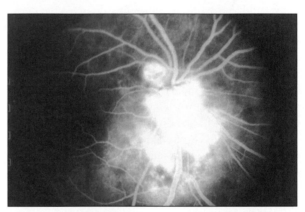

Fluorescein angiogram of the same patient reveals marked hyperfluorescence as a result of leakage in the region of the granuloma.

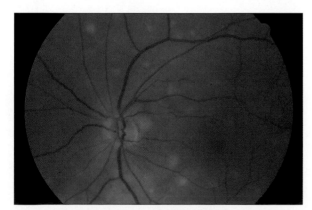

Sarcoidosis may mimic the inflammatory white dot syndromes with multifocal choroidal infiltrates. This patient had sarcoidosis confirmed by lung biopsy.

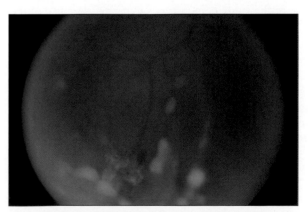

Characteristic vitreous findings include vitritis and vitreous "snowballs." This patient also had peripheral retinal neovascularization with hemorrhage.

SERPIGINOUS CHOROIDITIS

Serpiginous choroiditis is a chronic, progressive inflammatory condition affecting the choroid and retinal pigment epithelium (RPE). Recurrent attacks are the rule and can occur weeks to years after the initial event. Serpiginous choroiditis typically affects middle-aged individuals (30 to 60 years of age); there may be a slight male preponderance. Serpiginous choroiditis is bilateral but may be asymmetric.

Symptoms

Symptoms include blurred vision, central or paracentral scotomas, metamorphopsia, and visual field loss. Individuals may be asymptomatic before foveal involvement.

Clinical Features

The anterior segment is usually normal. If present, vitritis is mild. Serpiginous choroiditis involves the peripapillary region and macula. Acute lesions are slightly ill-defined, gray-white, jigsaw puzzle-shaped lesions at the level of the choriocapillaris and RPE. The active lesions may be associated with shallow subretinal fluid. Acute lesions are commonly located adjacent to atrophic scars. As the acute lesion clears, extensive atrophy of the choriocapillaris, RPE, and retina is seen. Areas of retinal pigment epithelial hyperpigmentation and subretinal fibrosis are common. Choroidal neovascularization may develop.

Ancillary Testing

Intravenous fluorescein angiography (IVFA) shows early hypofluorescence of the active lesions secondary to either an inflammatory occlusion of the choriocapillaris or blocked fluorescence by the edematous RPE. The late phase of the study demonstrates hyperfluorescence of the border of the active lesion that may extend centrally.

Indocyanine green angiography is divided into four stages: (1) hypofluorescent lesions in the subclinical or choroidal stage; (2) hypofluorescent lesions in the active stage, larger than those defined on IVFA; (3) hyperfluorescence in the healing/subhealing stage; and (4) hypofluorescent lesions with clearly defined margins in the inactive stage. Electroretinogram and electro-oculogram findings are usually normal.

Pathology/Pathogenesis

The etiology of serpiginous choroiditis is not completely understood. A possible immune-mediated mechanism has been proposed due to an increased frequency of HLA-B7 and retinal S-antigen associations. An association with varicella-zoster infection also has been postulated. Elevated von Willebrand factor has been reported, although the significance of this finding is unclear.

Treatment/Prognosis

The prognosis for serpiginous choroidopathy is guarded. Visual loss results from direct foveal involvement or the development of choroidal neovascularization. Rarely, individuals with foveal involvement may recover central vision, although visual recovery is usually incomplete.

Treatment involves the use of immunosuppressive agents such as prednisone, azathioprine, and cyclosporine. Acyclovir has been reported with limited success. Laser photocoagulation may be helpful in cases of choroidal neovascularization but has not been proven to limit the active inflammatory lesions.

Systemic Evaluation

Most individuals with serpiginous choroiditis are healthy and require no systemic evaluation.

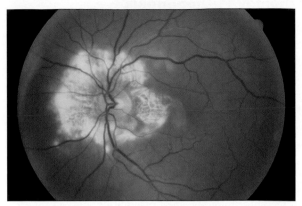

Serpiginous choroiditis involves the posterior fundus. Active choroiditis is characterized by slightly ill-defined, yellowish white areas adjacent to old chorioretinal atrophy.

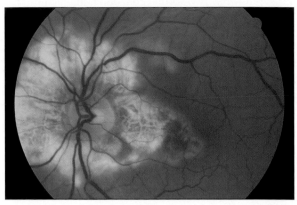

The active lesions become atrophic over the course of weeks. The atrophic regions may assume a jigsaw puzzle-like configuration.

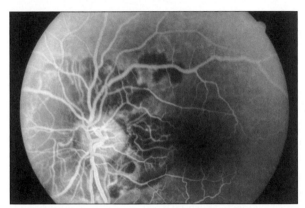

Fluorescein angiography of the active lesions reveals early hypofluorescence followed by late hyperfluorescence.

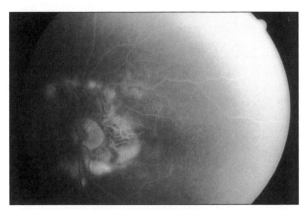

Late-phase angiogram of the same patient reveals late hyperfluorescence, which is most prominent along the border of the active lesion.

SYPHILIS

Ocular syphilis has two forms: congenital and acquired. Congenital syphilis is rare, accounting for less than 0.1% of all cases of syphilis. Acquired syphilis has been epidemic in the United States since the 1980s. Acquired syphilis has been called "the great imitator" and, indeed, ocular syphilis should be included in the differential diagnosis of *any* ocular inflammatory condition.

Symptoms

Patients with acquired ocular syphilis should be able to provide a history of a chancre at the site of inoculation (primary syphilis). Four to 10 weeks later, they should report a generalized rash, fever, malaise, headache, nausea, anorexia, and joint pain (secondary syphilis). At this second stage 10% of patients will have ocular involvement. Ocular symptoms typically include redness, mild pain, and blurred vision.

Clinical Features

In primary acquired syphilis, ocular findings are chancres of the eyelid and conjunctiva. In secondary syphilis, the eyelids can be involved with the generalized rash. Early in secondary syphilis, anterior uveitis may be the most common finding. Other findings include conjunctivitis, keratitis, iris nodules, episcleritis, and scleritis. Late in the secondary stage chorioretinitis, vitritis, and neuroretinitis may develop. Papillitis, exudative retinal detachment, and vasculitis are less common findings. Tertiary syphilis may demonstrate the neuro-ophthalmologic findings of Argyll Robertson pupils, end-stage optic atrophy, pseudo-retinitis pigmentosa, or cranial nerve palsies.

Ancillary Testing

Fluorescein angiography is nondiagnostic but may be helpful in posterior segment disease. For example, acute syphilitic posterior placoid chorioretinitis will show initial hypofluorescence followed by late staining at the level of the retinal pigment epithelium (RPE). Syphilitic retinal phlebitis and papillitis will demonstrate leakage and staining with fluorescein.

Pathology/Pathogenesis

Syphilis is a sexually transmitted disease caused by the spirochete *Treponema pallidum*. Some cases of ocular syphilis can probably be explained by direct spirochetal invasion of tissue. Other cases, such as interstitial keratitis, are more likely due to immune reactivity or cross-reactivity to spirochetal antigen.

Treatment/Prognosis

While penicillin is the treatment for syphilis, controversy still exists. One should refer to the most current treatment recommendations, and consultation with an infectious disease specialist may be helpful. During treatment, patients should be monitored for a Jarisch-Herxheimer reaction that can exacerbate existing ocular disease. After treatment the VDRL should be checked at 3, 6, and 12 months to ensure nonreactivity. If recognized and treated early, ocular syphilis can have a favorable prognosis.

Systemic Evaluation

Specific serologic tests for antitreponemal antibody are the fluorescent treponemal antibody absorption (FTA-ABS) test and the microhemagglutination assay—*Treponema pallidum* (MHA-TP). The FTA-ABS titers will remain elevated for life. Nonspecific serologic tests for *T pallidum* infection are the Venereal Disease Research Laboratories (VDRL) test and the rapid plasma reagin (RPR) test. These tests reflect disease activity and may be used to monitor therapy. Lumbar puncture should be considered. Also, coinfection with human immunodeficiency virus should be ruled out. Physicians must report every new case of syphilis to local health officials.

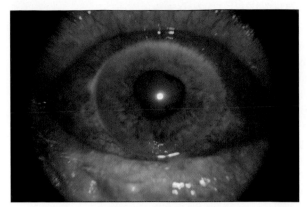

Syphilis is one of the masquerade syndromes; it can be associated with inflammation in any part of the eye. Anterior uveitis is a common manifestation.

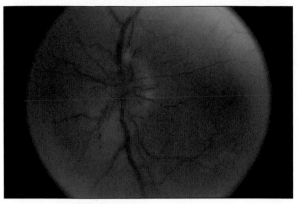

Patients with syphilis may develop optic neuritis, as seen in this patient with optic disc edema and hyperemia.

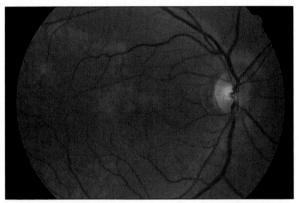

This patient with syphilis had yellowish white choroidal infiltrates in his right macula. There were areas of focal vasculitis involving primarily the retinal veins.

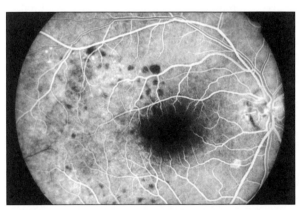

Fluorescein angiogram of the same patient revealed hypofluorescent spots corresponding to the choroidal lesions.

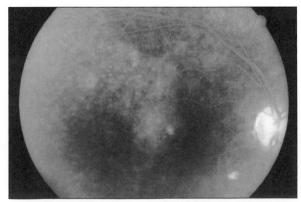

The late phase of the angiogram of the same patient demonstrated pinpoint areas of hyperfluorescence.

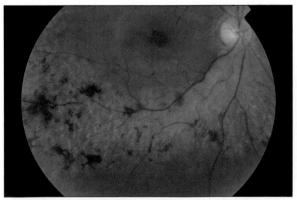

This patient with syphilis had a pseudo-retinitis pigmentosa appearance to her fundus. The pigmentary changes were more prominent in the perivascular distribution.

SYSTEMIC LUPUS ERYTHEMATOSUS

Systemic lupus erythematosus (SLE) is a multisystem, autoimmune disorder that most commonly affects women of childbearing age. The ocular manifestations are multiple and involve nearly every ocular and periocular structure. Approximately 3% to 10% of patients with SLE will have retinal disease.

Symptoms

Symptoms vary with degree of retinal involvement and may range from normal vision with cotton wool spots to severe, permanent visual loss with vaso-occlusive disease.

Clinical Features

Cotton wool spots with or without retinal hemorrhages are the most common retinal finding in patients with SLE. Severe vaso-occlusive disease (not a true vasculitis) is less common and may involve the central retinal artery, central retinal vein, branch retinal artery, or all retinal vessels. Systemic lupus erythematosus has also been associated with a frosted branch periphlebitis and exudative maculopathy.

Lupus choroidopathy is characterized by multifocal serous elevations of the neurosensory retina and/or retinal pigment epithelium in one or both eyes. Turbid subretinal fluid and subretinal fibrin may be seen.

Ancillary Testing

Fluorescein angiography may show retinal capillary nonperfusion, staining of inflamed retinal vessels, and retinal vascular occlusion. In patients with choroidopathy, fluorescein angiography may show delayed choroidal perfusion and leakage of dye into multifocal areas of neurosensory detachment.

Pathology/Pathogenesis

Systemic lupus erythematosus is characterized by polyclonal B-cell activation, a plethora of autoantibodies, and circulating immune complexes. Although the pathogenesis of SLE-associated retinopathy and choroidopathy is unclear, autoimmune mechanisms play a significant role. Immune complexes responsible for microangiopathy have been found in the walls of retinal and choroidal vessels. Histopathologically, tissue damage from immune complexes and associated cellular infiltration is seen as hematoxylin bodies and fibrinoid necrosis.

Treatment/Prognosis

No specific ocular treatment is necessary for cotton wool spots, but their presence correlates with active SLE. There is no known effective treatment for severe vaso-occlusive disease. Therapy with anticoagulation and high-dose corticosteroids may be considered. Panretinal photocoagulation may have a role in treating ischemia and preventing complications of neovascularization. The visual prognosis for vaso-occlusive retinal disease can be poor. Choroidopathy may be treated with corticosteroids, other immunosuppressive agents, or control of systemic hypertension, if present.

Systemic Evaluation

A complete physical examination looking for systemic manifestations of SLE should be done. Retinal vaso-occlusive disease has been correlated with central nervous system lupus, and may require neurologic consultation. Important laboratory tests include complete blood cell count, electrolyte panel, prothrombin time, partial thromboplastin time, lupus anticoagulant, anticardiolipin antibody, Veneral Disease Research Laboratories (VDRL) test, rapid plasma reagin (RPR) test, antinuclear antibody, anti-DNA, anti-smooth muscle antibodies, complement levels, and serum protein electrophoresis. Hypertension and renal disease may be significant factors in SLE-associated eye disease.

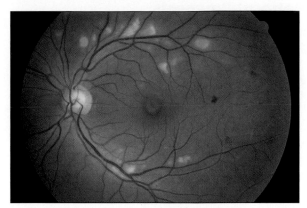

Cotton wool spots and intraretinal hemorrhages are the most common findings in patients with systemic lupus erythematosus.

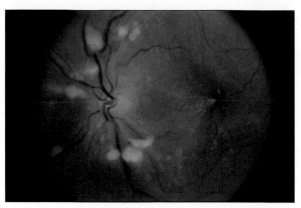

This patient had numerous peripapillary cotton wool spots as well as disc edema with a partial macular star. She had systemic lupus erythematosus with severe hypertension and renal disease.

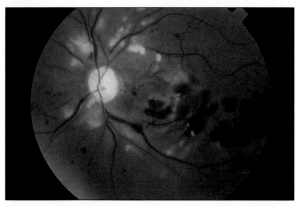

Some patients with systemic lupus erythematosus may suffer profound visual loss related to occlusion of the macular retinal vessels. There are prominent cotton wool spots and intraretinal hemorrhages associated with macular edema.

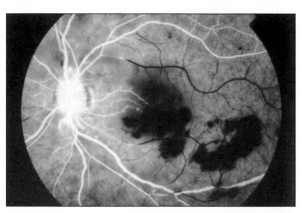

Fluorescein angiogram of the same patient confirms the macular ischemia.

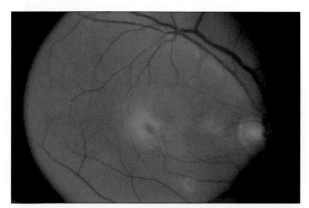

Lupus choroidopathy is characterized by multifocal, serous elevations of the retinal pigment epithelium and neurosensory retina. The whitish deposits are believed to be subretinal fibrin.

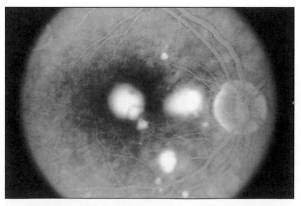

Fluorescein angiogram of lupus choroidopathy reveals multiple hyperfluorescent spots corresponding to areas of active leakage.

TOXOCARIASIS

Ocular toxocariasis is a common parasitic infestation in children and young adults caused by *Toxocara canis*. A common ascarid of dogs, *T canis* is the most frequent cause of visceral larval migrans and ocular toxocariasis. Interestingly, both diseases rarely occur together.

Symptoms

Patients typically present with unilateral visual loss, strabismus, or leukokoria. There is no discomfort. A delay between onset of symptoms and diagnosis is common and may average 1 year.

Clinical Features

Toxocara endophthalmitis classically presents in one of three ways: (1) chronic endophthalmitis, (2) posterior pole "granuloma," or (3) peripheral granulomatous inflammatory mass. Common to all presentations is a white and quiet eye. The degree of intraocular inflammation varies from mild, with a hazy vitreous, to severe, with granulomatous anterior uveitis, hypopyon, and dense vitreous membranes. It should be noted that the causative larva is 300 μm to 400 μm in size and cannot be seen clinically.

Ancillary Testing

In eyes with media opacification, ultrasonography is used to rule out other conditions in the differential diagnosis. An ultrasound can rule out short axial length in persistent hyperplastic primary vitreous, calcifications in retinoblastoma, and retinal detachment. If invasive testing is warranted, an anterior chamber tap can be used to test aqueous for enzyme-linked immunosorbent assay (ELISA) to *T canis*. When a hypopyon is aspirated, the presence of eosinophils is suggestive of the disease.

Pathology/Pathogenesis

Humans contract the disease primarily by ingestion of contaminated soil and not by direct contact with dogs. Infectious larvae migrate through the wall of the small intestine and are available for hematogenous spread to the eye. Damage to intraocular structures may occur from migration of the motile larva, toxicity due to secretory products of the worm, or the host inflammatory response. Histopathologically, the intraocular larvae incites an intense inflammatory reaction in which the larva is surrounded by eosinophils, mononuclear cells, histiocytes, epithelioid cells, and giant cells, forming a granuloma or abscess.

Treatment/Prognosis

Most cases of ocular toxocariasis present without significant inflammation or vitreoretinal pathology and require no treatment. Medical therapy is directed at controlling acute inflammation with local and systemic steroids. Because *T canis* larvae cannot replicate in humans, infection is not exacerbated by immune suppression. The benefit of antihelminthic agents is unproven. Vitreoretinal surgery can be used to manage complications such as vitreous opacification, retinal detachment, or epiretinal membrane. The visual prognosis largely depends on macular involvement and the potential for amblyopia.

Systemic Evaluation

Peripheral eosinophilia is rare in patients with ocular toxocariasis. A serum ELISA titer for *T canis* of 1:8 provides 90% specificity and 91% sensitivity and is highly suggestive (but not diagnostic) of ocular toxocariasis in the right clinical setting.

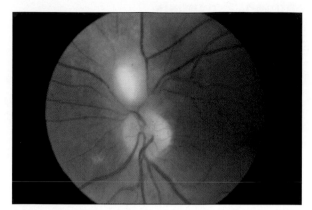

Toxocariasis may present with an inflammatory lesion in the posterior fundus. Peripapillary lesions are common. The associated vitritis may be mild or severe.

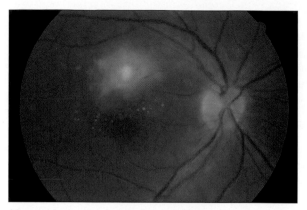

Macular lesions may result in visual loss. There may be associated subretinal fluid and subretinal deposits.

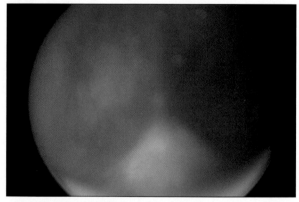

Peripheral Toxocara lesions are usually larger than the posterior lesions and often have fibrous extension with retinal folds extending to the posterior fundus.

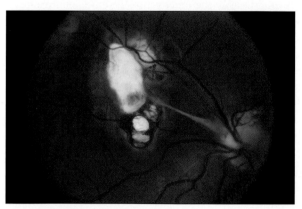

This patient had an old inflammatory scar with a fibrous band extending to the optic disc. The differential diagnosis includes toxoplasmosis.

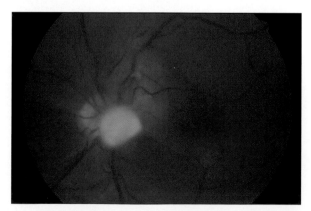

An unusual complication of ocular Toxocara infection is choroidal neovascularization. Note the grayish green subretinal lesion superotemporal to the optic disc.

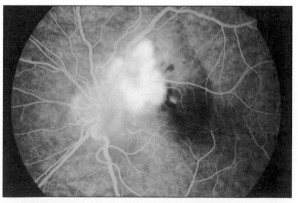

Fluorescein angiogram of the same patient reveals the area of classic choroidal neovascularization.

TOXOPLASMOSIS

Infection with *Toxoplasma gondii* is congenital or acquired. Ocular toxoplasmosis is usually a recurrent manifestation of congenital disease. Toxoplasmosis is the most common protozoal eye infection and the most frequent cause of focal necrotizing retinitis in healthy adults.

Symptoms

Symptoms are present in more than 90% of patients with active *Toxoplasma* retinochoroiditis. Most patients report floaters and reduced central vision.

Clinical Features

Focal necrotizing retinitis of the inner retina presents as a unilateral white-yellow retinal lesion with overlying vitritis (classic "headlight in the fog"). If the retinitis involves primarily the outer retina, a serous neurosensory retinal detachment may be present. A hyperpigmented chorioretinal scar can often be seen adjacent to the lesion or in the fellow eye. Associated retinal findings are hemorrhage or localized vasculitis. In some patients (often immunocompromised individuals), acute retinal necrosis with diffuse toxoplasmosis retinitis may be seen. Associated ocular findings are papillitis, mild granulomatous iritis, and scleritis.

Ancillary Testing

Ancillary testing is usually not necessary as the diagnosis of acute *Toxoplasma* retinitis is very likely in patients who demonstrate a focal retinitis in one eye and one or more chorioretinal scars. A fluorescein angiogram will show staining in the area of retinitis and late hyperfluorescence of the optic nerve. Visual field testing may reveal large defects due to optic nerve involvement.

Pathology/Pathogenesis

Human infection occurs by ingestion of *T gondii* oocysts from cats (acquired) or by maternal transplacental spread if the mother is infected during pregnancy (congenital). If the parasite reaches the eye, infection progresses from the retina to the choroid, producing a true retinochoroiditis. The host's immune response controls the infection as tachyzoites give way to bradyzoites and encystment. Tissue cysts may remain dormant for years. Ultimately, cysts rupture, releasing organisms into surrounding retina, with a recurrence of necrotic retinochoroiditis. Histopathologically, the inflammatory response is mononuclear with lymphocytes, macrophages, epithelioid cells, and plasma cells.

Treatment/Prognosis

In immunocompetent hosts, ocular toxoplasmosis is a self-limited disease. However, most active lesions that are 2 to 3 mm from the disc or fovea, which threaten or affect vision, or extramacular lesions with severe vitritis are treated. Classically, therapy consists of pyrimethamine, sulfadiazine, folinic acid, and corticosteroids. Clindamycin and trimethoprim-sulfamethoxazole have also been used. Oral corticosteroids should never be given without antibiotics. Topical corticosteroids and cycloplegics are used for anterior uveitis. The prognosis is favorable for most patients.

Systemic Evaluation

The enzyme-linked immunosorbent assay test can be used to detect IgG or IgM anti-*Toxoplasma* antibodies. Because of a high prevalence of seropositivity in the population, this is not a diagnostic test. The diagnosis of ocular toxoplasmosis is still presumptive, based on typical ocular findings in the setting of positive serology. It is important to rule out infection with human immunodeficiency virus as toxoplasmosis in patients with acquired immunodeficiency syndrome is a leading cause of death. Hematologic monitoring must be performed if treating with pyrimethamine.

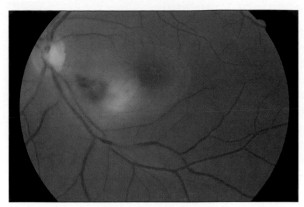

Ocular toxoplasmosis is characterized by full-thickness retinitis, usually located adjacent to a chorioretinal scar from previous infection. It is one of the most common causes of posterior uveitis.

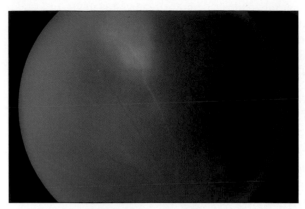

The description "headlight in the fog" refers to the appearance of the active toxoplasmosis retinitis through dense vitritis. Toxoplasmosis retinitis may be associated with vasculitis, as seen in this patient.

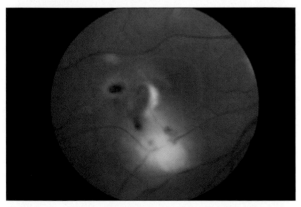

This pair of fundus photographs demonstrates the natural course of toxoplasmosis retinitis. There is active retinitis adjacent to pigmented chorioretinal scars.

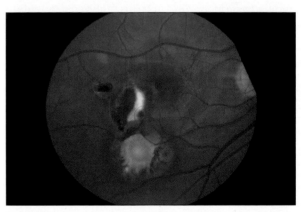

This photograph of the same patient taken 1 year later reveals an atrophic scar with mild pigmentation in the area of previous infection.

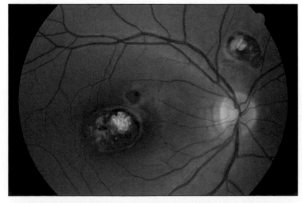

Congenital toxoplasmosis often involves the macula. The chororetinal scars may be large and pigmented with prominent scleral show.

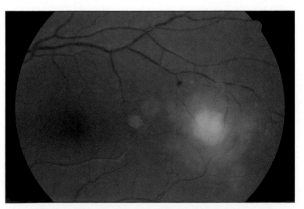

The fellow eye of the same patient reveals a focal area of active toxoplasmosis retinitis temporal to the macula.

TUBERCULOSIS

Ocular tuberculosis is rare, affecting 1% to 2% of patients with active disease. However, since 1984 reported cases of tuberculosis have been increasing, making this entity important to consider in the differential diagnosis of uveitis.

Symptoms

The clinical manifestations are varied, but patients may present with blurred vision, floaters, and occasionally redness, pain, and photophobia.

Clinical Features

Tuberculosis can involve both the anterior and posterior segments of the eye as well as the ocular adnexae and orbit. The most common ocular manifestations include phlyctenular keratoconjunctivitis, interstitial keratitis, granulomatous iridocyclitis, scleritis, choroidal granulomas, posterior uveitis, and retinal vasculitis.

Ancillary Testing

Fluorescein angiography and ultrasonography can be used to evaluate choroidal granulomas. On angiography, the lesions may be hyper- or hypofluorescent early; they stain late. B-scan ultrasonography typically shows an elevated mass with an absent scleral echo. A-scan ultrasonography shows low internal reflectivity. Fluorescein angiography will show staining of vessels in cases of retinal vasculitis.

Pathology/Pathogenesis

Mycobacterium tuberculosis is an acid-fast-staining obligate anaerobe with worldwide prevalence. Infection begins with inhalation of airborne organisms from patients with pulmonary tuberculosis. The majority of patients do not develop active disease, but the disease remains in a state of dormancy. Some patients develop rampant hematogenous spread resulting in miliary tuberculosis. In general, intraocular disease evolves from hematogenous spread (eg, choroidal tubercules). Surface ocular infection results from direct inoculation (eg, conjunctival nodule) or delayed hypersensitivity (eg, phlyctenule). Histopathologic examination of direct infection reveals caseating granulomas with Langerhans' giant cells and acid-fast bacilli.

Treatment/Prognosis

A patient with suggestive ocular findings and a positive purified protein derivative (PPD) test should be treated if there is other evidence of tuberculosis. The Centers for Disease Control and Prevention recommend that all newly diagnosed patients receive a four-drug regimen of isoniazid, rifampin, pyrazinamide, and either streptomycin or ethambutol for 6 to 9 months. Treatment should be coordinated with a specialist. Systemic corticosteroids should not be used in persons with ocular tuberculosis. Topical corticosteroids and cycloplegics may be used adjunctively.

Systemic Evaluation

Skin testing (PPD) is used to establish exposure to *M tuberculosis*. Because a positive skin test without active systemic disease is usually insufficient to make a presumptive diagnosis of intraocular tuberculosis, a full systemic evaluation should follow. This evaluation typically includes chest x-ray; sputum analysis; biopsy of liver, lymph nodes, or bone marrow; stool for acid-fast smear; and cultures of blood, urine, cerebrospinal fluid, or pleural fluid. It is important to rule out human immunodeficiency virus infection.

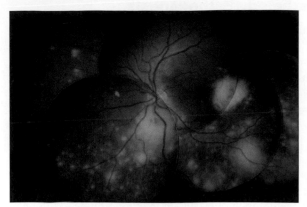

Fundus photograph montage of a patient with acquired immunodeficiency syndrome complicated by miliary tuberculosis. He had diffuse choroidal granulomas in each eye.

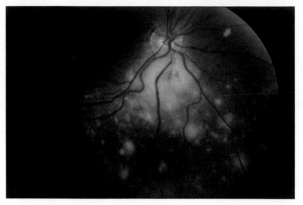

Higher-magnification photograph of the same patient confirms the subretinal location of the choroidal granulomas.

VOGT-KOYANAGI-HARADA SYNDROME

Vogt-Koyanagi-Harada (VKH) syndrome is a systemic inflammatory syndrome affecting primarily heavily pigmented individuals between the ages of 20 and 50 years. Asians, Spanish Americans, blacks, and Native Americans are most often affected.

Symptoms

Decreased vision may be associated with meningeal and ear symptoms, including neck stiffness, headache, tinnitus, and vertigo. Visual loss is usually bilateral but may be asymmetric. Iridocyclitis may cause photophobia, ciliary flush, and mild eye pain. Dysacusis, tinnitus, and hearing loss affect approximately 75% of patients with this disorder. Dermatologic involvement may include alopecia, poliosis, and vitiligo.

Clinical Features

Bilateral iridocyclitis with a granulomatous anterior chamber reaction is found with the initial onset of disease. Vitritis and exudative choroiditis lead to a decline in vision. Choroidal thickening is associated with overlying neurosensory retinal detachment. There are often multilobed serous detachments, which may coalesce into broad areas of serous retinal detachment. The optic nerve is hyperemic, and vitreous inflammatory cells are present.

Late in the course of disease, there may be optic disc neovascularization, choroidal neovascularization with hemorrhagic macular detachment, and depigmentation and clumping of the retinal pigment epithelium (RPE).

Ancillary Testing

Fluorescein angiography shows patchy delayed choroidal filling followed by pinpoint areas of hyperfluorescence at the level of the RPE. These pinpoint areas may leak into areas of serous retinal detachment. B-scan ultrasonography demonstrates thickening of the choroid, posterior serous retinal detachment, which may settle inferiorly, vitreous opacities, and posterior scleral thickening.

Lumbar puncture may show a cellular pleocytosis in the early stages of the disease.

Pathology/Pathogenesis

Although the pathogenesis is not completely understood, VKH syndrome is considered to be a cell-mediated autoimmune disease against melanocytes. A T-cell immune response may be directed against an antigenic component of the melanocyte, possibly tyrosinase or a tyrosinase-related protein.

Treatment/Prognosis

Corticosteroids are the first line of treatment to decrease the inflammatory disease. Systemic therapy is necessary, and the duration of treatment is often prolonged to prevent recurrence of disease. Visual outcomes with treatment are favorable. The retinal detachment usually resolves rapidly, with a slower resolution of anterior segment inflammation.

Immunosuppressive medications including cyclosporine and chlorambucil have been used when response to corticosteroids is inadequate.

Systemic Evaluation

Neurologic evaluation for associated meningeal disease is indicated. Neurologic symptoms may lead to changes in personality and even psychosis.

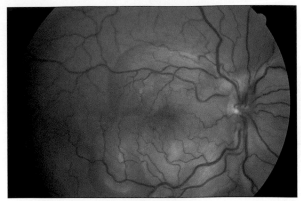

This patient with Vogt-Koyanagi-Harada syndrome had panuveitis with iridocyclitis, vitritis, and exudative choroiditis. Note the multilobular nature of the serous retinal detachments.

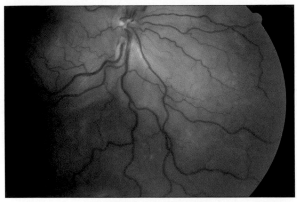

This fundus photograph of the same eye demonstrates turbid subretinal fluid and retinal pigment epithelial alterations.

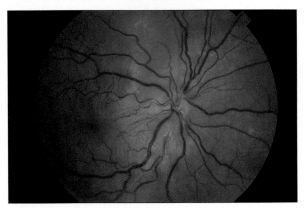

This patient with Vogt-Koyanagi-Harada syndrome has a serous neurosensory retinal detachment that is most notable superior to the optic disc.

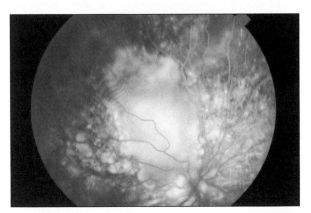

Fluorescein angiography reveals hyperfluorescence resulting from leakage in the region of the neurosensory retinal detachment.

TABLE 1

White Dot Syndromes

	APMPPE	Birdshot Chorioretinitis	DUSN
Age	Young (20s-40s)	Middle age (40s-60s)	Variable, may affect children
Sex	Men = Women	Women > Men	Men = Women
Laterality	Bilateral	Bilateral	Unilateral
Viral Illness	+/−	−	−
Onset	Abrupt	Insidious	Variable
Duration	Weeks-months; recurrence rare	Chronic, recurrent	Months-years Acute lesions: weeks-months
Symptoms	Blurred vision, scotomas, photopsias	Blurred vision, floaters, difficulty with night vision or color vision, photopsias	Severe loss of vision following apparent subacute visual loss
Vitreous Cells	Mild	Prominent	Mild
Findings	Multifocal, flat, gray-white placoid lesions at level of RPE posterior pole that fade rapidly in 7-12 days; may have mild optic disc swelling	Multiple, ill-defined cream-colored lesions at level of outer retina/RPE, patches of depigmentation, vascular leakage, CME	Early: +/− APD, disc edema, clusters of yellow-white spots at outer retina/RPE (in vicinity of worm) Late: APD, optic atrophy, RPE derangement, vessel attenuation
Fluorescein	Acute: block early, stain late Late: window defects	Normal; may have vascular leakage, CME	Acute: nonfluorescent early, stain late; +/− disc staining
ERG/EOG	+/− abnormal EOG	Abnormal ERG	Moderate to severe reduction of ERG (unilateral)
Sequelae	RPE alterations	CME, rare CNV	Optic atrophy, vessel attenuation, RPE atrophy
HLA	HLA-B7, HLA-DR2	HLA-A29 (strong)	—
Other	May have CNS vasculitis	+/− Hearing loss, vitiligo	—
Treatment	Observation; corticosteroids for CNS disease	Corticosteroids, cyclosporine	Direct photocoagulation; +/− thiabendazole
Prognosis	Excellent	Guarded; usually retain good vision in at least one eye	Poor (unless worm destroyed)
Etiology	Viral (?)	Autoimmune (?)	Nematodes: *Baylisascaris, Ancylostoma* (?)

TABLE 1

White Dot Syndromes

	MEWDS	Multifocal Choroiditis	Serpiginous Choroiditis
Age	Young (20s-40s)	Young; may affect children	Young, middle age (30s-60s)
Sex	Women > Men	Women > Men	Men > Women
Laterality	Unilateral	Bilateral	Bilateral but delayed/asymmetric
Viral Illness	+/−	+/−	−
Onset	Abrupt	Insidious	Variable
Duration	Weeks-months; recurrence rare	Chronic, recurrent	Chronic, recurrent; acute lesions weeks-months
Symptoms	Blurred vision, scotomas, photopsias	Blurred vision, floaters, scotomas, photopsias	Blurred vision, paracentral or central scotomas
Vitreous Cells	Mild	Prominent	Mild
Findings	Myopia, +/− APD, small white dots at level of outer retina/RPE, may coalesce to form patches, white/orange granularity to fovea; +/− disc edema, blind spot enlargement	Myopia, anterior uveitis (50%), active yellow-gray choroidal lesions replaced by punched-out scars; +/− disc swelling, CME; may present with CNV	Geographic zone of gray-white discoloration of RPE in peripapillary/macular area, centripedal extension with active peripheral edge and RPE and choriocapillaris atrophy in wake
Fluorescein	Early hyperfluorescence, late staining; "wreath-like" pattern	Acute: block early, stain late Late: window defects	Hypofluorescent early, borders stain late
ERG/EOG	Abnormal ERG	Normal-subnormal ERG	Normal
Sequelae	Very mild RPE alterations	Punched out scars; CNV (33%)	RPE mottling, scarring, loss of choriocapillaris, CNV (25%)
HLA	—	—	HLA-B7
Other	—	—	—
Treatment	Observation	Corticosteroids; photocoagulation for CNV	Immunosuppression, antiviral medications (?); photocoagulation for CNV
Prognosis	Excellent	Guarded	Guarded; may retain good vision in at least one eye
Etiology	Viral (?)	Viral (?)	Autoimmune, infectious (herpesvirus family) (?)

APD indicates afferent pupillary defect; APMPPE, acute posterior multifocal placoid pigment epitheliopathy; CME, cystoid macular edema; CNS, central nervous system; CNV, choroidal neovascularization; DUSN, diffuse unilateral subacute neuroretinitis; EOG, electro-oculogram; ERG, electroretinogram; MEWDS, multiple evanescent white dot syndrome; RPE, retinal pigment epithelium.

SELECTED REFERENCES

Acute Posterior Multifocal Placoid Pigment Epitheliopathy

1. Comu S, Verstraeten T, Rinkoff JS, Busis NA. Neurological manifestations of acute posterior multifocal placoid pigment epitheliopathy. *Stroke.* 1996;27:996–1001.

2. Gass JDM. *Stereoscopic Atlas of Macular Diseases.* 4th ed. St. Louis: Mosby, Inc; 1997:688–693.

3. Park D, Schatz H, McDonald HR, Johnson RN. Indocyanine green angiography of acute multifocal posterior placoid pigment epitheliopathy. *Ophthalmology.* 1995;102:1877–1883.

4. Polk TD, Goldman EJ. White dot chorioretinal inflammatory syndromes. *Int Ophthalmol Clin.* 1999;39:33–53.

5. Ryan SJ, Maumenee AE. Acute posterior multifocal placoid pigment epitheliopathy. *Am J Ophthalmol.* 1972;74:1006–1074.

6. Uyama M, Matsunsga T, Fukushima I, et al. Indocyanine green angiography and pathophysiology of multifocal posterior pigment epitheliopathy. *Retina.* 1999;19:12–21.

Acute Retinal Necrosis

1. Duker JS, Blumenkrantz MS. Diagnosis and management of ARN syndrome. *Surv Ophthalmol.* 1991;35:326–343.

2. Nishi M, Hanashiro R, Mori S, Masuda K, Mochizuki M, Hondo R. Polymerase chain reaction for the detection of the varicella-zoster genome in ocular samples from patients with acute retinal necrosis. *Am J Ophthalmol.* 1992;114:603–609.

3. Walters G, James TE. Viral causes of acute retinal necrosis syndrome. *Curr Opin Ophthalmol.* 2001;12:191–195.

Behçet's Disease

1. Baldassano VF Jr. Ocular manifestations of rheumatic diseases. *Curr Opin Ophthalmol.* 1998;9:85–88.

2. International Study Group for Behçet's Disease. Criteria for diagnosis of Behçet's disease. *Lancet.* 1990;335:1078–1080.

3. Michaelson JB, Dhisari FV. Behçet's Disease. *Surv Ophthalmol.* 1982;26:190.

4. Vaphiades MS, Lee AG, Kansu T. A bad eye and a sore lip. *Surv Ophthalmol.* 1999;44:148–152.

Birdshot Chorioretinopathy

1. Boyd SR, Young S, Lightman S. Immunopathology of the noninfectious posterior and intermediate uveitides. *Surv Ophthalmol.* 2001;46:209–233.

2. Gasch AT, Smith JA, Whitcup SM. Birdshot chorioretinopathy. *Br J Ophthalmol.* 1999;83:241–249.

3. Polk TD, Goldman EJ. White dot chorioretinal inflammatory syndromes. *Int Ophthalmol Clin.* 1999;39:33–53.

Cytomegalovirus Retinitis

1. Jacobson MA. Treatment of cytomegalovirus retinitis in patients with the acquired immunodeficiency syndrome. *N Engl J Med.* 1997;337:105–114.

2. Jacobson MA, Stanley H, Holtzer C, Margolis TP, Cunningham ET. Natural history and outcome of new AIDS-related cytomegalovirus retinitis diagnosed in the era of highly active anti-retroviral therapy. *Clin Infect Dis.* 2000;30:231–233.

3. Salmon-Ceron D. Cytomegalovirus infection: the point in 2001. *HIV Med.* 2001;2:255–259.

Diffuse Unilateral Subacute Neuroretinitis

1. Cunha de Souza E, Abujamra S, Nakashima Y, Gass JD. Diffuse bilateral subacute neuroretinitis: first patient with documented nematodes in both eyes. *Arch Ophthalmol.* 1999;117:1349–1351.

2. Gass JDM, Braunstein RA. Further observations concerning the diffuse unilateral subacute neuroretinitis syndrome. *Arch Ophthalmol.* 1983;101:1689–1697.

3. Gass JDM, Olsen KR. Diffuse unilateral subacute neuroretinitis. In: Ryan S, Lewis HL, eds. *Retina.* 3rd ed. St. Louis: Mosby, Inc; 2001:1669–1678.

Endophthalmitis

1. Ciulla TA, Starr MB, Masket S. Bacterial endophthalmitis prophylaxis for cataract surgery: an evidence-based update. *Ophthalmology.* 2002;109:13–24.

2. EVS Group. Results of the endophthalmitis vitrectomy study: a randomized trial of immediate vitrectomy and of intravenous antibiotics for the treatment of postoperative bacterial endophthalmitis. *Arch Ophthalmol.* 1995;113:1479–1496.

3. Kresloff MS, Castellarin AA, Zarbin MA. Endophthalmitis. *Surv Ophthalmol.* 1998;43:193–224.

4. Mamalis N, Nagpal M, Nagpal K, Nagpal PN. Endophthalmitis following cataract surgery. *Ophthalmol Clin North Am.* 2001;14:661–674.

5. Mandelbaum S, Forster RK. Exogenous endophthalmitis. In: Pepose JS, Holland GN, Wilhelmus KR, eds. *Ocular Infection and Immunity.* St. Louis: Mosby, Inc; 1996:1298–1320.

Human Immunodeficiency Virus Retinopathy

1. Holland GN, Gottlieb MS, Foos RY. Retinal cotton wool spots in acquired immunodeficiency syndrome. *N Engl J Med.* 1982;307:1702.

2. Kashiwase M, Sata T, Yamauchi Y, et al. Progressive outer retinal necrosis caused by herpes simplex virus type 1 in a patient with acquired immunodeficiency syndrome. *Ophthalmology.* 2000;107:790–794.

3. Schuman JS, Orellana J, Friedman AH, et al. Acquired immunodeficiency syndrome (AIDS). *Surv Ophthalmol.* 1987;31:384–410.

Intermediate Uveitis

1. Malinowski SM, Pulido JS, Folk JC. Long term visual outcome and complications associated with pars planitis. *Ophthalmology.* 1993;100:818–824.

2. Park WE, Mieler WF, Pulido JS. Peripheral scatter laser photocoagulation for neovascularization associated with pars planitis. *Arch Ophthalmol.* 1995;113:1277–1280.

Multifocal Choroiditis and Panuveitis

1. Dreyer RF, Gass JDM. Multifocal choroiditis and panuveitis: a syndrome that mimics ocular histoplasmosis. *Arch Ophthalmol.* 1984;102:1776–1784.

2. Folk JC, Pulido JS, Wolf MD. White dot chorioretinal inflammatory syndromes. In: *Focal Points: 1990 Clinical Modules for Ophthalmologists.* Vol 8, module 11. San Francisco: American Academy of Ophthalmology; 1990.

Multiple Evanescent White Dot Syndrome

1. Jampol LM, Sieving PA, Pugh D, et al. Multiple evanescent white dot syndrome, I: clinical findings. *Arch Ophthalmol.* 1984;102:671–674.

2. Lim JI, Kokame GT, Douglas JP. Multiple evanescent white dot syndrome in older patients. *Am J Ophthalmol.* 1999;127:725–728.

3. Luttrull JK, Marmor MF, Nanda M. Progressive confluent circumpapillary multiple evanescent white dot syndrome. *Am J Ophthalmol.* 1999;128:378–380.

4. Tsai L, Jampol LM, Pollock SC, Olk J. Chronic recurring multiple evanescent white dot syndrome. *Retina.* 1994;14:160–163.

Neuroretinitis

1. Cunningham ET, Koehler JE. Ocular bartonellosis. *Am J Ophthalmol.* 2000;130:340–349.

2. Dreyer RF, Hopen G, Gass JDM, Smith JL. Leber's idiopathic stellate neuroretinitis. *Arch Ophthalmol.* 1984;102:1140–1145.

3. Solley WA, Martin D, Newman NJ, et al. Cat scratch disease: posterior segment manifestations. *Ophthalmology.* 1999;106:1546–1553.

4. Wade NK, Levi L, Jones MR, et al. Optic disc edema associated with peripapillary serous retinal detachment: an early sign of systemic *Bartonella henselae* infection. *Am J Ophthalmol.* 2000;130:327–334.

Posterior Scleritis

1. Benson WE. Posterior scleritis. *Surv Ophthalmol.* 1988;32:297–316.

2. McCluskey PJ, Watson PG, Ligutman S, Haybittle J, Restori M, Branley M. Posterior scleritis: clinical features, systemic associations, and outcome in a large series of patients. *Ophthalmology.* 1997;106:2380–2386.

Presumed Ocular Histoplasmosis Syndrome

1. Gass JDM, Wilkinson CP. Follow-up study of presumed ocular histoplasmosis. *Trans Am Acad Ophthalmol Otolaryngol.* 1972;76:672–693.

2. Kleiner RC, Ratner CM, Enger C, Fine SL. Subfoveal neovascularization in ocular histoplasmosis syndrome: a natural history study. *Retina.* 1988;8:225–229.

3. Woods AC, Whalen HE. The probable role of benign histoplasmosis in the etiology of granulomatous uveitis. *Am J Ophthalmol.* 1960;49:205–220.

Sarcoidosis

1. Hunter DG, Regan CDJ. Retina lesions in sarcoid. In: Albert DA, Jakobiec FA, eds. *Principles and Practices in Ophthalmology.* Vol 3. Philadelphia: WB Saunders; 2000:2192–2197.

2. Marcus BF, Bovino JA, Burton TC. Sarcoid granuloma of the choroid. *Ophthalmology.* 1982;89:1326.

Serpiginous Choroiditis

1. Giovannini A, Mariotti C, Ripa E, Scassellati-Sforzolini B. Indocyanine green angiographic findings in serpiginous choroidopathy. *Br J Ophthalmol.* 1996;80:536–540.

2. Hooper PL, Kaplan HJ. Triple agent immunosuppression in serpiginous choroiditis. *Ophthalmology.* 1991;98:944–951.

3. Polk TD, Goldman, EJ. White dot chorioretinal inflammatory syndromes. *Int Ophthalmol Clin.* 1999;39:33–53.

Syphilis

1. Browning DJ. Posterior segment manifestations of active ocular syphilis, their response to a neurosyphilis regimen of penicillin therapy, and the influence of human immunodeficiency virus status on response. *Ophthalmology.* 2000;107:2015–2023.

2. Villanueva AV, Sahouri MJ, Ormerod LD, Puklin JE, Reyes MP. Posterior uveitis in patients with positive serology for syphilis. *Clin Infect Dis.* 2000;30:479–485.

Systemic Lupus Erythematosus

1. Jabs DA, Fine SL, Hochberg MC, Newman SA, Heiner GG, Stevens MB. Severe retinal vaso-occlusive disease in systemic lupus erythematosus. *Arch Ophthalmol.* 1986;104:558–563.

2. Jabs DA, Hanneken AM, Schachat AP, Fine SL. Choroidopathy in systemic lupus erythematosus. *Arch Ophthalmol.* 1988;106:230–234.

3. Neumann R, Foster DS. Corticosteroid-sparing strategies in the treatment of retinal vasculitis in systemic lupus erythematosus. *Retina.* 1995;15:201–212.

4. Ushiyama O, Ushiyama K, Koarada S, et al. Retinal disease in patients with systemic lupus erythematosus. *Ann Rheum Dis.* 2000;59:705–708.

Toxocariasis

1. Amin HI, MacDonald HR, Han DP, et al. Vitrectomy update for macular traction in ocular toxocariasis. *Retina.* 2000;20:80–85.

2. Gillespie SH, Dinning WJ, Voller A, Crowcroft NS. The spectrum of ocular toxocariasis. *Eye.* 1993;7:415–418.

Toxoplasmosis

1. Tabbara KF. Ocular toxoplasmosis: toxoplasma retinochoroiditis. *Int Opthalmol Clin.* 1995;35:15–29.

2. Uchio E, Ohno S. Ocular manifestations of systemic infections. *Curr Opin Ophthalmol.* 1999;10:452–457.

Tuberculosis

1. Dunn JP, Helm CJ, Davidson PT. Tuberculosis. In: Pepose JS, Holland GN, Wilhelmus KR, eds. *Ocular Infection and Immunity.* St. Louis: Mosby, Inc; 1996.

2. Helm CJ, Holland GN. Ocular tuberculosis. *Surv Ophthalmol.* 1993;38:229–256.

3. Centers for Disease Control and Prevention. Initial therapy for TB in the era of multidrug resistance: recommendations of the advisory council for the elimination of TB. *MMWR Morb Mortal Wkly Rep.* 1993;42:1–80.

Vogt-Koyanagi-Harada Syndrome

1. Nussenblatt RB, Palestine AG. Vogt-Koyanagi-Harada syndrome (uveomeningitic syndrome). In: Ryan SJ, ed. *Retina.* St. Louis: Mosby, Inc; 1989:723.

2. Read RW, Rao NA, Cunningham ET. Vogt-Koyanagi-Harada disease. *Curr Opin Ophthalmol.* 2000;11:437–442.

3. Snyder DA, Tessler HH. Vogt-Koyanagi-Harada syndrome. *Am J Ophthalmol.* 1980;90:69–75.

chapter 10

Trauma

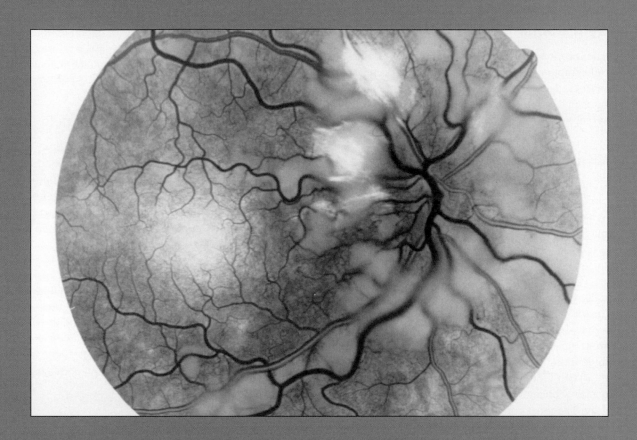

Timothy W. Olsen, MD

CHOROIDAL RUPTURE

A choroidal rupture occurs following blunt trauma to the globe. The term choroidal rupture is a misnomer in that the abnormality is a break in Bruch's membrane and the apposing retinal pigment epithelium. Choroidal ruptures have been reported in a variety of blunt injuries to the eye, including those involving contact with hands or fists, soccer balls, tennis balls, paint balls, or bungee cords; airbag deployment; and forceps delivery.

Symptoms

The location of the choroidal rupture determines the initial symptoms. If the rupture is outside of the central macula, the patient is likely to be asymptomatic. Ruptures that are juxtafoveal or subfoveal cause central visual loss or scotoma.

Clinical Features

Choroidal ruptures are commonly crescent shaped or circumlinear and typically form around the optic nerve. When multiple ruptures occur temporal to the disc, they may appear as a series of concentric lines, with the optic disc as its center. Choroidal ruptures that occur nasal to the disc have a less regular pattern.

Choroidal ruptures may be difficult to diagnose initially due to subretinal blood or commotio retinae. As the view clears, the rupture appears as a yellow-white streak, with large choroidal vessels visible. Visual acuity from the choroidal rupture alone may range from 20/20 to counting fingers.

With time, scar tissue fills in the choroidal rupture and may change its color or appearance to a shade of gray. The most common complication of choroidal rupture is a choroidal neovascular membrane. These membranes can occur from 1 month to several years after the injury. The choroidal neovascular membrane originates adjacent to the scar tissue and may bleed or grow into the subfoveal space.

Ancillary Testing

The initial fluorescein angiogram may demonstrate hypofluorescence as a result of subretinal hemorrhage overlying the choroidal rupture. The choroidal rupture itself usually exhibits a hyperfluorescent streak corresponding to the break in the Bruch's membrane-retinal pigment epithelial complex. A fluorescein angiogram is indicated if there is a suggestion of a choroidal neovascular membrane. Indocyanine green (ICG) angiography reveals hypofluorescence in the region of the choroidal rupture; ICG angiography may demonstrate more hypofluorescent streaks than expected clinically or by fluorescein angiography.

Pathology/Pathogenesis

Choroidal rupture is the indirect result of blunt trauma to the globe. When the globe is compressed in an anterior to posterior direction at the time of blunt injury, the sclera and retina may be elastic enough to resist injury, but the inelasticity of Bruch's membrane makes it susceptible to tearing.

Treatment/Prognosis

There is no treatment for the choroidal rupture itself. Occasionally, bleeding (vitreous or subretinal hemorrhage) associated with choroidal rupture will require pars plana vitrectomy. Treatment options for a choroidal neovascular membrane include laser photocoagulation or surgical excision. The role of photodynamic therapy is unclear.

Systemic Evaluation

No systemic evaluation is required for a choroidal rupture.

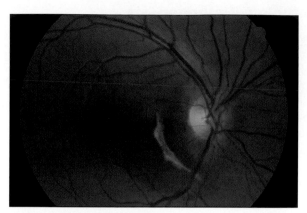

Acute choroidal rupture following a bungee-cord injury to the right eye. The choroidal rupture appears as a yellow-white streak concentric to the optic disc.

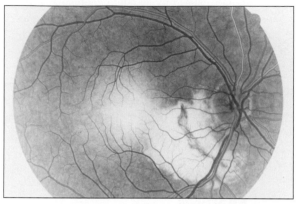

Fluorescein angiogram of the same patient reveals hyperfluorescence of the choroidal rupture and hypofluorescence corresponding to the surrounding subretinal hemorrhage.

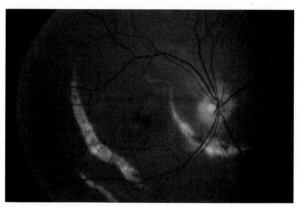

Multiple choroidal ruptures in a 15-year-old boy who was struck in the right eye with a rock 6 weeks earlier. He developed a subfoveal choroidal neovascular membrane.

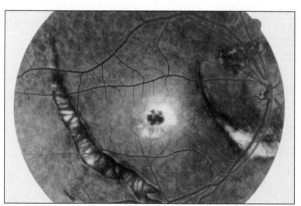

Fluorescein angiogram of the same patient reveals a classic subfoveal choroidal neovascular membrane. Note the visibility of the larger choroidal vessels within the temporal choroidal rupture.

COMMOTIO RETINAE

Commotio retinae, caused by an acute contusion of the neurosensory retina, is a condition of one or more gray-white patches of outer retina. This traumatic opacification of the outer retina is also known as Berlin's edema.

Symptoms

If the commotio retinae (or commotio) affects the center of the macula, the patient will notice a central scotoma and decreased central vision. Commotio outside the macula is generally asymptomatic.

Clinical Features

The color change to gray-white appears in the outer retina several hours after the injury. The optic disc and retinal vessels are uninvolved. In milder cases of commotio, the color change is subtle and less opaque than in more severe injuries. Milder injuries are accompanied by a return of central vision and a restoration of normal retinal color and function within days to weeks. In more severe cases, the commotio appears dense gray, often with associated retinal or preretinal hemorrhage. Severe commotio, or retinal contusion, can lead to permanent vision loss, if centered in the macula. The long-term clinical features of severe commotio include pigmentary derangement of the underlying retinal pigment epithelium (RPE) and a loss of the foveal reflex.

Ancillary Testing

The fluorescein angiographic findings of mild commotio are typically normal. In severe cases, due to damage to the RPE, hyperfluorescence may be seen in the area of commotio.

Pathology/Pathogenesis

Histologic data from animal studies have shown immediate fragmentation of photoreceptor outer segments and intracellular retinal edema in areas of commotio. This intracellular edema is thought to account for the gray color of the outer retina. Histopathologic examination of a human eye with commotio that was enucleated 24 hours after injury revealed damage to the photoreceptors similar to that seen in animals. The extent of damage to the photoreceptors may be the primary factor in the reversibility of visual loss.

Treatment/Prognosis

There is no treatment for commotio retinae. Patients may have complete recovery of visual loss or may be left with central visual deficits.

Systemic Evaluation

No systemic evaluation is required for commotio retinae. Ruptured globe, retinal detachment, and other ocular injuries must be excluded.

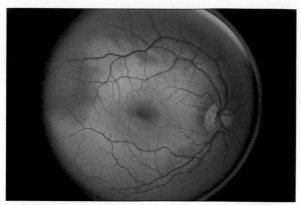

Commotio retinae in an 8-year-old boy who was struck in the right eye while wrestling. His vision was 20/200. There is prominent whitening of the outer retina throughout the macula.

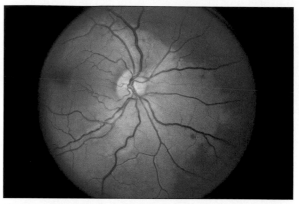

The borders between the normal and abnormal retina are fairly well defined. Note that the optic disc and retinal vessels are normal.

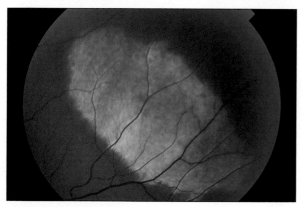

This patient has a prominent patch of commotio retinae. The borders are well defined.

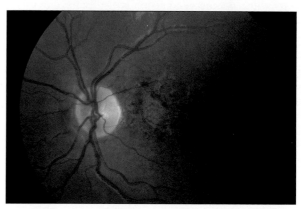

Although many individuals regain normal vision, retinal pigment epithelial alterations may limit visual recovery. Retinal pigment epithelial abnormalities include stippled hyperpigmentation and atrophy.

OPTIC NERVE AVULSION

In an avulsion of the optic nerve, the nerve is torn or partially torn posteriorly from its insertion into the retina at the level of the lamina cribrosa. This disinsertion or retraction of the nerve is due to a mechanical shearing force on the posterior aspect of the globe.

Symptoms

Patients present following head trauma that may be severe or seemingly minor. Visual acuity is often no light perception if the avulsion is complete; visual acuity may be better (20/100 to light perception) if the avulsion is partial. Patients have no pain associated with the avulsion; although, pain may be present due to external injuries.

Clinical Features

Patients with optic nerve avulsion typically have evidence of external trauma and will frequently have symptoms from an injury to the orbit. The normal optic disc is replaced by a depression or cavity, with surrounding and overlying hemorrhage. The amount of intraocular hemorrhage may be massive. The optic disc cavity is eventually replaced with glial tissue.

Ancillary Testing

Computed tomography may be necessary to rule out an intraorbital or intraocular foreign body. Neuroimaging is, however, unreliable in making the diagnosis of optic nerve avulsion.

Pathology/Pathogenesis

The optic nerve is "tethered" at its posterior entry site into the globe. The mechanism of injury at the level of the lamina cribrosa is likely due to a complete disruption of the ganglion cell axons as they exit the globe. Because the rectus and oblique muscles support the globe and hold it in a relatively static position, a sudden and rapid displacement of the nerve may shear the nerve from the posterior wall of the globe. In addition, a rapid forward pulling of the globe may also cause the nerve to avulse posteriorly. Rapid rotational eye movements have also been implicated as a primary mechanism for optic nerve avulsion.

Treatment/Prognosis

Treatment for optic nerve avulsion is supportive and conservative. The prognosis for vision is extremely poor. Final visual outcome is usually dependent on the initial visual acuity after injury. Surgical intervention is not warranted unless a rupture of the globe is suspected.

Systemic Evaluation

Careful attention to associated orbital, maxillofacial, cranial, and cervical injuries is warranted.

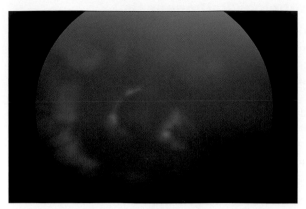

Acute optic nerve avulsion following a finger injury to the orbit. The optic disc is replaced by a large depression with hemorrhage extending throughout the retina and vitreous.

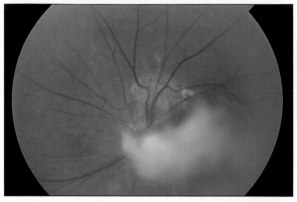

Following the acute injury, fibroglial proliferation occurs in and around the optic disc region and may extend into the vitreous cavity.

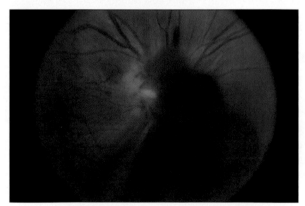

Fundus photograph following partial optic nerve avulsion. There is intraretinal, preretinal, and vitreous hemorrhage. Note the folds radiating from the optic disc.

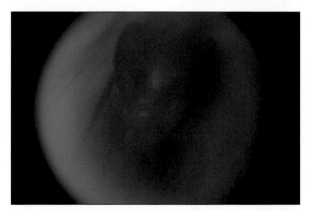

The vitreous hemorrhage may be diffuse or localized in the region of Cloquet's canal.

PURTSCHER'S RETINOPATHY

In 1910, Austrian ophthalmologist Otmar Purtscher described a retinopathy of bilateral peripapillary patches of retinal whitening and hemorrhages in patients who suffered massive head trauma. The term Purtscher's-like retinopathy has been used to describe similar fundus findings in association with other conditions, including pancreatitis, kidney disease, childbirth, cancer, and autoimmune disorders (systemic lupus erythematosus, scleroderma, dermatomyositis).

Symptoms

Patients generally experience rapid, painless, and profound visual loss in both eyes. Occasionally, the symptoms will be quite asymmetric or unilateral. The patients may note Amsler grid changes or central scotoma.

Clinical Features

A bilateral decrease in visual acuity and central visual field that corresponds to the degree of retinal involvement occurs in these patients. An afferent pupillary defect may be present if the condition is unilateral or asymmetric. The acute funduscopic appearance includes large patches of ischemic retinal whitening and intraretinal hemorrhages surrounding the optic disc. Optic nerve head swelling is typically absent. Over several weeks to months, the ischemic whitening fades, and the hemorrhages resolve. Late findings include arteriolar narrowing and nerve fiber layer atrophy in the ischemic area as well as optic nerve pallor.

Ancillary Testing

Visual acuity measurements and visual field testing may be helpful in documenting the extent of retinal involvement. Fluorescein angiography typically demonstrates a lack of capillary blood flow in the regions that correspond to the areas of ischemic retina. Indocyanine green angiography demonstrates areas of choroidal nonperfusion that may persist for months.

Pathology/Pathogenesis

The precise mechanism for Purtscher's retinopathy remains unknown. Microembolic theories remain the leading candidates for the pathogenesis of these ischemic retinal changes surrounding the optic disc. There is evidence that complement activation leading to leukocyte emboli may occlude the peripapillary retinal capillaries. Unilateral Purtscher-like retinopathy also has been described as a complication of local injury, either facial trauma or retrobulbar anesthesia.

Treatment/Prognosis

Treatment for Purtscher's retinopathy is supportive and directed at the underlying medical conditions. The ischemic retinal patches and retinal hemorrhages will resolve gradually. Final visual acuity depends on the level of retinal involvement and ranges from normal to severely reduced.

Systemic Evaluation

In the setting of trauma, other injuries should be evaluated and imaged as appropriate. In the absence of obvious trauma, a more thorough systemic evaluation should include testing for acute pancreatitis, disseminated intravascular coagulopathy, autoimmune disorders, pregnancy, renal function, thrombotic thrombocytopenic purpura, and hemolytic-uremic syndrome.

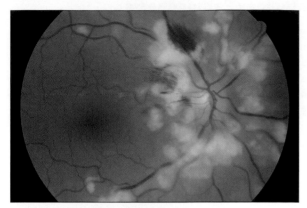

Purtscher's-like retinopathy in a woman with scleroderma. There are peripapillary superficial white patches, few intraretinal hemorrhages, and a normal optic disc.

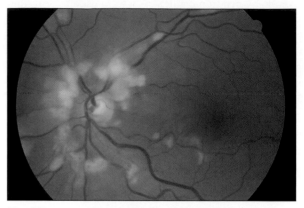

The fellow eye of the same patient demonstrates numerous superficial white patches concentrated around the optic disc. Note that the white patches obscure the underlying retinal vessels.

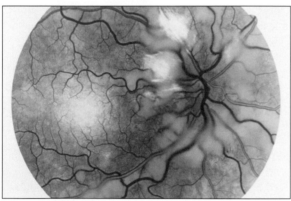

Fluorescein angiography of Purtscher's retinopathy reveals hypofluorescence corresponding to the white patches that results from blockage and capillary nonperfusion.

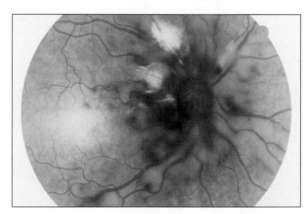

Venous phase angiogram demonstrates persistent hypofluorescence corresponding to the nonperfusion and areas of hyperfluorescence from retinal vascular leakage.

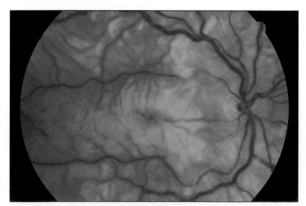

This 7-year-old boy had severe Purtscher's-like retinopathy following a presumed viral-induced dermatomyositis associated with acute renal failure. The fellow eye appeared similar.

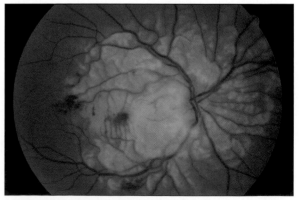

Unilateral Purtscher's-like retinopathy after a motor vehicle accident; the patient experienced chest compression injury and a long bone fracture. The visual loss was permanent.

SHAKEN BABY SYNDROME

Shaken baby syndrome (SBS) is a term used to describe a type of child abuse associated with severe ocular and systemic injuries but few if any external signs of abuse. The ophthalmologist's role in such cases is to document all ocular findings and note whether these findings are consistent with SBS. While no single ocular manifestation is pathognomonic of child abuse, ocular examination can provide significant and compelling information leading to the diagnosis.

Symptoms

The shaken baby may present to the emergency room in a comatose state from severe intracranial injuries. The alert child may have decreased visual function as indicated by inattentiveness to visual targets. The child may be irritable or agitated. Children may also present with seizure, failure to thrive, lethargy, vomiting, and respiratory difficulties.

Clinical Features

The child may have no signs of external trauma. Alternatively, the external ocular examination may reveal periorbital ecchymosis, eyelid lacerations, subconjunctival hemorrhages, corneal abrasions, hyphema, iris sphincter tears, and cataract.

Fundus features of SBS include extensive intraretinal, preretinal, and/or subretinal hemorrhages. Intraretinal hemorrhages occur throughout the entire retina, extending from the optic disc to the ora serrata. The preretinal hemorrhages and sub-internal limiting membrane hemorrhages are often round and dome shaped. Other fundus findings associated with acute SBS include vitreous hemorrhage, optic nerve swelling, retinal folds, retinoschisis, retinal dialysis or tears, and chorioretinal scars from previous trauma. While any of these retinal findings may occur in the SBS, none is pathognomonic.

Ancillary Testing

Ultrasonography may be useful in children with severe vitreous hemorrhage.

Pathology/Pathogenesis

Repeated acceleration-deceleration injury to the shaken infant may be the cause of the retinal hemorrhages, retinal folds, and retinoschisis seen in SBS. Bleeding may derive from vitreoretinal traction, in which the vitreous pulls on the retina and retinal blood vessels during rapid deceleration. Sudden shifts in intracranial venous pressure from chest trauma or head trauma may be a contributing factor.

Treatment/Prognosis

Treatment for the retinal hemorrhage is usually supportive. However, if a child has a large, nonclearing vitreous or preretinal hemorrhage that obstructs central vision, vitrectomy surgery should be considered to minimize amblyopia. In SBS, approximately 15% of infants die, 50% have significant morbidity, and 20% of survivors have poor vision. The causes of visual defects are more often lesions of the occipital cortex than the intraocular injuries. In terms of prognosis, mortality is correlated with the extent of visual loss and the area of retinal hemorrhages.

Systemic Evaluation

In a child under 3 years of age, the presence of retinal hemorrhages raises the possibility of child abuse and must be investigated. Ancillary testing is typically directed by the pediatrician. Testing may include neuroimaging to rule out associated central nervous system involvement such as subdural hematoma and subarachnoid hemorrhage and a careful radiographic search for bone fractures or other skeletal injuries. To exclude other causes of retinal hemorrhages, an appropriate workup includes (1) history taking regarding possible accidental trauma; (2) hemophilia; (3) von Willebrand's disease; (4) coagulopathies; and (5) vitamin K deficiency. The relationship between cardiopulmonary resuscitation and intraretinal hemorrhages is controversial.

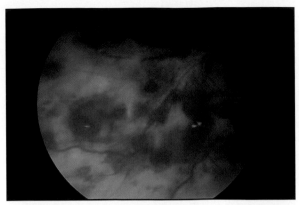

Shaken baby syndrome is characterized by widespread intraretinal hemorrhages, which are usually bilateral but may be unilateral or asymmetric.

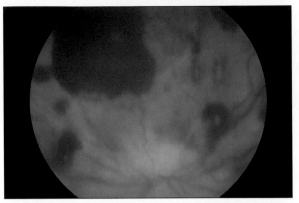

This child with shaken baby syndrome had vitreous hemorrhage obscuring the retinal details. Several white-centered intraretinal hemorrhages are present.

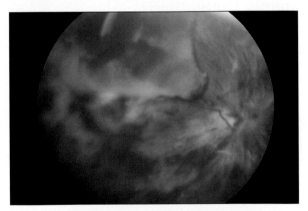

This infant had bilateral widespread intraretinal hemorrhages. In addition, an area of retinoschisis (upper left) is observed.

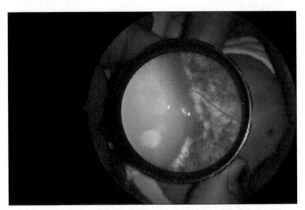

The fellow eye of the same patient demonstrates evidence of a traction retinal fold, which results from the strong relationship of the vitreous and the perimacular area in the young.

TERSON'S SYNDROME

Terson initially reported on the association of vitreous hemorrhage with an acute subarachnoid hemorrhage. Since then, Terson's syndrome has been applied to any form of intracranial hemorrhage with secondary vitreous or preretinal hemorrhage.

Symptoms

Patients with Terson's syndrome generally present to the ophthalmologist after an acute intracranial event, usually a ruptured intracranial aneurysm or a subdural hematoma. Patients are frequently obtunded initially and are not able to complain of acute visual loss. The ophthalmologist is often consulted when the patient regains consciousness and complains of poor vision or central scotoma. The visual loss may be unilateral or bilateral at presentation and typically ranges from 20/400 to light perception.

Clinical Features

The hemorrhages in this syndrome are localized to the sub-internal limiting membrane space of the macula or peripapillary region. These hemorrhages may break through into the vitreous and may or may not clear spontaneously. In general, there is no relative afferent pupillary defect unless there has been optic nerve damage from direct trauma or intracranial injury.

Ancillary Testing

No ancillary testing is necessary. Fluorescein angiography demonstrates hypofluorescence corresponding to the areas of preretinal hemorrhage.

Pathology/Pathogenesis

A rapid increase in intracranial pressure leading to impaired intraocular venous return is the most likely cause of the preretinal hemorrhage. The sudden rise in intracranial pressure due to intracranial hemorrhage or trauma may cause intraocular venous stasis, which in turn causes the superficial retinal capillaries to rupture. The resulting hemorrhage is typically within the sub-internal limiting membrane space.

Treatment/Prognosis

Many mild cases of preretinal hemorrhage, particularly those not involving the fovea, will resolve spontaneously. Larger hemorrhages that obscure the macula or result in nonclearing vitreous hemorrhage may require pars plana vitrectomy surgery. Removal of the internal limiting membrane can be performed without subsequent injury to the underlying neurosensory retina, and the blood can be easily evacuated. Surgical intervention can be delayed until the patient is medically and neurologically stable. The prognosis is generally good unless there has been hemorrhagic detachment of the neurosensory retina. In small children, failure to clear a large preretinal hemorrhage or a vitreous hemorrhage in a reasonable time period could lead to deprivation amblyopia of the affected eye.

Systemic Evaluation

Neurologic evaluation and imaging is urgent if hemorrhage of the sub-internal limiting membrane or spontaneous vitreous hemorrhage is noted in a conscious patient complaining of headache. An evaluation for bleeding tendencies or blood dyscrasia also may be warranted.

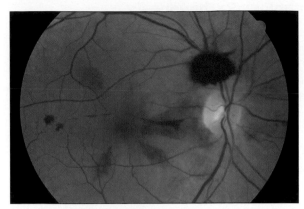

Terson's syndrome in a 35-year-old woman following a spontaneous subarachnoid hemorrhage. She had bilateral preretinal and vitreous hemorrhages.

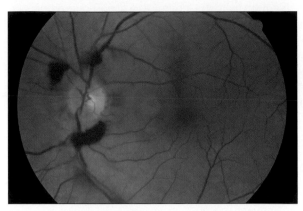

The preretinal hemorrhages were confined to the peripapillary and macular regions.

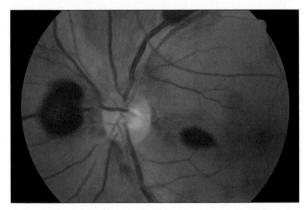

Preretinal and intraretinal hemorrhages in a patient with a ruptured intracranial aneurysm.

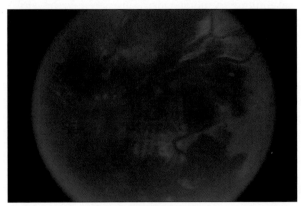

Severe preretinal and intraretinal hemorrhages in a patient with subarachnoid bleeding.

VALSALVA RETINOPATHY

Valsalva retinopathy is a rupture of superficial retinal capillaries that occurs when a rise in the intrathoracic or intra-abdominal pressure causes an associated rise in the intraocular venous pressure. This can occur during heavy or strenuous lifting, coughing, sneezing, vomiting, or straining. At times, no precipitating event can be identified.

Symptoms

Patients usually describe a sudden loss of central vision and a central scotoma.

Clinical Features

Patients with Valsalva retinopathy typically demonstrate a red, dome-shaped sub-internal limiting membrane mass that is round or oval. The elevation of the sub-internal limiting membrane may cause striae in the surrounding retina. As the blood resolves, the hemorrhage turns yellow. Further resorption of blood may lead to the presence of serous fluid. In the mildest case, patients have small, flat hemorrhages, which occur most commonly in the center of the macula. In addition to the more typical sub-internal limiting membrane hemorrhage, there may be vitreous hemorrhage, preretinal hemorrhage, intraretinal hemorrhages, and, less commonly, subretinal hemorrhage.

Ancillary Testing

Fluorescein angiography demonstrates hypofluorescence as a result of the blood blocking the underlying retinal and choroidal circulations. There are no other associated retinal vascular abnormalities.

Pathology/Pathogenesis

In a Valsalva maneuver, increased intrathoracic pressure is generated by forceful exhalation against a closed glottis. The increased intrathoracic pressure can cause increased intracranial venous pressure followed by decreased intraocular venous return. This results in the rupture of one or more inner retinal capillaries. Occasionally, Valsalva retinopathy is bilateral.

Treatment/Prognosis

Treatment is generally observation. In cases of non-clearing vitreous hemorrhage or large preretinal hemorrhage, vitrectomy may also be indicated. The YAG (yttrium-aluminum-garnet) laser may be used to disperse dense preretinal or sub-internal limiting membrane hemorrhages into the vitreous for more rapid clearance. Most hemorrhages clear spontaneously.

Systemic Evaluation

A systemic workup should include testing for blood dyscrasia, high blood pressure, and coagulopathy, particularly in patients with a family history or personal history of bleeding tendencies.

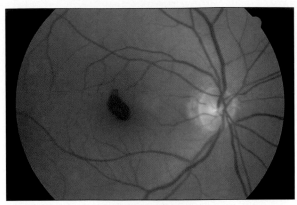

Small preretinal hemorrhage in a woman following a severe coughing episode. She presented with an acute central scotoma in her right eye.

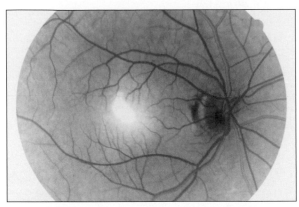

The fluorescein angiogram of the same patient revealed hypofluorescence without any other retinal vascular abnormality.

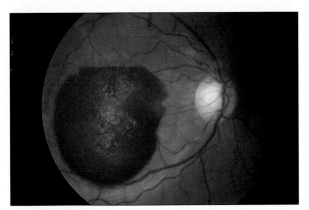

This 38-year-old man had a persistent preretinal hemorrhage in his right eye reducing his vision to hand motions.

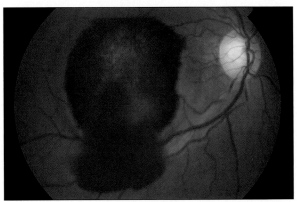

YAG laser was applied to the inferior aspect of the hemorrhage. This immediate posttreatment photograph reveals dispersion of the hemorrhage into the vitreous. His vision returned to 20/20.

SELECTED REFERENCES

Choroidal Rupture

1. Aguilar JP, Green WR. Choroidal rupture: a histopathologic study of 47 eyes. *Retina.* 1984;4:269–275.
2. Gross JG, King LP, de Juan E, Powers P. Subfoveal neovascular membrane removal in patients with traumatic choroidal rupture. *Ophthalmology.* 1996;103:579–585.
3. Kohno T, Miki T, Shiraki K, Kano K, Hirabayashi-Matsushita M. Indocyanine green angiographic features of choroidal rupture and choroidal vascular injury after contusion ocular injury. *Am J Ophthalmol.* 2000;129:38–46.
4. Wyszynski RE, Grossniklaus HE, Frank KE. Indirect choroidal rupture secondary to blunt ocular trauma: a review of eight eyes. *Retina.* 1988;8:237–243.

Commotio Retinae

1. Liem AT, Keunen JE, Van Norren D. Reversible cone photoreceptor injury in commotio retinae of the macula. *Retina.* 1995;15:58–61.
2. Mansour AM, Green WR, Hogge C. Histopathology of commotio retinae. *Retina.* 1992;12:24–48.
3. Sipperly JO, Quigley HA, Gass JDM. Traumatic retinopathy in primates: the explanation of commotio retinae. *Arch Ophthalmol.* 1978;96:2267–2273.

Optic Nerve Avulsion

1. Fard AK, Merbs SL, Pieramici DM. Optic nerve avulsion from a diving injury. *Am J Ophthalmol.* 1997;124:562–564.
2. Foster BS, March GA, Lucarelli MJ, Samiy N, Lessell S. Optic nerve avulsion. *Arch Ophthalmol.* 1997;115:623–630.
3. Friedman SM. Optic nerve avulsion secondary to a basketball injury. *Ophthalmic Surg Lasers.* 1999;30:676–677.
4. Roth DB, Warman R. Optic nerve avulsion from a golfing injury. *Am J Ophthalmol.* 1999;128:657–658.

Purtscher's Retinopathy

1. Jacob HS, Goldstein IM, Shapiro I, Craddock PR, Hammerschmidt DE, Weissmann G. Sudden blindness in acute pancreatitis: possible role of complement-induced retinal leukoembolization. *Arch Intern Med.* 1981;141:134–136.
2. Lemagne JM, Michiels X, Van Causenbroeck S, Snyers B. Purtscher-like retinopathy after retrobulbar anesthesia. *Ophthalmology.* 1990;97:858–861.
3. Purtscher O. Noch unbekannte Befunde nach Schadeltrauma. *Berl Dtsch Ophthalmol Ges.* 1910;36:294–301.

Shaken Baby Syndrome

1. Han DP, Wilkinson WS. Late ophthalmic manifestations of the shaken baby syndrome. *J Pediatr Ophthalmol Strabismus.* 1990;27:299–303.
2. Kivlin JD. Manifestations of the shaken baby syndrome. *Curr Opin Ophthalmol.* 2001;12:158–163.
3. Kivlin JD, Simons KB, Lazoritz S, Ruttum MS. Shaken baby syndrome. *Ophthalmology.* 2000;107:1246–1254.

Terson's Syndrome

1. Gnanaraj L, Tyagi AK, Cottrell DG, Fetherston TJ, Richardson J, Stannard KP, et al. Referral delay and ocular surgical outcome in Terson syndrome. *Retina.* 2000;20:374–377.
2. Kuhn F, Morris R, Witherspoon CD, Mester V. Terson syndrome: results of vitrectomy and the significance of vitreous hemorrhage in patients with subarachnoid hemorrhage. *Ophthalmology.* 1998;105:472–477.
3. Schultz PN, Sobol WM, Weingeist TA. Long-term visual outcome in Terson syndrome. *Ophthalmology.* 1991;98:1814–1819.

Valsalva Retinopathy

1. Kadrmas EF, Pach JM. Vitreous hemorrhage and retinal vein rupture. *Am J Ophthalmol.* 1995;120:114–115.
2. Ulbig MW, Mangouritsas G, Rothbacher HH, Hamilton AM, McHugh JD. Long-term results after drainage of premacular subhyaloid hemorrhage into the vitreous with a pulsed Nd:YAG laser. *Arch Ophthalmol.* 1998;116:1465–1469.

chapter 11

Peripheral Retinal Diseases

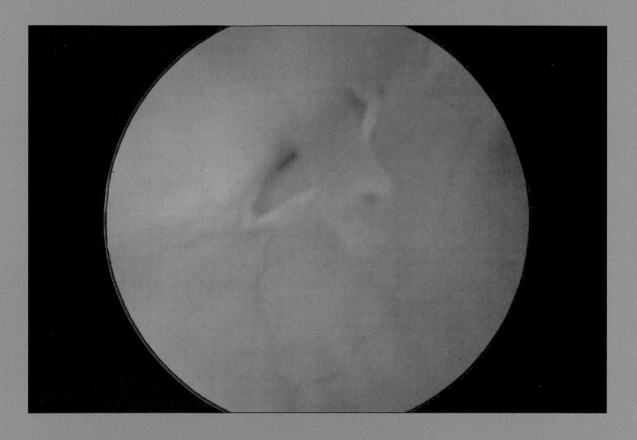

Norman E. Byer, MD

CYSTIC RETINAL TUFTS

Cystic retinal tufts are associated with approximately 10% of clinical retinal detachments. They are tiny congenital developmental abnormalities that can occur in association with small asymptomatic retinal breaks in young people, or with symptomatic traction tears at the time of posterior vitreous detachment (PVD).

Symptoms

No symptoms are associated with cystic retinal tufts.

Clinical Features

Clinically, lesions appear as tiny (0.1 to 1.0 mm) yellowish or chalky-white retinal tufts in the equatorial region. When scleral indentation is applied, the base is seen to have sloping borders as the lesion merges with the adjacent retina, in contrast with true retinal tears, which tend to have a sharper, more acute angle. Also, the flaps of true retinal tears are translucent, and one can see through them to a partial degree, whereas cystic retinal tufts are opaque. In some cases, an asymptomatic localized form of vitreous detachment can produce a tiny traction retinal tear or a round break, with overlying free operculum. In such cases, a tiny rim of subretinal fluid may occur around the retinal break.

Ancillary Testing

No other testing is required.

Pathology/Pathogenesis

Cystic retinal tufts represent a developmental anomaly that is characterized by an abnormal deposition of glial tissue at the vitreoretinal interface, which is strongly adherent to both vitreous and retina. This glial cap shows crypts of formed vitreous within its substance. Therefore, at the time of a generalized posterior vitreous detachment, which occurs in around 25% to 30% of persons during life (or more following cataract surgery), cystic retinal tufts may become the sites of new, symptomatic, traction retinal tears.

Treatment/Prognosis

Because of the high prevalence of this lesion in the population, the risk of retinal detachment for any patient with cystic retinal tufts is far less than 1%. It is therefore not necessary or proper to recommend treatment for a patient with uncomplicated lesions. However, if PVD has caused a new traction tear, with or without retinal detachment, this must be promptly treated by currently accepted techniques. (See "Retinal Detachment" and "Retinal Breaks" later in this chapter.)

Systemic Evaluation

There are no systemic associations with cystic retinal tufts.

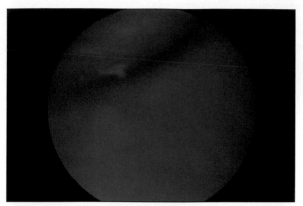

Cystic retinal tuft is seen with scleral indentation, showing sloping borders of flap.

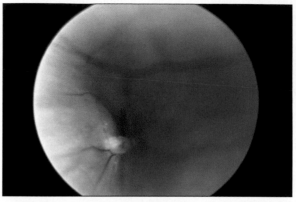

Cystic retinal tuft, with scleral indentation, shows typical chalky-white deposit on flap.

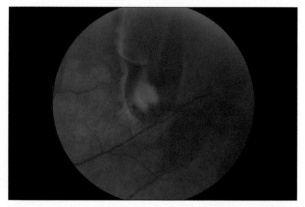

Tandem traction retinal tear shows chalky-white apex of flap.

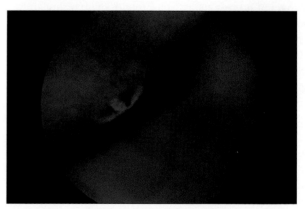

Cystic retinal tuft is seen with scleral indentation.

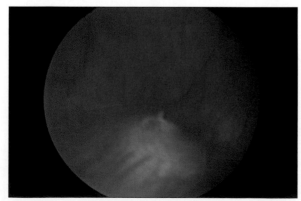

Cystic retinal tuft occurs with preexisting tiny traction tear and chalky-white apex on flap in 20-year-old man.

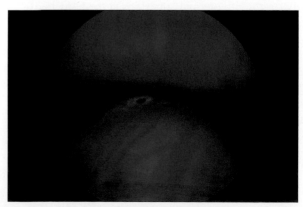

Same eye 6 years later shows complete avulsion of former attached flap. Still no symptoms and no posterior vitreous detachment were present.

LATTICE DEGENERATION

Lattice degeneration is a very common, inherited, congenital abnormality of the peripheral retina. It usually shows an autosomal dominant pattern and occurs in about 8% of healthy individuals of both sexes.

Symptoms

No known symptoms are associated with this condition, per se. Occasionally, after age 45, if an acute posterior vitreous detachment (PVD) occurs, a retinal tear may be observed at a lattice lesion; the tear then may produce symptoms of this event (floaters or light flashes).

Clinical Features

Lattice degeneration is almost always discovered inadvertently, either in the course of a routine eye examination or in conjunction with symptoms of a PVD. When discovered it presents as small round, oval, or linear islands that are whitish, pigmented, or reddish, and generally are located in the equatorial zone and parallel with it. To discover all such lesions, it is necessary to use indirect ophthalmoscopy combined with scleral indentation.

Occasionally, white lines ("lattice") crisscross the lesion, and/or tiny atrophic round retinal holes may be seen. Very infrequently, a traction retinal tear may be found on the posterior edge of the lesion. This tear always denotes a previous PVD, which, in the absence of recent visual floaters or light flashes, is probably long-standing.

Pathology/Pathogenesis

Lattice degeneration is located histologically at the vitreoretinal interface and is always associated with abnormally strong vitreoretinal adhesions at the borders of each lesion. These adhesions represent the chief clinical danger of this disease because of their ability to lead to retinal tears and detachment after PVD. Typical histologic features include a discrete area of thinning of the retina, a newly formed fibrocellular membrane lining the surface on the vitreous side, exaggerated vitreoretinal attachments at the borders of the lesion, and a discrete overlying space from which the vitreous is absent. Also, there may be sclerotic vascular changes sometimes in the vicinity of the lesion.

Treatment/Prognosis

During the lifetime of a patient with lattice degeneration, the likelihood of having a retinal detachment on this basis is in the range of 1% to 2%. Among patients having lattice degeneration and a PVD, approximately 24% will suffer a retinal tear as a result, but only 16% will develop a tear at the site of a visible lattice lesion. Among patients with lattice degeneration associated with tiny atrophic holes, only 2% will be in danger of a later retinal detachment. If a new traction tear or a retinal detachment develops, these should be promptly treated with current techniques. (See "Retinal Detachment" and "Retinal Breaks" later in this chapter.) The current literature regarding prevention of retinal detachment does not provide sufficient information to strongly support prophylactic treatment of lesions other than symptomatic flap tears.

Systemic Evaluation

No systemic evaluation is required.

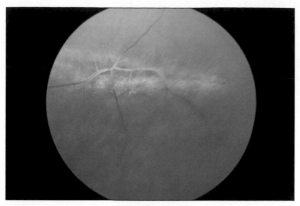

Lattice degeneration is observed with white lines (without scleral indentation).

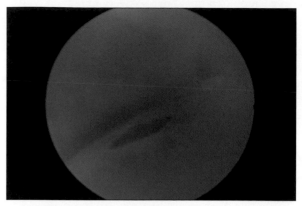

Lattice degeneration occurs with reddish crater, without white lines (with scleral indentation).

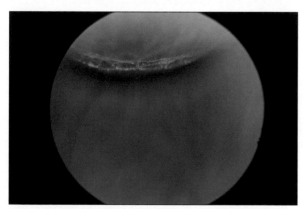

Superior lattice degeneration is seen in snail-track form (with scleral indentation).

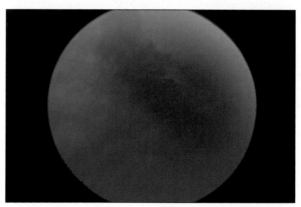

Lattice degeneration with massive pigmentation is caused by secondary changes in pigment epithelium (without scleral indentation).

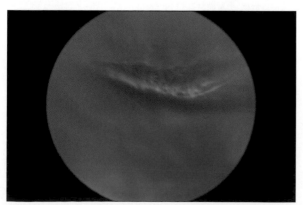

Lattice degeneration is shown with combined features of reddish crater and snail-track appearance (with scleral indentation).

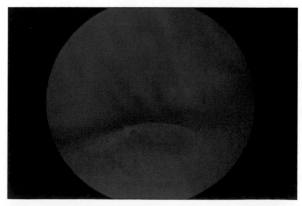

Lattice degeneration appears with tiny atrophic hole and subclinical retinal detachment of long duration (with scleral indentation).

RETINAL BREAKS

The evaluation of retinal breaks is very important with respect to the effective prevention of clinical rhegmatogenous retinal detachment. The most serious retinal breaks (actual discontinuities) are traction breaks, including both tears with attached flaps and tears with free opercula (ie, completely avulsed flaps). Such flaps, when clinically significant, almost always occur as a direct result of posterior vitreous detachment (PVD).

Symptoms

When PVD occurs it is often associated with symptoms either of new vitreous floaters (one or more) or of lightning streaks or, rarely, loss of peripheral visual field. Some tiny peripheral tears occur in association with cystic retinal tufts, without symptoms and without PVD as their cause. A third category of retinal breaks is atrophic holes, usually tiny and round, resulting almost always from lattice degeneration. These holes are not symptomatic and only rarely lead to clinical retinal detachment (around 2%).

Clinical Features

In patients with recent history of visual floaters or light flashes, who are older than 45 years (or, if highly myopic, even at much younger ages), a prompt and thorough examination with indirect ophthalmoscopy and scleral indentation is mandatory. If a tear is found it usually will show an attached retinal flap on the peripheral side. If it is recent (within a few days) it may also show several scattered intraretinal hemorrhages, or less frequently some degree of vitreous blood that has gravitated inferiorly.

Atrophic retinal holes are not symptomatic and are not associated with hemorrhage. They are usually, but not always, contained within a lattice lesion.

Ancillary Testing

No specific ancillary testing is required. B-scan ultrasongraphy may be helpful in cases of cataract or vitreous hemorrhage, for which visualization of the fundus is difficult.

Pathology/Pathogenesis

Retinal tears result from traction exerted by the detaching posterior vitreous on preexisting abnormal vitreoretinal adhesions. This traction produces a tear in normal retinal tissue adjacent to the point of traction, and may result in a remaining attached flap of retinal tissue, or a completely avulsed retinal fragment. Symptomatic tears are the result of PVD. Asymptomatic tiny tears (either with an attached flap or a free operculum) usually result from cystic retinal tufts. Atrophic holes are caused by very slowly progressive thinning of retinal tissue within lesions of lattice degeneration.

Prognosis and Treatment

If associated with attached flaps, about 50% of symptomatic traction tears will lead to clinical retinal detachment (less in tears with free, avulsed opercula). Therefore, all such tears should be promptly surrounded with either laser or cryotherapy applications. Retinal tears that are discovered in eyes without recent symptoms (less than 3 months), even if a PVD is present, do not need to be treated, since there is no clinical proof of significant danger of retinal detachment.

Retinal tears not associated with recent symptoms, in the absence of a PVD, are generally due to cystic retinal tufts. These tears also do not require treatment because they have a negligible risk of detachment. Atrophic retinal holes have no relationship to vitreoretinal symptoms and an extremely low risk of retinal detachment in primary eyes, and do not require treatment. In fellow eyes, the risk may be somewhat higher, but it has not been shown to be significantly reduced by prophylactic treatment.

Systemic Evaluation

No systemic evaluation is recommended.

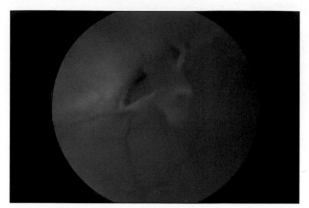

Large traction retinal tear is visible (with scleral indentation).

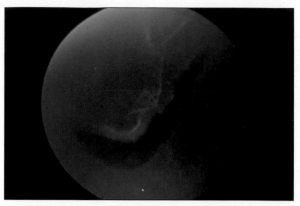

Large traction retinal tear occurs secondary to posterior vitreous detachment at border of lattice lesion.

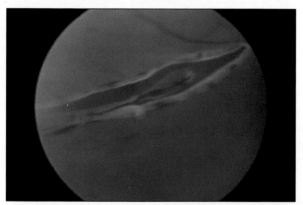

Very large traction retinal tear is associated with torn central vessel and retinal hemorrhages.

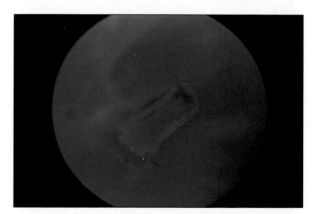

Traction retinal tear with floating operculum is completely avulsed from old chorioretinal scar.

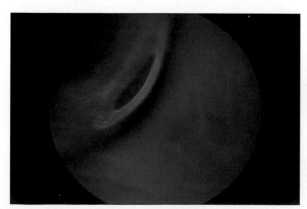

Large atrophic retinal hole in a lattice lesion is not associated with posterior vitreous detachment.

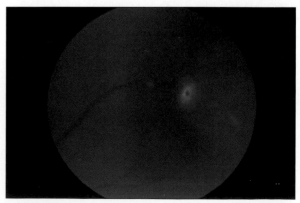

Tiny traction retinal tear with free operculum, secondary to cystic retinal tuft and of long duration, is observed.

RETINAL DETACHMENT

Traditionally, retinal detachment has been a leading category in ophthalmology as a cause for loss of vision. It is an end result of many diverse types of pathology including development abnormalities, inflammation, vasculopathy, diabetes, tumors, trauma, and others in which it is a secondary development. However, the traditional, most common, and most treatable condition denoted by this term is primary, idiopathic, rhegmatogenous retinal detachment, which is discussed here.

Symptoms

Symptoms consist typically of visual "floaters," light flashes, blurred vision, or visual field defects. Any such symptoms should immediately alert the ophthalmologist to perform a visual and retinal examination on both eyes of the patient, with full pupillary dilation, using indirect ophthalmoscopy and scleral indentation, combined with vitreous examination using a Goldmann three-mirror contact lens. Occasionally, if the area of retinal detachment is small or limited to the periphery, symptoms may be minimal or absent.

Clinical Features

In primary rhegmatogenous retinal detachments, at least one retinal break always occurs, usually a retinal tear in association with a posterior vitreous detachment. An elevated portion of the retina is visible and has an altered appearance, being more grayish or less orange, and with less distinct choroidal vessels visible beneath it.

The surface of the retina may show a lack of uniformity, with depressions, "wrinkled" appearance, or small intraretinal hemorrhages near the retinal break. The vitreous may show a variable amount of dispersed blood or a deposit of red blood, usually inferiorly. When scleral indentation is performed, the appearance of the retina may change so that the elevation is not as high, or so that the shape or apparent size of the retinal break is changed.

Ancillary Testing

The diagnosis and localization of retinal detachment requires careful ophthalmoscopic examination. B-scan ultrasonography may be useful in cases of inadequate visualization of the fundus such as cataract or vitreous hemorrhage.

Pathology/Pathogenesis

In a rhegmatogenous retinal detachment, part of the vitreous fluid that has become liquefied passes through the retinal break into the subretinal space, elevating the visual retina above the layer of the pigment epithelium. When this occurs it causes some degree of diminution of vision varying from slight to severe.

Treatment/Prognosis

Successful treatment depends on the accurate finding and permanent closure of all retinal breaks in the area of the detachment. Closure is achieved with cryotherapy and usually some means of producing a permanent scleral buckle, such as the placement of a localized or encircling silicone exoplant, which may be solid or sponge, in the area of the retinal breaks. Also, other degenerative spots (eg, lattice degeneration) should be treated at the same time. Pars plana vitrectomy may be indicated for certain cases of retinal detachment.

Systemic Evaluation

No systemic evaluation is required in patients with rhegmatogenous retinal detachment.

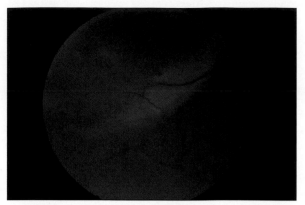

Superior retinal detachment with tiny traction tear is shown.

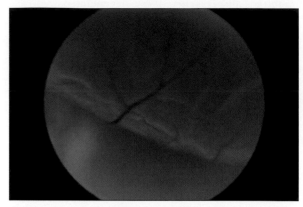

Superior retinal detachment is observed.

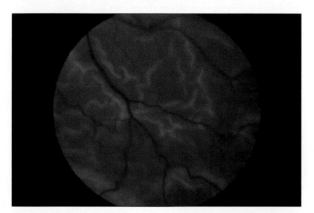

Retinal detachment shows wrinkled retinal surface.

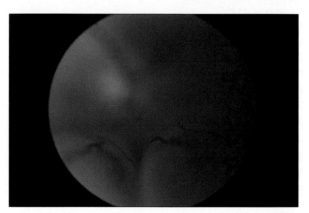

Inferior retinal detachment demonstrates bullous folds.

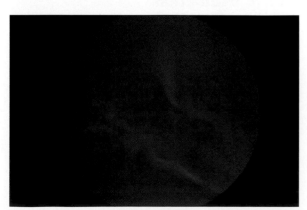

Bullous retinal detachment has hidden traction tear.

SENILE (ADULT-ONSET) RETINOSCHISIS

Senile retinoschisis is a hereditary, degenerative intraretinal disease. It leads to the splitting of a portion of the retina into two separate layers, in which area vision is permanently lost. Senile retinoschisis can rarely be present in the late teens but attains a much increased prevalence after age 40 years. It is present in approximately 7% of individuals over that age.

Symptoms

In almost all cases, there are no symptoms produced by retinoschisis. In rare instances, the patient may note visual field loss. However, even in the presence of very large lesions that have progressed to a point as close as 2 disc diameters (DD) from the macula, it is unusual for a patient to be aware of any interference with vision.

Clinical Features

Senile retinoschisis, in addition to appearing without symptoms, is usually of subtle appearance. Therefore, it very frequently escapes detection, even in a complete eye examination. It is found most frequently in the lower outer quadrant but may occur in any location.

Retinoschisis presents as a uniform, dome-shaped elevation of the retina, with a convex posterior border. It is seen most often, and by far the best, when indirect ophthalmoscopy combined with careful scleral indentation is used. Often, it is first noticed because of either the multitudes of very minute yellow-white flecks present on the retinal surface or a few whitish lines having a vascular configuration. During scleral indentation the lesion behaves like a fluid-filled space, tending to rise as a unit with indentation. This finding is in contrast to a rhegmatogenous retinal detachment, in which indentation tends to change the height of the elevation, making it appear flatter. The outer layer is difficult to see, but in about 15% of cases it may contain a retinal break. Also, in some cases, the outer layer may then be partly elevated above the layer of the pigment epithelium.

Ancillary Testing

No other tests are necessary in retinoschisis.

Pathology/Pathogenesis

Histologically, the splitting process begins in the outer plexiform or inner nuclear layers of some portion of the peripheral retina, as a microscopic degeneration of neuroretinal and glial supporting elements. The involved area then begins to collect a viscous substance, which contains mucopolysaccharide. As this process very gradually progresses, the involved retina becomes two separate degenerated layers, with complete severing of neuronal elements, resulting in total and permanent loss of visual function in the involved area.

Treatment/Prognosis

Long-term natural history studies have established that the overall risk of clinical retinal detachment is very low—around 0.05% (1 in 2000 cases). A unique form of "schisis-detachment" exists, in which a portion of intraretinal fluid passes through an outer layer retinal hole and elevates the outer layer partially. Fortunately, this complication occurs without symptoms and remains localized and nonprogressive, and does not justify any kind of surgical or other treatment. The rare occurrence of a symptomatic, progressive rhegmatogenous retinal detachment must be surgically treated, usually by an external scleral buckling procedure and by closing all through-and-through and outer wall retinal breaks.

The risk of progression of retinoschisis into the macula is extremely rare. Also, there is an unexplained tendency of the splitting process, even when it approaches to within 2 to 3 DD from the fovea, to become stationary at that point and not to progress farther. Attempts to surgically halt the progress of retinoschisis posteriorly have not been very successful, and there are three excellent reasons against it: (1) various serious postsurgical complications have been reported; (2) even if thought successful, this disease frequently appears again elsewhere, because it is multicentric in origin; and (3) no lost vision can ever be restored by surgery, even if the operation was regarded as successful.

Systemic Evaluation

No systemic evaluation is necessary.

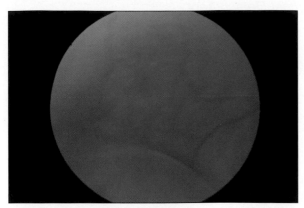

Subtle uniform, concentric retinal elevation represents retinoschisis inferiorly (with scleral indentation).

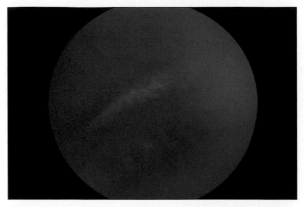

Retinoschisis, lower outer quadrant, shows a multitude of yellowish flecks on the surface of the inner layer (with scleral indentation).

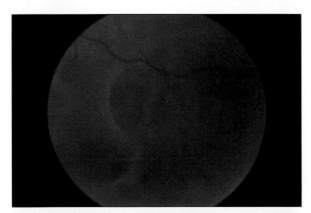

Retinoschisis with oval, vertical, outer-layer retinal break and adjoining yellowish fold indicates the location of the outer layer (with scleral indentation).

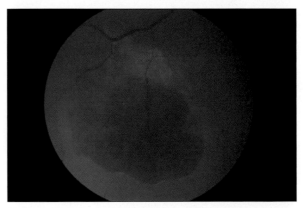

Retinoschisis is shown with large outer layer break (without scleral indentation). Note overlying intact vessels of the inner layer.

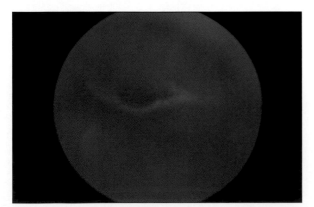

Retinoschisis is observed with "schisis-detachment" (with scleral indentation). Yellow transverse line represents the outer layer. Note just above the yellow line on the left, the outer layer lies against the inner layer on the left, but on the right, the schisis cavity is seen separating the two layers.

SELECTED REFERENCES

Cystic Retinal Tufts

1. Byer NE. Cystic retinal tufts and their relationship to retinal detachment. *Arch Ophthalmol.* 1981;99:1788–1790.

2. Foos RY. Vitreous base, retinal tufts and retinal tears: pathogenic relationships. In: Pruett RC, Regan CDJ, eds. *Retina Congress.* New York: Appleton-Century-Crofts; 1972:259–279.

Lattice Degeneration

1. Byer NE. Changes in and prognosis of lattice degeneration of the retina. *Trans Am Acad Ophthalmol Otolaryngol.* 1974;78:114–125.

2. Byer NE. Lattice degeneration of the retina—Review. *Surv Ophthalmol.* 1979;23:213–248.

3. Byer NE. Long-term natural history of lattice degeneration of the retina. *Ophthalmology.* 1989;96:1396–1401.

4. Wilkinson CP. Evidence-based analysis of prophylactic treatment of asymptomatic retinal breaks and lattice degeneration. *Ophthalmology.* 2000;107:12–15.

Retinal Breaks

1. Byer NE. Rethinking prophylactic treatment of retinal detachment. In: Stirpe M, ed. *Acta of Third International Congress on Vitreoretinal Surgery: Advances in Vitreoretinal Surgery.* New York: Ophthalmic Communications Society, Inc; 1991.

2. Byer NE. What happens to untreated asymptomatic retinal breaks, and are they affected by posterior vitreous detachment? *Ophthalmology.* 1998;105:1045–1049.

3. Wilkinson CP. Evidence-based analysis of prophylactic treatment of asymptomatic retinal breaks and lattice degeneration. *Ophthalmology.* 2000;107:12–15.

Retinal Detachment

1. Michels RG, Wilkinson CP, Rice TA. *Retinal Detachment.* 2nd ed. St. Louis: Mosby, Inc; 1996.

Senile (Adult-Onset) Retinoschisis

1. Byer NE. Clinical study of senile retinoschisis. *Arch Ophthalmol.* 1968;79:36–44.

2. Byer NE. Long-term natural history study of senile retinoschisis with implications for management. *Ophthalmology.* 1986;93:1127–1137.

3. Foos RY. Senile retinoschisis—Relationship to cystoid degeneration. *Trans Am Acad Ophthalmol Otolaryngol.* 1970;74:33–50.

chapter 12

Diseases of the Vitreous

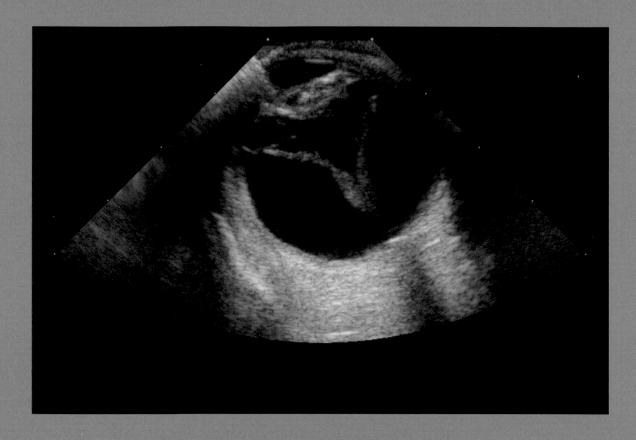

G. William Aylward, MD

AMYLOIDOSIS

Amyloidosis is a condition of abnormal protein deposition in one or more organ systems of the body. The ocular form of amyloidosis occurs only with familial amyloidotic polyneuropathy (FAP), a rare genetic disorder, and follows an autosomal dominant transmission pattern.

Symptoms

Patients with ocular amyloidosis in the vitreous report blurred vision in one or both eyes. The condition is bilateral but may be asymmetric. Patients may occasionally report dry eye symptoms, which are due to lacrimal gland involvement. Although FAP is a genetic disorder, patients do not become symptomatic until the fourth or fifth decade of life.

Clinical Features

Vitreous opacities are the ocular hallmark of amyloidosis. These vitreous opacities typically appear whitish-gray, thick, and fibrillar and may completely obscure the view to the retina. Other posterior segment features of amyloidosis include sheathing of the retinal vessels, perivascular infiltrates, and superficial gray retinal patches. The infiltrates and gray patches are thought to be intraretinal amyloid.

The anterior segment features of amyloidosis involve the conjunctiva and pupil. Patients with amyloidosis may have perilimbal microaneuryms on the conjunctiva. An unusual feature of this condition is a scalloped or irregular pupillary margin that may be due to denervation of the pupillary sphincter muscle. Patients may also have anisocoria or decreased pupillary reaction to light. On the posterior lens surface, a clinical feature termed pseudopodia lentis can be seen. Pseudopodia lentis appears as a cluster of small white dots that are thought to be the footplates of the amyloid fibers.

The differential diagnosis of amyloidosis includes asteroid hyalosis, large cell lymphoma, posterior uveitis, old vitreous hemorrhage, and chronic endophthalmitis.

Ancillary Testing

Electroretinography and electro-oculography may show subnormal findings; however, these tests are not usually required to make the diagnosis. A biopsy can be performed of either the conjunctiva or the vitreous. Analysis of the vitreous samples should include bacterial and fungal cultures for endophthalmitis, cytology for lymphoma, and histopathologic analysis for the presence of amyloid.

Pathology/Pathogenesis

Amyloid is a homogeneous, acellular protein. A vitreous biopsy specimen stains positively with Congo red stain (a marked green color) and exhibits birefringence when viewed under a polarizing light microscope. Amyloid in the vitreous is also eosinophilic, with hematoxylin and eosin staining. The pathogenesis of amyloidosis is related to the aberrant formation of a single protein. Instead of the normal folding of a mature protein, amyloid forms abnormal sheets or folds of protein called "beta pleats."

Treatment/Prognosis

Pars plana vitrectomy is now the standard method for obtaining a biopsy specimen as well as for clearing the vitreous opacities. The prognosis for improved vision is good following surgery, although amyloid can recur in 20% to 25% of patients.

Systemic Evaluation

Patients with clinical signs consistent with ocular amyloidosis should be asked about their family history and ancestry, as FAP is much more common in people of Portuguese descent. Biopsies may be done of the vitreous, conjunctiva, skin, rectum, and sural nerve. Patients who have FAP should have cardiac evaluation for possible cardiomyopathy or thickening of the atrial or ventricular wall.

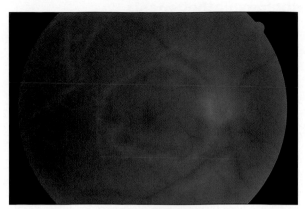

This 61-year-old man complained of reduced vision and floaters. His examination revealed prominent whitish gray vitreous opacities obscuring the view of the retina.

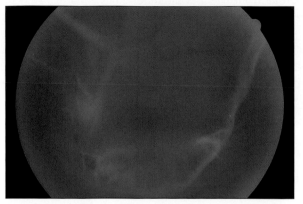

The fellow eye had similar vitreous findings. Note the prominent vitreous strands. A diagnostic and therapeutic pars plana vitrectomy confirmed the presence of amyloid.

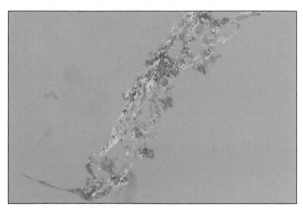

Cytologic examination of the vitreous fluid removed during pars plana vitrectomy of his left eye demonstrated positive Congo red/Sirius red staining for amyloid.

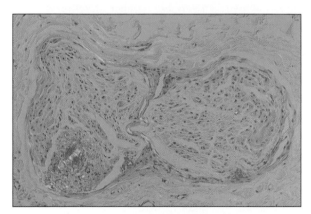

The same patient had peripheral neuropathy. Sural nerve biopsy revealed marked loss of the myelinated axons and focal areas of amyloid deposition in the endoneurium, mainly involving the blood vessel walls.

ASTEROID HYALOSIS

Asteroid hyalosis is a common vitreous abnormality characterized by innumerable deposits throughout the vitreous. The term asteroid refers to the refractile appearance of the deposits as seen with slit lamp biomicroscopy. Asteroid hyalosis is observed most commonly in the older population and affects men and women equally. Asteroid hyalosis is usually unilateral but may be bilateral or asymmetric.

Symptoms

Most patients with asteroid hyalosis are asymptomatic or complain of mild floaters. The report of floaters is rare, even in patients with extensive vitreous involvement.

Clinical Features

Patients with asteroid hyalosis have normal visual acuity. Examination reveals a variable number of yellowish white, oval or round deposits within the collagen framework of the vitreous that may form clumps or strands. The deposits are highly refractile in some patients.

Ancillary Testing

Fluorescein angiography is helpful in evaluating retinal abnormalities when the asteroid deposits prevent direct visualization of the fundus. Ultrasonography also may be useful in evaluating the fundus when asteroid deposits are prominent.

Pathology/Pathogenesis

The cause of asteroid hyalosis is unknown. Historically, asteroid bodies were believed to be calcium soaps. More recent reports employing electron spectroscopic imaging reveal a homogeneous distribution of calcium, phosphorus, and oxygen similar to hydroxyapatite.

Treatment/Prognosis

Most patients with asteroid hyalosis are asymptomatic and do not require treatment. In rare cases where patients have visual alterations related to the asteroid deposits or where visualization of the fundus is essential, pars plana vitrectomy may be useful.

Systemic Evaluation

Although the majority of patients with asteroid hyalosis are otherwise healthy, asteroid hyalosis has been associated with diabetes mellitus. The relationship between asteroid hyalosis and diabetes is unclear and remains controversial.

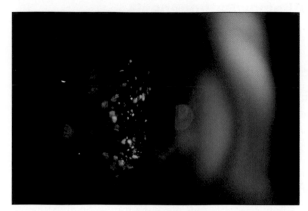

Asteroid hyalosis is viewed by slit lamp biomicroscopy. The yellowish white deposits may be quite refractile in some patients. The deposits move in synchrony with the vitreous.

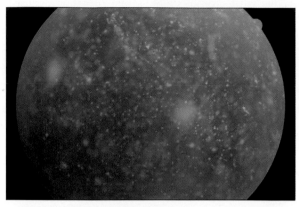

Asteroid hyalosis is viewed through the fundus camera. The deposits are variable in shape and size and tend to have a softer, yellowish appearance.

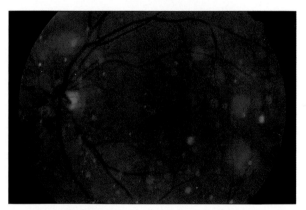

In some instances, the extent of asteroid deposits may interfere with visualization of the fundus. This patient had reduced vision in her left eye attributed to asteroid hyalosis.

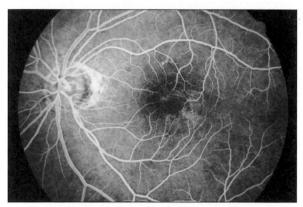

Fluorescein angiography of the patient was extremely helpful in determining the cause of visual loss. It revealed idiopathic juxtafoveal retinal telangiectasis.

IDIOPATHIC VITRITIS

Idiopathic vitritis, or idiopathic senile vitritis, is a cause of symptomatic floaters and loss of vision. It occurs in patients, more commonly women, in their sixth decade or older.

Symptoms

Patients present with floaters and blurriness in one or both eyes.

Clinical Features

The visual acuity in this condition is variable and often asymmetrical, but is rarely worse than 20/200. There are no signs of anterior segment inflammation. Vitreous cells are the hallmark of this disorder. Cystoid macular edema (CME) is typically present, as is a more diffuse retinal edema. Mild disc swelling can also be seen. Examination of the peripheral fundus may reveal narrowed and sheathed vessels, but snowbanking/peripheral exudation is not a feature. A mild epiretinal membrane is often present in the macula. The differential diagnosis includes large cell lymphoma (primary ocular or central nervous system lymphomas), pars planitis, vitiliginous chorioretinitis, and retinitis pigmentosa sine pigmenti.

Ancillary Testing

Fluorescein angiography is helpful in confirming the presence of CME. In cases with marked disc swelling, computed tomographic scanning may be necessary to rule out papilledema.

Pathology/Pathogenesis

The cause of idiopathic vitritis is unknown.

Treatment/Prognosis

Little is known about the prognosis of this disorder. The macular edema may respond to anti-inflammatory treatment, including corticosteroids, but the treatment must be given chronically.

Systemic Evaluation

No systemic associations are known in idiopathic vitritis, but magnetic resonance imaging of the brain may be necessary to rule out a primary central nervous system lymphoma. HLA-A29 testing may be performed in patients suspected of having birdshot chorioretinopathy.

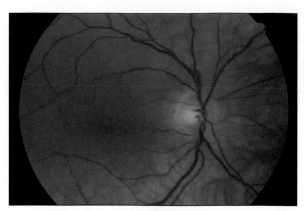

This 64-year-old woman complained of floaters and mild visual loss worse in her left eye. Her examination revealed mild vitreous inflammation bilaterally. She had not undergone cataract surgery.

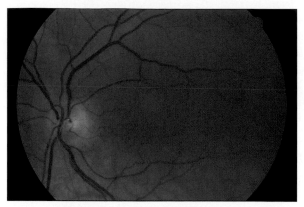

The ophthalmoscopic examination was similar in each eye. Loss of the normal foveal reflexes and cystoid macular edema were observed with fundus contact lens evaluation.

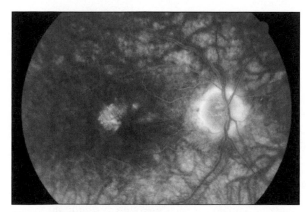

Fluorescein angiography of the same patient revealed localized hyperfluorescence in the right macula consistent with cystoid macular edema.

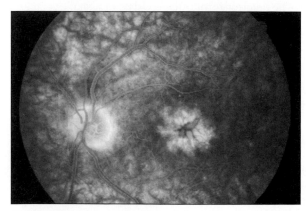

Fluorescein angiography of the left eye demonstrated a more classic petaloid pattern of hyperfluorescence.

PERSISTENT HYPERPLASTIC PRIMARY VITREOUS

Persistent hyperplastic primary vitreous (PHPV) is a congenital, sporadic condition characterized by abnormal regression of the embryonic vascular structures, the posterior hyaloid artery, and the tunica vasculosa lentis. It occurs most commonly in full-term infants. Depending on the structures involved, PHPV may be classified into anterior, posterior, and combined (anterior and posterior) forms.

Symptoms

Anterior PHPV presents in the neonatal period as leukokoria. Posterior PHPV may be detected later in childhood at an evaluation of reduced vision or strabismus.

Clinical Features

In the majority of patients, PHPV is a unilateral condition. The anterior form often consists of a shallow anterior chamber and a vascularized fibrous membrane (the tunica vasculosa lentis) behind the lens. The lens is smaller than normal, and may become cataractous. Swelling of the lens may cause secondary angle-closure glaucoma. The abnormal vessels in the membrane may bleed, leading to vitreous hemorrhage, or contract, leading to retinal detachment. Microphthalmos is typically present.

In posterior PHPV, traction retinal folds may extend along the surface of the macula; a vitreous stalk on the optic disc and vitreous membranes may also be present. The most common form of the condition, a combination of the anterior and posterior forms, includes one or more of the above abnormalities along with a vascularized stalk extending from the posterior lens surface to the optic disc. The differential diagnosis of PHPV includes retinopathy of prematurity, familial exudative vitreoretinopathy, and toxocariasis.

Ancillary Testing

Ultrasound examination can be helpful in determining microphthalmos. The B-scan may also show a stalk of tissue (containing the posterior hyaloid artery) extending from the posterior lens surface to the optic nerve. The retina may be attached or may exhibit traction elevation in the area of the attached hyaloid stalk. Doppler testing may be used to detect blood flow in the hyaloid artery.

Pathology/Pathogenesis

In the first trimester of pregnancy, the internal ocular structures are supplied by the tunic vasculosa lentis. Failure of this vascular structure to regress leads to the clinical findings in anterior PHPV. Abnormal adherence of the regressing primary vitreous to the developing retina leads to the formation of traction retinal folds.

Treatment/Prognosis

Prognosis for eyes with PHPV is poor. If the eye does not have severe microphthalmia, surgical removal of the lens and retrolenticular membrane may help prevent angle-closure glaucoma. Postoperative care includes rigorous amblyopia therapy and glaucoma management. Treatment is more successful in anterior PHPV than in the posterior form.

Systemic Evaluation

There are no known associations with systemic disease or with maternal disease during pregnancy.

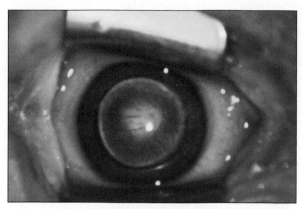

This young girl presented with leukokoria. Examination revealed a vascularized fibrous membrane behind the lens consistent with persistent hyperplastic primary vitreous.

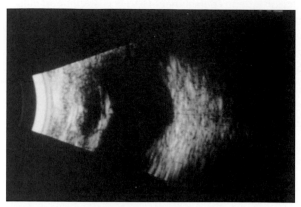

B-scan ultrasonography of the same patient demonstrates a dense signal posterior to a clear intraocular lens.

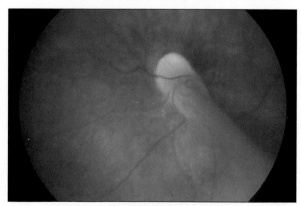

Fundus photograph of a patient with posterior persistent hyperplastic primary vitreous demonstrating a retinal fold.

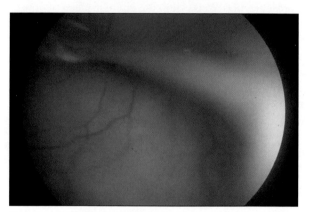

Fundus photograph of a patient with persistent hyperplastic primary vitreous reveals a prominent fold inserting into a mass of vitreous membranes.

POSTERIOR VITREOUS DETACHMENT

Posterior vitreous detachment (PVD) is a common condition in which the vitreous separates from the inner surface of the retina. A PVD is a frequent cause of urgent consultations. It affects men and women equally and occurs in the sixth and seventh decades of life, or earlier in patients with myopia.

Symptoms

The symptoms of PVD include a sudden onset of one or more floaters (often described by the patient as veils or cobwebs). Patients often report small, crescent-shaped flashing lights in the temporal periphery that are stimulated by eye movement and are more easily seen under dark-adapted conditions.

Clinical Features

The presence of a Weiss ring, the circular piece of condensed vitreous that has separated from the optic nerve, confirms the clinical diagnosis of PVD. An optically empty space behind the posterior hyaloid is also suggestive of PVD. There may be associated nerve fiber layer hemorrhage on the optic disc or retina. On clinical examination alone, it is difficult to be certain if the posterior vitreous separation is truly complete. It is possible for the vitreous to be detached over the optic nerve but remain attached in the macula. In patients with PVD, the presence of a vitreous hemorrhage or pigment in the anterior vitreous (tobacco dust or Shaffer's sign) is highly correlated with the presence of a retinal tear.

Ancillary Testing

Fundus examination should be supplemented by 360° indirect ophthalmoscopy with scleral depression, or three-mirror contact lens examination of the periphery, or both, in order to exclude a retinal tear. Incomplete vitreous separation (with the posterior vitreous still attached in the macula) may be seen on optical coherence tomography or B-scan ultrasonography. Ultrasound examination is very helpful in confirming the diagnosis of PVD when vitreous hemorrhage is present.

Pathology/Pathogenesis

Degradation of the vitreous collagen matrix (syneresis) accompanied by thinning of the posterior hyaloid results in a sudden disruption of the posterior hyaloid membrane. This breakdown allows fluid from the vitreous body to enter the preretinal space, and dissect the relatively weak adhesion between the vitreous and the inner retina.

Treatment/Prognosis

No treatment is required for PVD. Patients who present with an acute PVD and have no associated findings are at a relatively low risk for developing a retinal tear. The risk of developing a retinal tear is greatest in patients who present with PVD and vitreous hemorrhage and/or peripheral vitreoretinal traction. In these latter patients, a follow-up visit should be scheduled for 3 to 6 weeks after the onset of symptoms. All patients with PVD should be warned of the signs and symptoms of retinal tear and detachment.

Systemic Evaluation

There are no known systemic associations of PVD.

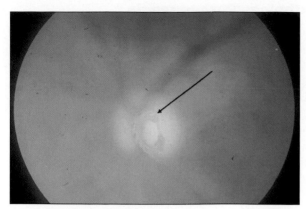

A Weiss ring (arrow) is seen suspended in front of the optic disc. Note that the retinal details are blurred because the focal plane of the Weiss ring is anterior to the optic disc/retina.

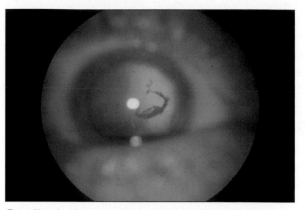

Retroillumination reveals a prominent Weiss ring in a patient with a posterior vitreous detachment.

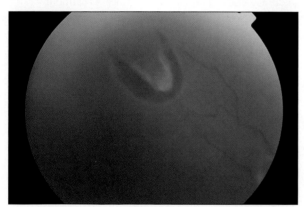

Patients with acute posterior vitreous detachment are at risk for developing retinal tears. Acute, symptomatic horseshoe tears should be treated to reduce the risk of retinal detachment.

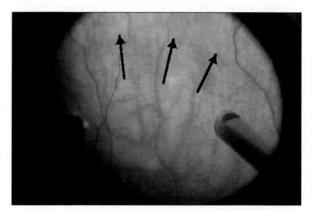

This photograph was taken during pars plana vitrectomy. It demonstrates the advancing line of vitreous separation as the posterior hyaloid is peeled off the retina.

PROLIFERATIVE VITREORETINOPATHY

Proliferative vitreoretinopathy (PVR) is a modified wound-healing response that occurs in eyes with rhegmatogenous retinal detachment. It can occur following primary retinal detachments (especially in patients in whom there is a delay in repairing the detachment), or following surgical repair of retinal detachment.

Symptoms

Contracting PVR membranes can reopen treated retinal breaks, or cause new breaks, thus leading to retinal re-detachment and associated sudden visual loss. In the absence of retinal breaks, PVR is asymptomatic, unless there are membranes on the macula, causing symptoms of metamorphopsia and central blurring.

Clinical Features

The clinical features of PVR have been classified according to severity and location. Grade A consists of vitreous haze and pigment in the vitreous. In grade B there is wrinkling of the retina with vascular tortuosity. In grade C, full-thickness retinal folds (star folds) have developed. The extent of the folds in clock hours and the location (anterior or posterior) are dictated by numbers and the letters A and P. The notation CP2, for example, means two clock hours of posterior full-thickness retinal folds.

Ancillary Testing

In the presence of dense media opacity, ultrasound examination can be helpful in determining the configuration of the retinal detachment.

Pathology/Pathogenesis

Proliferative vitreoretinopathy results in the formation of fibrocellular contractile membranes on both surfaces of the detached neurosensory retina, on the posterior vitreous face, and in the vitreous base. Inflammation and breakdown of the blood-ocular barrier are followed by migration and proliferation of retinal pigment epithelial cells. Membranes are formed by cells laying down collagen under the influence of growth factors and adhesion molecules. Finally, contraction of the membranes occurs, leading to retinal shortening.

Treatment/Prognosis

Proliferative vitreoretinopathy is a serious complication of retinal detachment surgery, and may lead to severe loss of vision. Anterior PVR compromises the function of the ciliary body, leading to hypotony. Treatment requires vitrectomy surgery to relieve traction, treatment of retinal breaks, and the insertion of a tamponade agent (either long-acting gas or silicone oil). Success rates of treatment vary according to the severity of the disease, but functional results are often poor.

Systemic Evaluation

There are no known systemic associations of PVR.

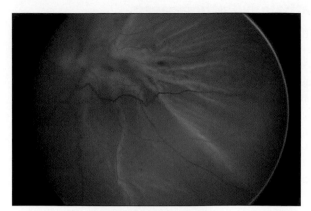

Proliferative vitreoretinopathy is characterized by full-thickness retinal folds radiating from an area of fibrocellular proliferation.

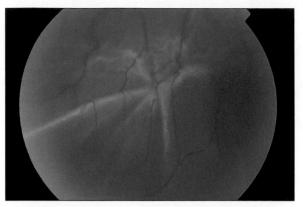

The classic finding in patients with proliferative vitreoretinopathy is a star fold, as seen in this patient following a retinal detachment.

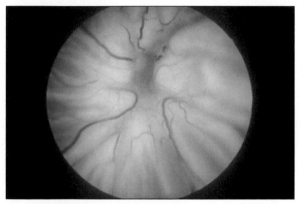

This fundus photograph demonstrates an early funnel-shaped retinal detachment in a patient with proliferative vitreoretinopathy.

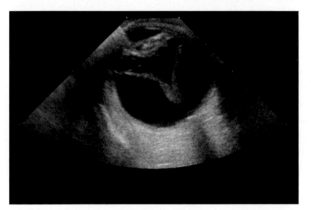

B-scan ultrasound of the same patient reveals a characteristic pattern of a funnel-shaped retinal detachment.

VITREOUS HEMORRHAGE

Vitreous hemorrhage is a significant cause of sudden vision loss. Vitreous hemorrhage can be due to a wide variety of causes including proliferative diabetic retinopathy, posterior vitreous detachment (PVD) with or without retinal tear or retinal detachment, and other retinal vascular, hereditary, and inflammatory diseases.

Symptoms

Most patients experience an acute loss of vision. It is not unusual for the hemorrhage to occur at night and the visual loss is first noticed by the patient on waking. Some patients, particularly patients with diabetes, report seeing a distinct red stream as the bleeding occurs. Associated symptoms of flashing lights may indicate an underlying PVD or retinal tear.

Clinical Features

On slit lamp examination, red blood cells may be seen on the posterior lens surface and in the anterior vitreous directly behind the lens. Blood may be present in the vitreous cavity (intravitreal hemorrhage) or behind the vitreous (subhyaloid hemorrhage). If the vitreous hemorrhage does not resolve within a few weeks, the blood will lose its hemoglobin and will become gray or white in color. Occasionally, red blood cells migrate into the anterior chamber, and these cells may obstruct the trabecular meshwork, causing a rise in intraocular pressure.

Vitreous hemorrhage is often accompanied by other retinal findings including posterior vitreous detachment, retinal tear or detachment, vein occlusion, proliferative diabetic retinopathy, trauma, macroaneurysm, or macular degeneration.

Ancillary Testing

Ultrasound examination is invaluable in the assessment of eyes with significant vitreous hemorrhage. Detection of a posterior vitreous detachment, submacular hemorrhage, and even large retinal tears is possible with B-scan echography. Serial ultrasound examinations are required to follow up patients in the absence of an adequate view of the retina.

Pathology/Pathogenesis

A PVD with or without a retinal tear or retinal detachment can cause vitreous hemorrhage by exerting traction on a retinal blood vessel. Abnormal retinal vessels in diabetic retinopathy, retinal vein occlusions, or other proliferative retinopathies can bleed because of vitreous traction on the preretinal blood vessels. Other causes of vitreous hemorrhage include choroidal neovascularization with "breakthrough bleeding," X-linked juvenile retinoschisis, and subarachnoid hemorrhage (Terson's syndrome).

Treatment/Prognosis

Vitreous hemorrhage will generally clear spontaneously, and vision will return as long as the underlying cause is treated. Nonclearing vitreous hemorrhage may be treated with elective pars plana vitrectomy, although urgent intervention is required in the presence of retinal detachment.

System Evaluation

Vitreous hemorrhage is often associated with diabetes and hypertension; these conditions should be tested for in the absence of a definite underlying cause.

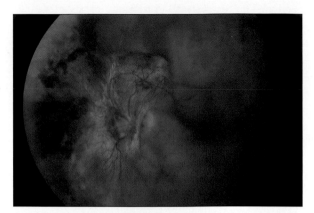

Proliferative diabetic retinopathy is a common cause of vitreous hemorrhage. The vitreous provides a scaffold for the proliferation of the new vessels. Contraction of the vitreous may lead to vitreous hemorrhage or traction retinal detachment.

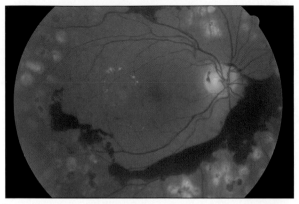

In patients with regressed neovascularization following laser photocoagulation, posterior vitreous detachment may lead to vitreous hemorrhage.

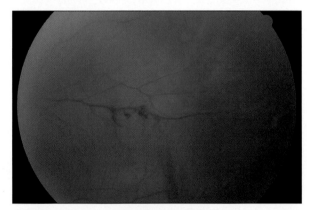

Posterior vitreous detachment (PVD) may be associated with vitreous even in the absence of retinal tear or detachment. This patient with an acute PVD has a vitreous hemorrhage extending from a retinal vessel.

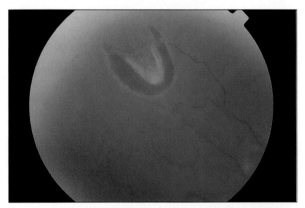

The presence of a vitreous hemorrhage in the setting of acute posterior vitreous detachment raises the suspicion of a retinal tear or detachment.

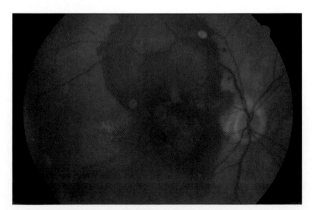

Breakthrough vitreous bleeding may occur in patients with exudative age-related macular degeneration and massive subretinal hemorrhage.

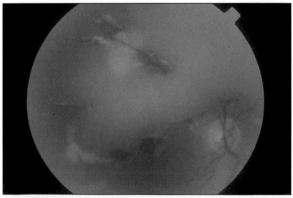

Fundus photograph of a patient with chronic vitreous hemorrhage related to proliferative diabetic retinopathy. Note the yellow coloration of the vitreous hemorrhage due to changed hemoglobin.

SELECTED REFERENCES

Amyloidosis

1. Doft BH, Machemer R, Skinner M, et al. Pars plana vitrectomy for vitreous amyloidosis. *Ophthalmology.* 1987;94:607–611.

2. Gorevic PD, Rodrigues MM. Ocular amyloidosis. *Am J Ophthalmol.* 1994;117:529–532.

Asteroid Hyalosis

1. Moss SE, Klein R, Klein BE. Asteroid hyalosis in a population: the Beaver Dam eye study. *Am J Ophthalmol.* 2001;132:70–75.

2. Parnes RE, Zakov ZN, Novak MA, Rice TA. Vitrectomy in patients with decreased visual acuity secondary to asteroid hyalosis. *Am J Ophthalmol.* 1998;125:703–704.

3. Winkler J, Lunsdorf H. Ultrastructure and composition of asteroid bodies. *Invest Ophthalmol Vis Sci.* 2001;42:902–907.

Idiopathic Vitritis

1. Brinton GS, Osher RH, Gass JDM. Idiopathic vitritis. *Retina.* 1983;3:95–98.

2. Gass JDM. *Stereoscopic Atlas of Macular Diseases: Diagnosis and Treatment.* 4th ed. St. Louis: Mosby, Inc; 1997:708–709.

3. Johnson LA, Wirostko E. Chronic idiopathic vitritis: ultrastructural properties of bacteria-like bodies within vitreous leukocyte phagolysosomes. *Am J Clin Pathol.* 1986;86:19–24.

Persistent Hyperplastic Primary Vitreous

1. Dass AB, Trese MT. Surgical results of persistent hyperplastic primary vitreous. *Ophthalmology.* 1999;106:280–284.

2. Goldberg MF. Persistent fetal vasculature (PFV): an integrated interpretation of signs and symptoms associated with persistent hyperplastic primary vitreous (PHPV). LIV Edward Jackson Memorial Lecture. *Am J Ophthalmol.* 1997;124:587–626.

3. Reese AB. Persistent hyperplastic primary vitreous. *Am J Ophthalmol.* 1955;40:317–331.

Posterior Vitreous Detachment

1. Byer NE. Natural history of posterior vitreous detachment with early management as the premier line of defense against retinal detachment. *Ophthalmology.* 1994;101:1503–1513.

2. Novak MA, Welch RB. Complications of acute symptomatic posterior vitreous detachment. *Am J Ophthalmol.* 1984;97:308–314.

3. Preferred Practice Pattern. Management of posterior vitreous detachment, retinal breaks, and lattice degeneration. #110022 American Academy of Ophthalmology; 1998.

4. Tanner V, Harle D, Tan J, et al. Acute posterior vitreous detachment: the predictive value of vitreous pigment and symptomatology. *Br J Ophthalmol.* 2000;84:1264–1268.

Proliferative Vitreoretinopathy

1. Asaria RH, Kon CH, Bunce C, et al. How to predict proliferative vitreoretinopathy: a prospective study. *Ophthalmology.* 2001;108:1184–1186.

2. Charteris CG. Proliferative vitreoretinopathy: pathobiology, surgical management and adjunctive treatment. *Br J Ophthalmol.* 1995;79:953–960.

3. Machemer R, Aaberg TM, Freeman HM, et al. An updated classification of retinal detachment with proliferative vitreoretinopathy. *Am J Ophthalmol.* 1991;112:159–165.

Vitreous Hemorrhage

1. DeBernardo C, Blodi B, Byrne SF. Echographic evaluation of retinal tears in patients with spontaneous vitreous hemorrhage. *Arch Ophthalmol.* 1992;110:511–514.

2. Sarrafizadeh R, Hassan TS, Ruby TS, et al. Incidence of retinal detachment and visual outcome in eyes presenting with posterior vitreous separation and dense fundus-obscuring vitreous hemorrhage. *Ophthalmology.* 2001;108:2273–2278.

chapter 13

Histopathology of Retinal Diseases

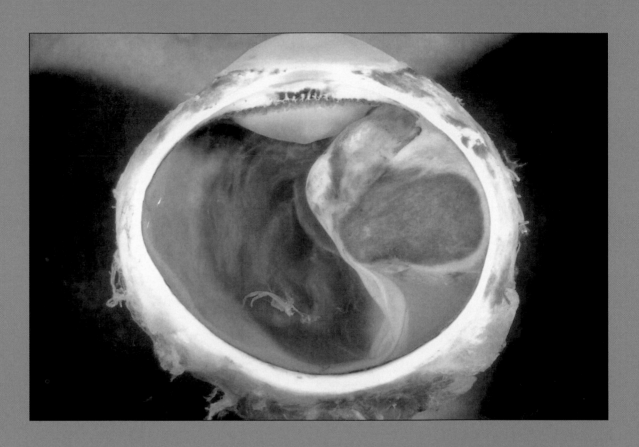

Robert H. Rosa, Jr, MD

MACULAR DISEASES

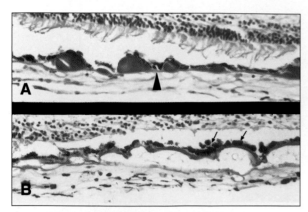

Age-related macular degeneration (AMD). Drusen, the hallmark of AMD, are extracellular deposits located beneath the retinal pigment epithelium (RPE) on the inner surface of Bruch's membrane (arrowhead). Note the intact RPE and photoreceptor cell layer over the drusen (A). A drusenoid detachment of the RPE is present (B). Also seen are focal areas of hypertrophy of the RPE (arrows), loss of the photoreceptor inner and outer segments, and attenuation of the outer nuclear layer over the retinal pigment epithelial detachment.

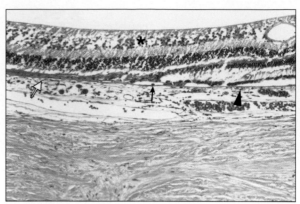

Nonexudative age-related macular degeneration (AMD). Geographic atrophy is observed in more advanced nonexudative AMD. The macular region is identified by the thick ganglion cell layer (>2 to 3 cells thick) (asterisk). Note the abrupt transition (arrow) between normal retina (right of arrow) and geographic atrophy (left of arrow). Geographic atrophy is characterized histologically by loss of the photoreceptor cell layer, retinal pigment epithelium, and choriocapillaris (open arrow). Note the intact choriocapillaris (arrowhead) beneath the normal retina.

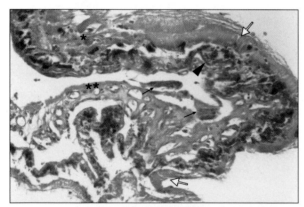

Exudative age-related macular degeneration (AMD). In selected cases, choroidal neovascularization (CNV) might be amenable to surgical extraction. Most of the membranes exhibit two components histologically: subretinal (asterisk) and sub-retinal pigment epithelial (double asterisk). In this surgically excised membrane, photoreceptor outer segments (open arrows) focally line the inner surface of the membrane. Basal laminar deposit (BLD)—a histologic marker for AMD—is a periodic acid-Schiff-positive granular material beneath the retinal pigment epithelium (arrowhead). The role of inflammation in AMD is unknown; however, multinucleated giant cells (arrows) have been reported in association with CNV and BLD in AMD.

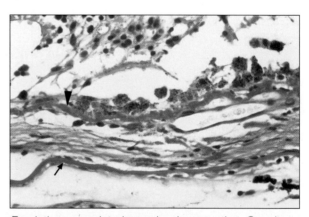

Exudative age-related macular degeneration. Occult choroidal neovascularization (CNV) (between arrowhead and arrow) is typically located beneath the retinal pigment epithelium (RPE) and within Bruch's membrane. The arrowhead identifies basal laminar deposit, which rests on the RPE basement membrane and localizes the inner surface of Bruch's membrane. The arrow identifies the outer surface of Bruch's membrane. Note the disorganization of the outer retina and RPE and loss of the photoreceptors overlying the CNV.

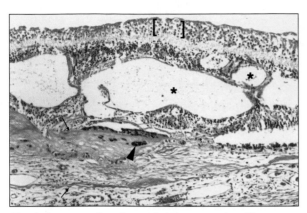

Exudative age-related macular degeneration. The macular region is identified by the thickness of its ganglion cell layer (>2 to 3 cells thick) (between brackets). Note the cystoid macular edema with cystic spaces in the outer plexiform and, to a lesser extent, inner nuclear layers (asterisks). A disciform macular scar (between arrows) is present and composed of subretinal fibrovascular tissue, occasional chronic inflammatory cells, and hyperplastic retinal pigment epithelium (arrowhead). The bottom arrow identifies the outer aspect of Bruch's membrane.

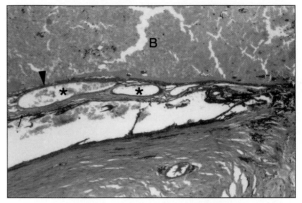

Idiopathic polypoidal choroidal vasculopathy (IPCV). Pathologic studies indicate that choroidal neovascularization (CNV) is a common finding in IPCV. In one study, cavernous vascular channels (asterisks) and CNV were present between the retinal pigment epithelium (arrowhead) and the outer aspect of Bruch's membrane (arrow) in the peripapillary region. On serial stepped sections, the cavernous vascular channels were contiguous with branches of the short ciliary arteries. Note the dense subretinal blood (B), which is characteristic of this disease.

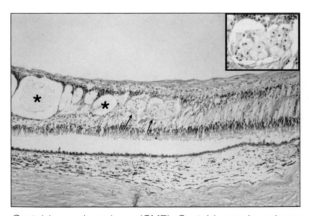

Cystoid macular edema (CME). Cystoid macular edema is a common finding in various vascular and inflammatory conditions of the eye. Proteinaceous material originating from incompetent or hyperpermeable retinal capillaries accumulates in the outer plexiform layer (called Henle's layer in the macular region), forming cysts (asterisks) that may extend into the inner nuclear layer. Aggregates of lipid-laden macrophages (arrows, inset) may be observed and correspond clinically to hard exudates.

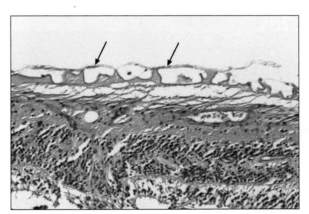

Epiretinal membrane (ERM). The cellular constituents of idiopathic ERMs typically include fibrous astrocytes and fibrocytes (often with myoblastic differentiation, which accounts for the contractile properties of the membrane) and occasionally Müller cells. In association with a retinal break or detachment, retinal pigment epithelium may also be observed in an ERM. Note the contraction features of the internal limiting membrane caused by this thin, hypocellular ERM (arrows). Clinically, retinal striae and cellophane maculopathy would be apparent on ophthalmoscopy in such a case.

RETINAL VASCULAR DISEASES

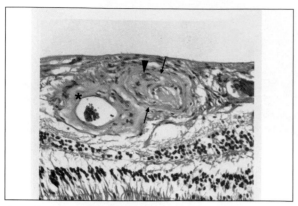

Branch retinal vein occlusion (BRVO). In a remote BRVO, the thrombus (between arrows) becomes organized (fibrotic) and often exhibits recanalization (arrowhead). Note the thickened, hyalinized wall (asterisk) of the adjacent arteriole, indicating the systemic risk factor of hypertension in BRVO.

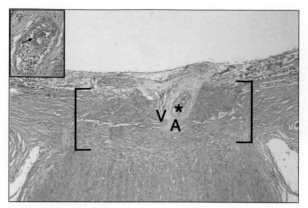

Central retinal artery occlusion (CRAO). The majority of emboli to the retina are cholesterol emboli or Hollenhorst plaques. Platelet-fibrin thrombi are often observed in CRAO in association with calcific or cholesterol emboli. Note the central retinal artery (A) and vein (V) in the region of the lamina cribrosa (between brackets). An organized thrombus is present in the central retinal artery (asterisk). At higher magnification (inset), recanalization (arrow) of the central retinal artery is apparent.

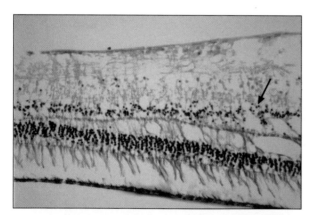

Central retinal artery occlusion (CRAO). In acute CRAO, ischemic infarction of the inner two thirds of the retina occurs. Histopathologic changes include edema or thickening of the inner retina and coagulative necrosis, accounting for the retinal whitening seen clinically. Note the fragmented or pyknotic nuclei (arrow) in the inner nuclear layer. The photoreceptor cell layer (including the outer nuclear layer and the inner and outer segments) is intact, as its nutrients and oxygen are supplied by diffusion from the choroid.

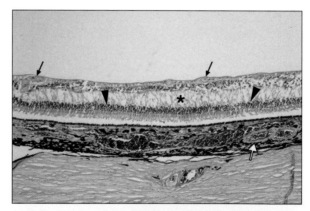

Inner ischemic retinal atrophy and hypertensive retinal and choroidal vascular changes. Inner ischemic retinal atrophy is a common histopathologic finding after central and branch retinal artery and vein occlusions. It is characterized by marked thinning of the inner retina, with loss of the nerve fiber, ganglion cell, and inner plexiform layers, and the inner one third to two thirds of the inner nuclear layer. Note the intact outer plexiform layer (asterisk) and the intact subjacent photoreceptors (arrowheads). Note also the difference between the relative thickness of the inner and outer nuclear layers. Hypertensive changes (arteriolar sclerosis—thickening of the blood vessel wall) are present in the inner retina (arrows) and choroid (open arrow).

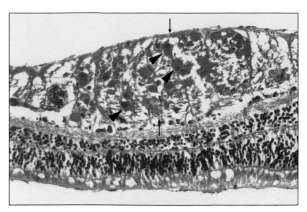

Cotton wool spot. This nerve fiber layer infarct is characterized by fusiform thickening of the nerve fiber layer of the retina (between arrows) and cytoid bodies (arrowheads). Cytoid bodies are swollen ganglion cell axons with a nucleoid (eosinophilic aggregate of cytoplasmic organelles) and stagnant axoplasmic flow.

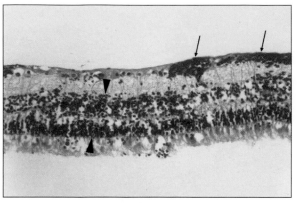

Intraretinal hemorrhages. Flame-shaped hemorrhages correlate pathologically with blood in the nerve fiber layer (arrows). Dot and blot hemorrhages are localized to inner and outer nuclear layers and the outer plexiform layer (between arrowheads). These types of hemorrhages are nonspecific and are seen in various ocular conditions including diabetic, hypertensive, and radiation retinopathies, shaken baby syndrome, and retinopathy of blood dyscrasias.

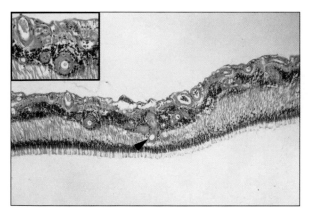

Retinal telangiectasis. Irregular retinal capillary dilation and variable thickening of the blood vessel walls characterize this retinal vascular disorder (inset). Note the numerous variably sized blood vessels in the inner retina in this case. In one area, a dilated blood vessel extends into the outer plexiform layer (arrowhead).

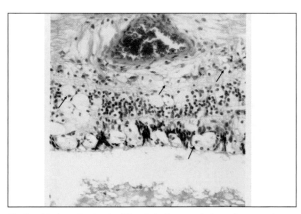

Retinal telangiectasis (Coats' disease). In advanced stages of this vascular anomaly, extensive intra- and subretinal exudation can occur. Note the numerous lipid-laden macrophages (arrows) in all layers of the retina and in the subretinal eosinophilic proteinaceous exudate.

RETINAL VASCULAR DISEASES (CONT'D)

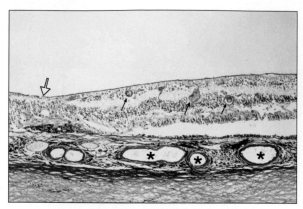

Diabetic retinopathy. An early change in the fundus of diabetic patients is the formation of microaneurysms (arrows), which are outpouchings of the retinal capillaries with basement membrane thickening. Note the focal laser scar (open arrow) characterized by thinning of the retina, gliosis, loss of the normal lamellar architecture, and retinal pigment epithelial hyperplasia. Hypertensive changes (arteriolar sclerosis—thickening of the blood vessel wall) are present in the choroid (asterisks).

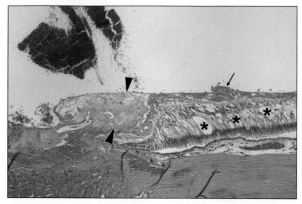

Neovascularization of the optic disc (NVD) and retina (NVE). Retinal and optic disc neovascularization occurs as a pathologic response to retinal ischemia and may be associated with several systemic and localized ocular diseases—including diabetic retinopathy, sickle cell retinopathy, and central and branch retinal vein occlusion. This eye with diabetic retinopathy exhibits NVD (between arrowheads), NVE (arrow), cystoid edema (asterisks), and vitreous hemorrhage.

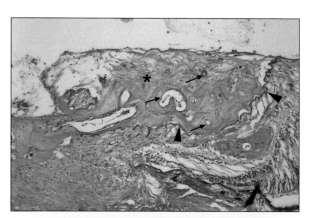

Neovascularization of the optic disc. Condensed vitreous (asterisk) with blood vessels (arrows) is present overlying the optic disc and internal limiting membrane (ILM) (arrowhead) of the peripapillary retina. Note the apparent contraction and folds in the ILM.

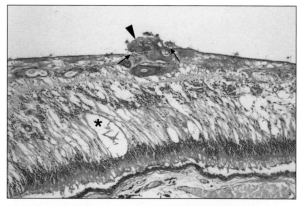

Neovascularization of the retina. Retinal neovascularization is usually contiguous with the venous circulation of the retina. Small defects in the internal limiting membrane (between arrows) are observed at the site of origin. Note the condensed vitreous (arrowhead), which serves as a matrix or scaffold for the proliferation of the new vessels at the vitreoretinal interface. A few cysts are present in the outer plexiform layer (asterisk).

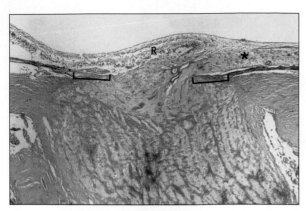

Retinopathy of prematurity (ROP). Temporal dragging of the optic disc and macula may occur in ROP secondary to contraction of neovascularization of the retina near the equator. Note the displacement of the optic disc (asterisk) onto the temporal retinal pigment epithelium (RPE) and choroid. The nasal peripapillary retina (R) is displaced temporally and rests on the optic nerve. Nasal and temporal peripapillary scleral crescents (brackets) are present with absence of the RPE in these areas.

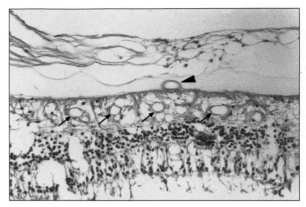

Retinopathy of prematurity (ROP). Intraretinal microvascular abnormalities (IRMA) and neovascularization of the retina (NVE) may be observed in ROP. A form of intraretinal neovascularization, IRMA is also seen in diabetic retinopathy. Note the ghost-like vessels (arrows) within the nerve fiber layer consistent with IRMA and the condensed epiretinal vitreous with similar vessels (arrowhead) representing NVE.

INTRAOCULAR TUMORS

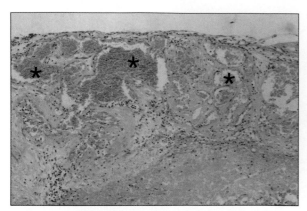

Retinal cavernous hemangioma. This retinal vascular hamartoma is composed of thin-walled, variably sized, interconnecting aneurysms (asterisks) in the inner retina. Variable fibroglial proliferation may occur on the anterior surface of the tumor, causing a whitish color change in the fundus.

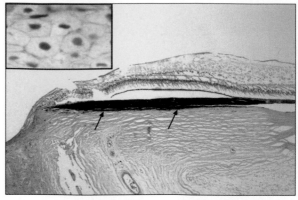

Melanocytoma. These intensely pigmented nevi (also called magnocellular nevi) classically involve the optic disc, but can arise from any part of the uvea. In this juxtapapillary choroidal melanocytoma (arrows), the cytologic details are obscured by heavy pigmentation of the nevus cells. Bleached or depigmented sections (inset) are necessary to evaluate the cytologic features of the tumor cells. Note the characteristic plump polyhedral cells with a low nuclear-to-cytoplasmic ratio and bland nuclei.

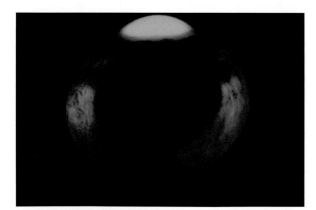

Ocular melanoma. Transillumination is a key component of the pathologic gross examination of an enucleated eye with melanoma. Transillumination allows for localization of the tumor margins and orientation for gross sectioning. It may also be employed clinically to evaluate anterior tumors.

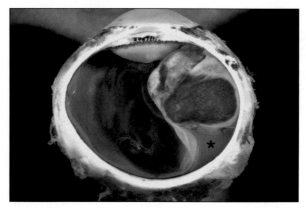

Ocular melanoma. Ciliochoroidal melanomas may be quite large and exhibit variable pigmentation and focal hemorrhage. The tumor may abut the posterior surface of the lens and induce cataractous changes. A secondary exudative retinal detachment (asterisk) can occur.

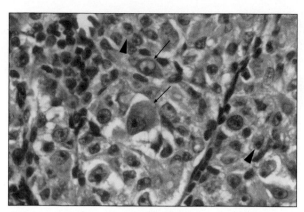

Ocular melanoma. Tumor cell type is an important prognostic indicator. A predominantly epithelioid cell tumor carries the greatest risk for metastasis and mortality. Most tumors are mixed cell types (containing both epithelioid and spindle cells). Note the large round cells with round nuclei, prominent nucleoli, abundant cytoplasm, and distinct cell borders (arrows), which are classic epithelioid cells. Intermediate epithelioid cells (arrowheads) are similar but smaller cells with indistinct cell borders.

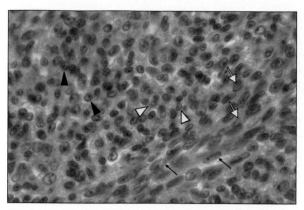

Ocular melanoma. Spindle cells are frequently identified in ciliochoroidal melanoma. Spindle B cells (arrows) are plump cells with spindle-shaped nuclei, prominent nucleoli, and indistinct cell borders. Spindle A cells (open arrows) exhibit thinner spindle-shaped nuclei, with a central chromatin strip or nuclear fold. Note the spindle B (arrowheads) and spindle A (open arrowheads) cells in cross section.

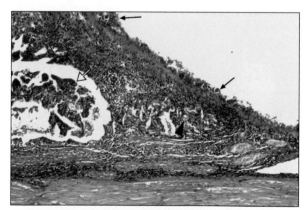

Choroidal metastasis. The lung is the most common primary site for choroidal metastasis in males. Note the disrupted retinal pigment epithelium, with drusen formation (arrows), elevated Bruch's membrane, and scattered chronic inflammatory cells within the choroid. Two lobules of metastatic adenocarcinoma of the lung are present within the choroid: one with a papillary configuration (open arrow) and the other with apparent mucin production (arrowhead).

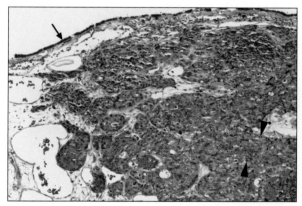

Choroidal metastasis. The breast is the most common primary site for choroidal metastasis in females. Note the marked thickening of the choroid beneath the relatively intact retinal pigment epithelium and choriocapillaris (arrow) by this metastatic carcinoma of the breast. The tumor exhibits a lobular pattern, with frequent mitotic figures (arrowheads).

INTRAOCULAR TUMORS (CONT'D)

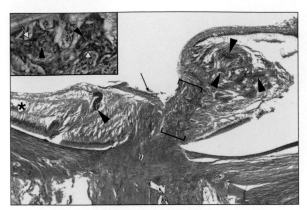

Combined hamartoma of the retina and retinal pigment epithelium (RPE). Prominent components of this hamartoma include blood vessels and hyperplastic RPE, which account for the exudation and pigmentation often observed in these lesions. Note the marked thickening of the peripapillary retina, the pigmented epipapillary membrane (arrow), focal cystoid edema (asterisk), numerous blood vessels (arrowheads), and hyperplastic RPE (between brackets). The inset shows hyperplastic RPE (open arrows) surrounding small vascular channels (arrowheads) at higher magnification.

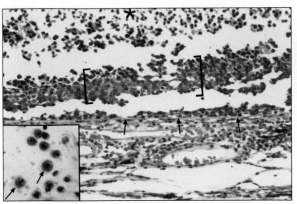

Intraocular/central nervous system lymphoma. This tumor (also called reticulum cell sarcoma) often originates at the level of the retinal pigment epithelium (RPE) internal to (on top of) Bruch's membrane (arrows). The tumor cells may cause detachment of the RPE or replace the RPE. Note the multilayered infiltrate of viable tumor cells (between brackets) and the retinal necrosis (asterisk) overlying the viable tumor cells. The tumor cells have large and hyperchromatic nuclei and occasional prominent nucleoli. Note the intact choroid, with an infiltrate of chronic inflammatory cells. The inset shows a diagnostic vitreous biopsy specimen with large atypical lymphoid cells (arrows) that have nuclear membrane abnormalities and prominent nucleoli characteristic of ocular lymphoma.

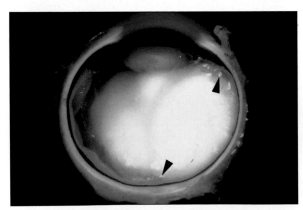

Retinoblastoma. Large tumors may fill much of the vitreous cavity, producing leukokoria. Note the chalky white precipitates (arrowheads) that represent calcium deposition within the tumor. These calcific deposits can be detected by B-scan ultrasonography.

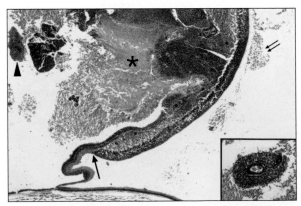

Retinoblastoma. This tumor can originate in any layer of the retina. Note the abrupt transition (arrow) between normal retina and tumor near the ora serrata. Because of its rapid growth, the tumor may outgrow its vascular supply, and extensive areas of necrosis (asterisk) and vitreous seeding (double arrow) are observed in some tumors. In some areas, residual viable tumor cells are present surrounding a blood vessel (inset). This configuration resembles a rosette and is called a pseudorosette (inset). Note the basophilia (dark blue color) in the blood vessel walls (inset) secondary to deposition of nuclear DNA released by necrotic tumor cells.

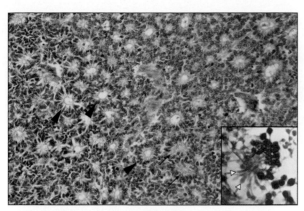

Retinoblastoma. Common histologic findings in this tumor are rosettes, including Homer Wright rosettes (arrows), Flexner-Wintersteiner rosettes (arrowheads), and fleurettes (inset) (in order of increasing retinal differentiation). Note the stubby inner segments (open arrow) that characterize the fleurette.

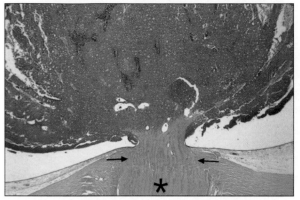

Retinoblastoma. The extent of tumor invasion into the optic nerve on pathologic examination is significant in establishing the prognosis and in dictating further treatment. In this case, the tumor invades the prelaminar optic nerve (anterior aspect of the optic disc), and the prognosis for survival is excellent. The prognosis for survival becomes increasingly poor with posterior extension of the tumor to the lamina cribrosa (between arrows), retrolaminar optic nerve (asterisk), and surgical margin (in order of decreasing survival).

INFLAMMATORY DISEASES

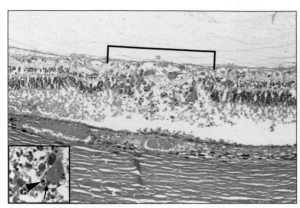

Cytomegalovirus retinitis. Cytomegalovirus retinitis may cause focal full-thickness necrosis of the retina (bracket). Note the abrupt transition between the normal retina and the area of retinitis. The characteristic histopathologic finding is the cytomegalo cell (inset), with eosinophilic intranuclear (arrowhead) and intracytoplasmic (arrow) viral inclusions.

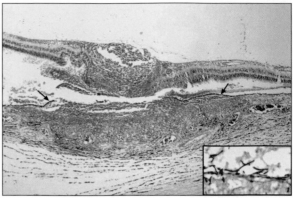

Endogenous fungal endophthalmitis. The chorioretinitis in these cases is often posterior and multifocal. In this fungal chorioretinal abscess, there is full-thickness retinal inflammation with necrosis, intra- and subretinal hemorrhage, focal retinal pigment epithelial detachment by inflammatory cells (arrows), and a dense infiltrate of acute and chronic inflammatory cells (including granulomatous inflammation) within the choroid. Special stains for fungi (Gomori's methenamine silver) show numerous branching, septated fungal hyphae (inset) consistent with Aspergillus sp.

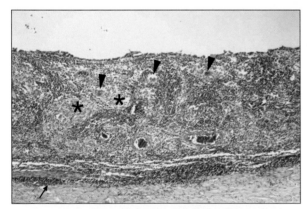

Sympathetic ophthalmia. In this condition, the choroid is often markedly thickened, with a dense infiltrate of chronic inflammatory cells including epithelioid cells (asterisks), multinucleated giant cells (arrowheads), and numerous lymphocytes. The chronic inflammatory reaction may also involve the ciliary vessels and nerves (arrow) and the retinal vasculature. Note the intact choriocapillaris beneath the retinal pigment epithelium.

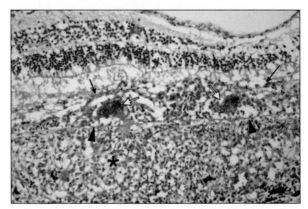

Sympathetic ophthalmia. Granulomatous inflammation is characteristic of this ocular disease. A Dalen-Fuchs nodule is an aggregate of epithelioid cells and/or multinucleated giant cells (open arrows) interposed between the retinal pigment epithelium (arrows) and Bruch's membrane (arrowheads). Note the dense infiltrate of histiocytes in the choroid (asterisk).

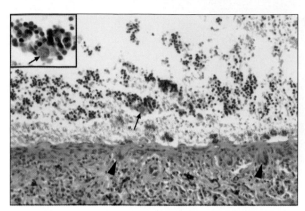

Ocular toxoplasmosis. In human immunodeficiency virus infection, Toxoplasma gondii *may produce a necrotizing retinitis and granulomatous choroiditis. Note the extensive necrosis of the retina and retinal pigment epithelium, with loss of the normal lamellar architecture of the retina. A T* gondii *tissue cyst (arrow, inset) is present. Marked chronic granulomatous inflammation with epithelioid and multinucleated giant cells (arrowheads) are present in the choroid, with loss of the choriocapillaris.*

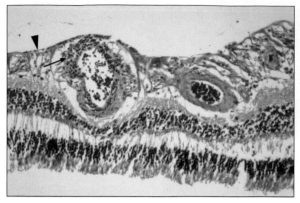

Vascular sheathing. In various local and systemic diseases (including central retinal vascular occlusion, sympathetic ophthalmia, collagen vascular disease, and sarcoidosis), inflammatory cells may surround or enter the retinal blood vessel walls. Note the chronic inflammatory cell infiltrate (arrow) within the wall of this branch retinal vein and the spillover of inflammatory cells onto the internal limiting membrane (arrowhead).

TRAUMA

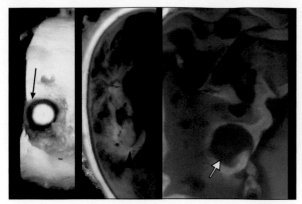

Child abuse (shaken baby syndrome). Ophthalmic examination in the live patient and pathologic examination of the eyes post mortem may be critical in establishing the diagnosis of child abuse. At times, the only pathologic findings at autopsy are observed in the eyes. Careful examination of the optic nerve sheath in cross section may reveal blood in the subdural and arachnoid spaces (arrow). Crater-like retinal folds (arrowhead) in the macular region are virtually pathognomonic of shaken baby syndrome and are often associated with sub-internal limiting membrane (ILM) hemorrhages. Scattered blot and sub-ILM hemorrhages (open arrow) may be observed in the midperipheral and peripheral retina.

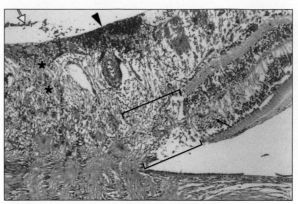

Papilledema. Histologically, papilledema is characterized by lateral displacement of the juxtapapillary retina from the optic nerve head by swollen nerve fiber bundles (between brackets) and by thickening or swelling of the nerve fibers in the anterior aspect of the optic nerve head (asterisks). Note the associated intraretinal (arrow) and nerve fiber layer (arrowhead) hemorrhages and trace vitreous hemorrhage (open arrow) in this case of shaken baby syndrome. Similar pathologic findings may be observed in other causes of papilledema, including pseudotumor cerebri, central nervous system mass lesions, and malignant hypertension.

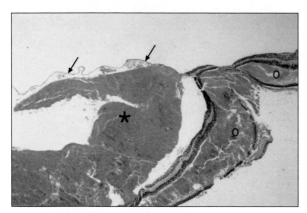

Sub-internal limiting membrane (ILM) hemorrhage. This type of retinal hemorrhage most often appears clinically as a large blot hemorrhage and occasionally as a boat-shaped hemorrhage. Note the large amount of blood (asterisk) beneath the retinal ILM (arrows). A dense hemorrhage is also present in the outer plexiform layer (O) in this case of shaken baby syndrome.

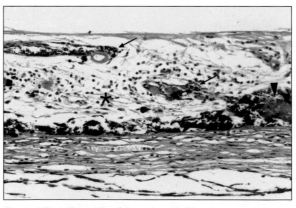

Traumatic retinopathy (pseudo-retinitis pigmentosa [RP]). Traumatic retinopathy and RP share similar histologic findings, including marked loss of the photoreceptor cell layer; focal gliosis (asterisk); pigment migration into the retina, often around blood vessels (arrows); variable retinal pigment epithelial attenuation, hypertrophy, and hyperplasia; and drusen formation (arrowhead). Note also the loss of the normal lamellar architecture of the retina and indistinct choriocapillaris.

PERIPHERAL RETINAL DISEASES

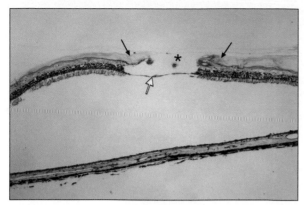

Lattice degeneration of the retina. This common peripheral retinal degeneration is characterized histologically by liquefied vitreous (asterisk) over the area of retinal degeneration bordered by condensed vitreous (arrows). The inner retina is primarily affected. An inner lamellar hole with an operculum (beneath asterisk) and a thin outer retinal membrane (open arrow) can progress to an atrophic full-thickness hole.

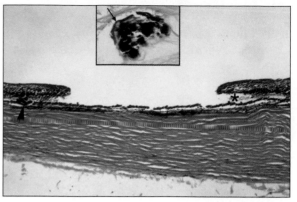

Operculated retinal tear. These tears in the peripheral retina carry a low risk for progression to retinal detachment. Note the rounded, gliotic margins of the full-thickness retinal defect. Localized subretinal fluid (asterisk) and focal retinal pigment epithelial hyperplasia (arrowhead) are present. The inset shows an operculum with internal limiting membrane (arrow) and neuroglia, which was observed a short distance from the retinal hole in this photomicrograph.

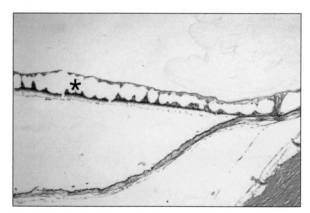

Typical peripheral cystoid degeneration of the retina with focal retinoschisis. This peripheral retinal degeneration is almost universally present in autopsy and enucleated eyes of patients over 8 years old. It begins near the ora serrata with cysts in the outer plexiform and inner nuclear layers. These cysts may coalesce to form areas of retinoschisis (asterisk).

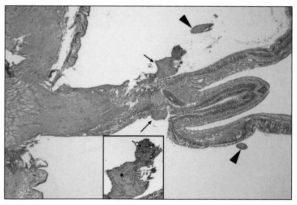

Retinal detachment (RD) with proliferative vitreoretinopathy (PVR). Retinal detachment may be complicated by PVR. In PVR, preretinal and subretinal fibroglial and retinal pigment epithelial proliferation may be observed. Note the open funnel, total RD with retinal folds, subretinal fibroglial strands (arrowheads), and a subretinal napkin-ring membrane (arrows). The subretinal napkin-ring membrane (inset) is composed of fibroglial tissue (asterisk) with hyperplastic retinal pigment epithelium (open arrow).

SELECTED REFERENCES

1. Eagle RC Jr. *Eye Pathology: An Atlas and Basic Text.* Philadelphia: WB Saunders Co; 1999.

2. Sassani JW, ed. *Ophthalmic Pathology With Clinical Correlations.* Philadelphia: Lippincott-Raven Publishers; 1997.

3. Spencer WH, ed. *Ophthalmic Pathology: An Atlas and Textbook.* 4th ed. Philadelphia: WB Saunders Co; 1996.

4. Yanoff M, Fine BS. *Ocular Pathology.* Barcelona: Mosby-Wolfe; 1996.

The author would like to express sincere gratitude to Frank Horak in the Scott and White Photography Department for his expertise and invaluable assistance in digital imaging.

chapter 14

Clinical Trials in Retina

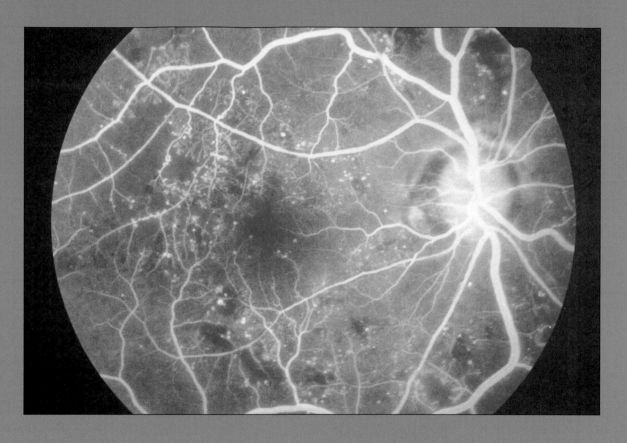

Peter J. Kertes, MD

THE DIABETIC RETINOPATHY STUDY

The role of laser photocoagulation in the treatment of diabetic retinopathy remained controversial following its first description by Meyer-Schwickerath in the 1950s. In 1971, the Diabetic Retinopathy Study (DRS), which was organized under the leadership of Mathew Davis, MD, began to address these fundamental controversies definitively. The study was the first of many well-designed, prospective, and randomized clinical trials that guide the current practice of ophthalmology.

Study Objectives

The question posed by the DRS was, "Does photocoagulation surgery reduce the risk of severe visual loss in diabetic retinopathy?" The DRS set out to better establish the natural course of untreated diabetic retinopathy. It also was designed to compare the effects of treatment techniques involving extensive scatter photocoagulation and focal treatment of new vessels on the surface of the retina with either xenon arc or argon laser energy.

Treatment Groups/Trial Design

Eligible patients had diabetic retinopathy in both eyes, with proliferative diabetic retinopathy (PDR) in at least one eye, or severe, nonproliferative changes in both eyes. Severe nonproliferative changes were defined as the presence of at least three of the following:

- cotton wool spots
- intraretinal microvascular abnormalities (IRMAs)
- extensive retinal hemorrhages
- venous beading

Eligible eyes had to have a visual acuity ≥20/100 in each eye. Eyes with a traction retinal detachment that threatened the macula were excluded, as were eyes with a history of previous laser photocoagulation treatment. One eye of each participating patient was randomly selected to receive photocoagulation, and the fellow eye was followed independently without photocoagulation. The mode of laser treatment was also randomly assigned as either xenon arc or argon laser.

A total of 1727 patients were enrolled from 15 centers; 858 eyes were randomized to receive argon laser photocoagulation and 869 were randomized to receive xenon arc.

The primary outcome measure was development of severe visual loss, that is, visual acuity <5/200 at two or more consecutive 4-month follow-up visits. Secondary outcome measures included regression of diabetic retinopathy and side effects related to treatment.

Summary of Results and Implications for Clinical Practice

The findings of the DRS mandate prompt scatter laser photocoagulation in eyes with high-risk PDR. High-risk characteristics are defined as the presence of three or more of the following:

- vitreous or pre-retinal hemorrhage;
- new vessel growth;
- new vessel growth on or within 1 disc diameter (DD) of the optic disc (NVD); or
- severe new vessels (NVD ≥ one-fourth to one-third of a disc area or, in the absence of NVD, an area ≥ one-half disc area of retinal neovascularization elsewhere [NVE]).

The DRS scatter laser photocoagulation treatment protocol reduced the risk of severe visual loss by greater than 50%. Ongoing follow-up of some of the original study participants confirmed that the beneficial effects of extensive scatter photocoagulation persist for at least 15 years after treatment and suggested that these beneficial effects are permanent.

In high-risk PDR, the benefits of photocoagulation were clear. In eyes with severe nonproliferative diabetic retinopathy (NPDR) or PDR without high-risk characteristics, however, the DRS findings were not clear. They did not provide a clear choice between prompt treatment and careful follow-up with deferral of treatment until high-risk characteristics developed. The risk of severe visual loss in these eyes appeared to be relatively low. Subsequent analysis of the data accumulated in the DRS found that the incidence of severe visual loss in eyes of older-onset diabetic patients randomized to deferral of photocoagulation exceeded that of younger-onset diabetics. In eyes of older-onset diabetics, the analysis suggested that laser treatment should be seriously considered, even though these eyes may not fulfill the original criteria for high-risk characteristics.

The DRS also found that treated eyes were more likely to suffer an initial loss of two to four lines of visual acuity. This loss was largely secondary to increased macular edema. As more untreated eyes suffered significant visual loss over time, this difference no longer existed after 1 year.

Treatment also resulted in peripheral visual field loss, an effect that was more often seen in eyes randomized to xenon arc treatment than in those randomized to receive argon laser scatter photocoagulation.

THE EARLY TREATMENT DIABETIC RETINOPATHY STUDY

The Diabetic Retinopathy Study (DRS) clearly demonstrated the benefits of panretinal laser photocoagulation in proliferative diabetic retinopathy (PDR) with high-risk characteristics. The DRS did not, however, address the question of timing or extent of panretinal laser photocoagulation in diabetic retinopathy. Also, it did not clarify the role of laser photocoagulation in early PDR. While diabetic macular edema had been recognized as an important source of visual loss in diabetic retinopathy, the role of laser treatment in this setting had yet to be verified by a randomized, controlled clinical trial. The Early Treatment Diabetic Retinopathy Study (ETDRS) addressed these issues. In addition, the literature of the day was replete with papers extolling both the risks and benefits of adjunctive aspirin use in the management of diabetic retinopathy. The results of the ETDRS would finally settle the issue.

Study Objectives

The ETDRS set out to answer three questions:

- When in the course of diabetic retinopathy is it most effective to initiate panretinal photocoagulation?

- Is photocoagulation effective in the management of diabetic macular edema?

- Is aspirin treatment effective in altering the course of diabetic retinopathy?

Treatment Groups/Trial Design

Eligible patients were diabetics with mild, moderate, or severe nonproliferative diabetic retinopathy (NPDR) or early PDR in both eyes. As the DRS had clearly shown the benefit of scatter laser photocoagulation in eyes with high-risk PDR, such patients were excluded from the ETDRS.

The ETDRS defined macular edema as thickening of the retina and/or hard exudates within 1 disc diameter (DD) of the center of the macula. Clinically significant macular edema (CSME) was defined as the presence of one or more of the following:

- retinal thickening at or within 500 μm of the center of the macula;

- hard exudates at or within 500 μm of the center of the macula, if associated with adjacent retinal thickening; or

- a zone or zones of retinal thickening 1 disc area in size, at least part of which is within 1 DD of the center of the fovea.

Eyes were stratified into three different categories and randomized accordingly:

1. Eyes with moderate to severe NPDR or early PDR and no macular edema were assigned randomly to either early photocoagulation or deferral of photocoagulation until high-risk characteristics appeared. Those assigned to early photocoagulation were further randomized to either

   - immediate full scatter panretinal photocoagulation or

   - immediate mild scatter panretinal photocoagulation.

2. Eyes with macular edema and "less severe" retinopathy were assigned randomly to either early photocoagulation or deferral of photocoagulation. Those assigned to early photocoagulation were further randomized to one of the following four groups:

   - immediate focal photocoagulation with deferral of mild scatter panretinal photocoagulation until severe NPDR develops;

   - immediate focal photocoagulation with deferral of full scatter panretinal photocoagulation;

   - immediate mild scatter panretinal photocoagulation with deferral of focal photocoagulation for (at least) 4 months, and focal treatment given only if CSME is present; or

   - immediate full scatter panretinal photocoagulation with deferral of focal photocoagulation.

3. Eyes with macular edema and "more severe" retinopathy were assigned randomly to either early photocoagulation or deferral of photocoagulation. Those assigned to early photocoagulation were further randomized to one of these four groups:

   - immediate mild scatter panretinal photocoagulation with immediate focal photocoagulation;

   - immediate mild scatter panretinal photocoagulation with deferral of focal photocoagulation;

   - immediate full scatter panretinal photocoagulation with immediate focal photocoagulation; or

   - immediate full scatter panretinal photocoagulation with deferral of focal photocoagulation.

Further randomization of patients to either aspirin (650 mg daily) or placebo in a double-masked manner at enrollment resulted in approximately one half of the patients in each group receiving aspirin.

A total of 3928 study patients were enrolled at 23 clinical centers between April 1980 and August 1985.

Outcome Measures

Outcome measures to assess the benefits of early photo-coagulation were severe visual loss (visual acuity <5/200 at two consecutive follow-up visits) and vitrectomy rate. The outcome measure to assess the effect of photocoagulation on macular edema was moderate visual loss (loss of 15 or more letters).

Outcome measures to assess the role of aspirin were mortality, development of cardiovascular disease, progression to high-risk retinopathy, development of vitreous hemorrhage, and development of cataract. Secondary outcome measures included changes in the visual field, as measured by Goldmann perimetry; and changes in color vision, evaluated with the Farnsworth-Munsell 100-hue test.

Summary of Results and Implications for Clinical Practice

The ETDRS addressed the question of timing and extent of panretinal laser photocoagulation in eyes with severe NPDR or early PDR. The findings showed that scatter photocoagulation before the development of high-risk PDR did not significantly alter the end point of severe visual loss. The ETDRS data, however, do suggest that patients with type 2 diabetes and severe NPDR or early PDR are more likely to benefit from early scatter laser treatment than are patients with type 1 diabetes. Eyes approaching high-risk characteristics should be considered for scatter photocoagulation. Such treatment should not be delayed if the eye already has high-risk characteristics. Once this threshold to treat has been reached, scatter photocoagulation should be given as a "full" treatment.

Focal photocoagulation of CSME substantially decreased the risk of moderate visual loss and was recommended for all eyes with CSME and mild to moderate NPDR. Focal treatment should also be performed in eyes with CSME and severe NPDR or early PDR, preferably before or in conjunction with scatter photocoagulation. Laser photocoagulation applied in the form of "focal" or "grid" treatment decreases the frequency of persistent macular edema, reduces the risk of moderate visual loss, increases the chance of visual improvement, lessens the loss of color vision, and is associated with only minor visual field loss.

The study also concluded that aspirin offered no benefit in preventing progression of diabetic retinopathy or cataract, or in reducing systemic morbidity and mortality in the ETDRS population of diabetic patients. However, no hazardous ocular or systemic effects of taking aspirin were noted in diabetic patients who required aspirin for cardiovascular disease or other medical conditions.

THE DIABETIC RETINOPATHY VITRECTOMY STUDY

The Diabetic Retinopathy Study (DRS) clearly demonstrated the benefits of scatter laser photocoagulation in reducing visual loss from the complications of proliferative diabetic retinopathy (PDR). In spite of this, many patients continued to suffer severe visual loss, either because vitreous hemorrhage or severe cicatricial neovascularization developed before adequate laser treatment could be offered, or because laser photocoagulation failed to adequately prevent progression to traction retinal detachment or severe vitreous hemorrhage.

Vitrectomy surgery was developed in the early 1970s, and reports emerged on successful visual restoration in patients with nonclearing diabetic vitreous hemorrhage. As the procedure gained a broader acceptance, it was offered to a greater number of patients with complications of PDR. Although the surgery was successful in many eyes, it was not without substantial complications, and a significant percentage of eyes lost all light perception. A debate emerged surrounding the timing and role of vitrectomy surgery in severe PDR.

Study Objectives

The Diabetic Retinopathy Vitrectomy Study (DRVS) consisted of three studies designed to evaluate the natural course and effect of surgical intervention on severe PDR and its complications. These study groups were as follows:

- Group N: a natural history study designed to provide data on the outcome of conventional management at the time of the study;

- Group NR: a study that assessed the merits of early surgical intervention in eyes with severe PDR but without severe visual loss; and

- Group H: a randomized trial that compared the outcome of surgical intervention in eyes with severe visual loss resulting from vitreous hemorrhage when surgery was done either shortly after the occurrence of hemorrhage or deferred for one year.

Group N: Course of Visual Acuity in Severe PDR with Conventional Management

Study Objectives

The study intended to follow up a large number of eyes with severe PDR over a 2-year period to determine their visual outcome. It also hoped to identify a subgroup of patients in whom the prognosis with conventional management was so poor that a randomized trial of vitrectomy in eyes still retaining useful vision was justified.

Treatment Groups/Trial Design

Eyes with severe iris neovascularization or neovascular glaucoma, a history of previous vitrectomy, or photocoagulation done within 3 months of study entry were excluded. Group N eyes were further subdivided into three subgroups defined by the predominant retinopathy present at study entry:

- Group NN (142 eyes) consisted of eyes with severe new vessels covering at least 4 disc areas of retina. At least one edge of the neovascular membrane was elevated, consistent with partial posterior vitreous detachment. The vitreous was relatively clear, and the visual acuity was 10/50 or better.

- Group ND (290 eyes) was composed of eyes with traction retinal detachment and vision of 10/50 or better, unless vitreous hemorrhage was thought to be the cause of visual loss, in which case visual acuities of 10/200 were permitted. The retinal elevation was at least 4 disc areas in extent, and the macula was attached. Retinal elevation could be less than 4 disc areas if one or more of the vitreoretinal adhesions causing the elevation was present within 30° of the center of the macula and if there were new vessels with blood in them (active new vessels) or if red vitreous hemorrhage was present (fresh hemorrhage).

- Group NH (hemorrhage) was composed of eyes

1. in which vitreous and preretinal hemorrhage obscured at least one half of the field in at least three of the seven standard photographic fields; or

2. in which there were thought to be at least 4 disc areas of new vessels, some of which were obscured by hemorrhage.

Patients were treated with the conventional methods of the time. Scatter laser photocoagulation was done at the discretion of the treating ophthalmologist. If a severe vitreous hemorrhage developed during the follow-up period, eligible patients could be entered into the randomized treatment trial (group H). Pars plana vitrectomy was allowed if

- the patient was not entered into the group H trial and a severe hemorrhage persisted for 1 year;

- traction retinal detachment progressed to involve the fovea; or

- rhegmatogenous retinal detachment developed.

Outcome Measures

The primary outcome measure was best-corrected visual acuity assessed at 1 and 2 years after study entry. Poor vision was defined as a visual acuity <5/200. Good vision was defined as a visual acuity of 10/20 or better.

Summary of Results and Implications for Clinical Practice

- A total of 744 eyes of 622 patients were enrolled in the trial.

- In almost all groups, change in vision was greater between baseline and year 1 than between years 1 and 2.

- Both initial visual acuity and the activity of retinopathy predicted further visual loss.

- At the 2-year visit, 156 eyes had poor vision for which the cause was recorded: 35% had a retinal detachment; 31% had vitreous hemorrhage.

- Twenty-five percent of all eyes had undergone vitrectomy.

There was a clear trend toward worse outcome, depending on the severity of retinopathy. The prognosis in eyes with a traction retinal detachment sparing the macula did not justify surgical intervention for this indication, irrespective of retinopathy activity. Analysis of data allowed the definition of a subgroup of eyes with a sufficiently poor prognosis to justify a randomized trial of vitrectomy in eyes still retaining useful vision (group NR).

GROUP NR: EARLY VITRECTOMY FOR SEVERE PDR IN EYES WITH USEFUL VISION

Study Objectives

In this study, early vitrectomy was compared to the conventional strategy of surgical intervention after severe visual loss occurred secondary to macular detachment, vitreous hemorrhage, or other complications of PDR, in eyes with severe active proliferative disease and useful vision.

Treatment Groups/Trial Design

Eyes eligible for this study had a visual acuity of 10/200 or better, with extensive active neovascular or fibrovascular proliferation. Four subgroups of new vessel severity (NVC 1 to 4) were defined for treatment in the analysis of outcome. A total of 370 eyes were randomly assigned to early vitrectomy or to conventional management.

For eyes assigned to early vitrectomy, repeat vitrectomy was allowed if recurrent hemorrhage reduced vision to 10/200 and failed to clear in 1 month, and was strongly encouraged after 4 months. Postoperative

scatter laser photocoagulation was done for progressive iris neovascularization and was allowed for active retinal neovascularization in special cases.

In the conventional management group, vitrectomy was carried out for the following indications:

- Development of a macular detachment with a visual acuity ≤10/100

- Visual loss of three lines or more since randomization

- Ultrasonographic evidence of a macular detachment when the retina was obscured by new vitreous hemorrhage

- Severe vitreous hemorrhage that reduced visual acuity to ≤5/200 for ≤6 months

- Decrease of acuity from ≥10/50 at entry to ≤10/100 during follow-up, when the decrease was attributed to traction on the optic nerve, peripapillary retina or macula, or fibrous proliferation in front of the macula that could possibly be reduced by surgery. Photocoagulation was permitted during follow-up at the discretion of the study ophthalmologists.

Outcome Measures

The principal outcome measures evaluated at annual follow-up visits following randomization for 4 years were as follows:

- Visual acuity ≥10/20 (good vision)

- Visual acuity ≤5/200 (poor vision)

- No light perception.

Summary of Results and Implications for Clinical Practice

After 4 years of follow-up, while the proportion of eyes with a poor visual outcome was similar in the two groups, the percentage of eyes with a visual acuity of ≥10/20 was 44% in the early vitrectomy group and 28% in the conventional management group. Baseline visual acuity was predictive of poor vision, and prior photocoagulation increased the chances of good vision. As new vessel severity increased, the outcome with conventional management worsened for each end point.

The study thus recommended consideration for early vitrectomy in eyes with useful vision and advanced active PDR with extensive new vessel growth. The eyes best suited for early surgery were those with both fibrous proliferation and at least moderately severe new vessel growth in which extensive scatter laser photocoagulation had already been carried out or was precluded by vitreous hemorrhage.

Group H: Early Vitrectomy for Severe Vitreous Hemorrhage

Study Objectives

As vitreous hemorrhage was the most common indication for diabetic vitrectomy, surgeons had long realized that after removal of a long-standing vitreous hemorrhage significant traction retinal detachment was often discovered. However, following surgery, proliferation did not recur once all the membranes had been removed. Surgeons thus hypothesized that vitreous and membrane removal soon after the occurrence of vitreous hemorrhage might improve surgical outcomes. The question asked was, "In patients with severe acute visual loss from vitreous hemorrhage, will there be better outcomes with immediate vitrectomy or with deferral of surgery for 1 year?"

Treatment Groups/Trial Design

Eligible eyes met the following criteria:

- a history of sudden visual loss consistent with a severe vitreous hemorrhage within six months prior to randomization;

- a visual acuity from 5/200 to light perception on two baseline visits; and

- a vitreous hemorrhage that did not allow visualization of any major retinal vessel or other landmark for a distance ≥3 DD.

A total of 616 eyes were randomized to early vitrectomy done within a few days of randomization or deferral of surgery for 1 year after randomization if vision remained ≤5/200 secondary to persistent vitreous hemorrhage.

Outcome Measures

The primary outcome measure was visual acuity, with special attention paid to landmark visual acuities 10/20, 10/100, and no light perception.

Summary of Results and Implications for Clinical Practice

After 2 years of follow-up, 25% of the early vitrectomy group had a visual acuity ≥10/20, as compared to 15% in the deferral group. Type 1 diabetic patients accounted for most of this advantage, with 36% in the early vitrectomy group achieving a visual acuity ≥10/20 vs 12% in the deferral group. No such advantage was seen among type 2 diabetic patients (16% in the early vitrectomy group vs 18% in the deferral group). These results

persisted for 4 years and were most significant in type 1 diabetic patients with a disease duration less than 20 years. No light perception was more common in the early vitrectomy group through 18 months, but was essentially equivalent at 24 months (early 25% vs deferred 19%).

Much information was garnered about the natural history of severe vitreous hemorrhage in the 1 year that patients in the conventional management group were followed up. During this time span, hemorrhage cleared spontaneously in 21.7%, and 11% required a vitrectomy for development of traction retinal detachment. The vitreous hemorrhage cleared nearly twice as often in type 2 diabetic patients compared to type 1 diabetic patients (29.2% vs 16.4%).

After 4 years of follow-up, the deferral group had more neovascular glaucoma, but fewer patients with retinal detachment. Of all operated-on eyes, 23% required additional procedures, most commonly a vitreous washout for recurrent vitreous hemorrhage.

Summary of Clinical Recommendations

Diabetic vitrectomy may achieve both anatomic and physiologic goals. Anatomically, the goal of surgery is to remove any vitreous opacities and fibrovascular traction so that detached retina may reattach. Physiologically, vitreous and fibrovascular tissue removal controls and generally halts the process of further fibrovascular proliferation and PDR.

In eyes with severe vitreous hemorrhage, early vitrectomy may be advantageous, especially in type 1 diabetic patients with a disease duration of less than 20 years. Diabetic vitrectomy, however, should not be undertaken lightly, as significant potential complications exist. There is a greater argument and urgency for early surgery in the setting of uncontrolled fibrovascular proliferation or when scatter laser photocoagulation is incomplete.

Eyes with severe active neovascularization with moderate or no hemorrhage may also benefit from early surgery in an effort to control the proliferative process. Scatter laser treatment should be carried out in the usual fashion, because the eyes that responded best to early vitrectomy were those in which extensive laser treatment had been carried out before surgery, and those in which photocoagulation was precluded by the presence of vitreous hemorrhage.

Traction retinal detachments sparing the fovea are, in and of themselves, not an indication for diabetic vitrectomy until the fovea becomes detached, provided that the proliferative process is not severe and no other indications for surgical intervention are present.

THE DIABETES CONTROL AND COMPLICATIONS TRIAL

Although well-designed population-based studies, such as the Wisconsin Epidemiologic Study of Diabetic Retinopathy (WESDR), showed a strong stepwise relation between glycosylated hemoglobin and the incidence and progression of diabetic retinopathy, the role of glycemic control and hyperglycemia in the pathogenesis of diabetic retinopathy was far from settled. As continuous subcutaneous insulin infusion (CSII) systems became available in the 1970s, reports of studies emerged describing the early worsening of retinopathy in persons assigned to the CSII group, as compared to the conventional insulin treatment group. It was clear that a randomized, controlled clinical trial was needed to evaluate, in an experimental design, whether intensive insulin treatment, resulting in better glycemic control, as compared to more conventional insulin treatment, would reduce the incidence and progression of diabetic microvascular complications. The findings would also describe the risks associated with intensive insulin treatment.

Study Objectives

The Diabetes Control and Complications Trial (DCCT) was "designed to compare intensive with conventional diabetes therapy with regard to their effects on the development and progression of early vascular and neurologic complications of insulin dependent diabetes mellitus (IDDM)." The study also was intended to make recommendations regarding the benefits and risks associated with intensive insulin therapy. The study's two main questions were as follows:

- Will intensive therapy prevent the development of diabetic retinopathy in patients with no retinopathy (primary prevention)? and

- Will intensive therapy affect the progression of early retinopathy (secondary intervention)?

Other issues investigated in the DCCT involve the magnitude of the effect of intensive insulin treatment on progression and regression of retinopathy, the degree to which this affects changes over time, and the relation of the effect to the level of severity of the retinopathy at baseline.

Treatment Groups/Trial Design

For inclusion in the primary prevention group, patients needed to meet the following criteria:

- duration of IDDM from 1 to 5 years;

- no retinopathy;

- visual acuity of 20/25 or better in each eye; and

- urinary excretion of less than 40 mg of albumin in 24 hours.

For inclusion in the secondary prevention group, patients needed to have the following:

- duration of IDDM from 1 to 15 years;

- the presence of very mild to moderate nonproliferative retinopathy (NPDR) in at least 1 eye;

- visual acuity of 20/32 or better in each eye; and

- urinary excretion rates of less than 200 mg of albumin per 24 hours.

Eligible patients were randomized to either conventional or intensive insulin therapy. Conventional therapy consisted of 1 or 2 daily injections of insulin, daily self-monitoring of urinary and blood glucose levels, and education about exercise and diet. Intensive therapy consisted of administration of insulin 3 or more times daily by injection or by an external pump. Self-monitoring of blood glucose levels was performed 4 times daily, and adjustment of the insulin dosage made accordingly. The goal of intensive therapy was essentially to maintain a level of glycemia in the non-diabetic range.

Outcome Measures

The most important primary outcome measure was a sustained, that is, at two consecutive six-month visits, three-step progression of diabetic retinopathy. Other ocular end points included

- the incidence of microaneurysms;

- development of severe NPDR or proliferative retinopathy (PDR);

- clinically significant macular edema; and

- the incidence of visual loss.

Some of the non-ocular outcomes measured in the study were the development of microalbuminuria or gross proteinuria and the incidence of clinical neuropathy. Neuropsychological and quality-of-life outcomes were also included.

Summary of Results and Implications for Clinical Practice

Intensive insulin treatment, as practiced in the DCTT, resulted in statistically significant reductions over a 9-year period in the following:

- the incidence of retinopathy (27%) and sustained three-step progression (76%) in the primary prevention group;

- progression to severe NPDR or worse (61%); and

- the need for laser treatment for macular edema or PDR (59%) in the secondary intervention group compared to conventional treatment.

Although intensive treatment may result in an initial worsening in some eyes with retinopathy, after 3 years of being on the regimen, the rate of sustained progression was lower and improvement was observed in eyes that had progression of retinopathy. The investigators also found that severe hypoglycemia was two to three times more common in the group randomized to intensive insulin treatment.

The DCCT investigators concluded that "intensive therapy should form the backbone of any health care strategy aimed at reducing the risk of visual loss from diabetic retinopathy" in persons with IDDM. Their analysis showed that intensive therapy would result in a "gain of 920,000 years of sight, 691,000 years free from end-stage renal disease, and 678,000 years free from lower extremity amputation, and 611,000 years of life at an additional cost of 4.0 billion dollars over the lifetime" of the 120,000 persons with IDDM in the United States who meet DCCT eligibility criteria.

THE BRANCH VEIN OCCLUSION STUDY

Branch vein occlusion (BVO) is a common disorder among retinal vascular diseases that is second only to diabetic retinopathy as a cause of decreased vision. The Branch Vein Occlusion Study (BVOS), which enrolled patients from July 1977 through February 1984, has elucidated the natural course and optimal management of patients with BVO.

Study Objectives

The BVOS sought to answer three questions regarding the complications of BVO:

- Could peripheral scatter argon laser photocoagulation prevent the development of neovascularization?

- Could peripheral scatter argon laser photocoagulation prevent vitreous hemorrhage?

- Could macular argon laser photocoagulation improve visual acuity in eyes with macular edema reducing vision to 20/40 or worse?

Treatment Groups/Trial Design

Four groups of eyes with BVOs were studied:

- Group I eyes were those at risk for the development of neovascularization that had a recent (3 to 18 months since onset) BVO involving a retinal area of at least 5 disc diameters (DD) with no neovascularization. Eyes were randomized either to peripheral scatter argon laser photocoagulation or to no laser treatment. All eyes were followed up to determine whether treatment with this type of photocoagulation prevented the development of neovascularization.

- Group II eyes were those at risk for the development of vitreous hemorrhage that had a recent (3 to 18 months since onset) BVO with retinal neovascularization present. Eyes were randomized either to peripheral scatter argon laser photocoagulation or to no laser treatment. All eyes were followed up to determine whether this type of photocoagulation prevented vitreous hemorrhage.

- Group III eyes were those at risk for visual loss from macular edema that had a recent (3 to 18 months since onset) BVO with macular edema reducing visual acuity to 20/40 or worse. Eyes were randomized either to a grid type of argon laser photocoagulation within the involved macular region or to no laser treatment. These eyes were followed up to determine whether this form of treatment improved the visual acuity in eyes with macular edema that reduced the vision to 20/40 or worse.

- Group X were those eyes that were determined to be at high risk for the development of neovascularization and had a recent (3 to 18 months since onset) BVO with capillary nonperfusion involving an area of retina at least 5 DD in diameter and without neovascularization. Recruitment of this group of patients only began after the sample size required for the group I patients had been reached and recruitment for that group terminated. The purpose for the group X patients was to maintain a pool of patients with a high risk of developing neovascularization and who would therefore become eligible for group II. Group X patients were also followed up for natural course information.

Outcome Measures

For groups I and II, outcomes were the occurrence of retinal neovascularization and vitreous hemorrhage. For group III eyes, the primary outcome measure was a gain of two or more lines of visual acuity at two or more consecutive four-month follow-up visits.

Summary of Results and Implications for Clinical Practice

The following are the recommendations for management of acute BVO based on the BVOS data:

Vision Reduced to 20/40 or Worse

- Wait for sufficient clearing of retinal hemorrhage to obtain high-quality fluorescein angiography.

- Evaluate fluorescein angiography for macular edema vs macular nonperfusion.

- If macular edema explains visual loss, and vision continues to be 20/40 or worse without spontaneous improvement after 3 months of observation, recommend grid-pattern macular photocoagulation.

- If macular nonperfusion explains visual loss, no treatment is available to improve vision.

Area of Retinal Involvement Greater Than 5 DD

- Wait for sufficient clearing of retinal hemorrhage to obtain high-quality fluorescein angiography.

- Evaluate fluorescein angiography for nonperfusion. If there is more than 5 DD of nonperfusion, follow up at 4-month intervals for development of neovascularization.

- If neovascularization develops and is confirmed, perform sector scatter laser photocoagulation in involved quadrant.

THE CENTRAL VEIN OCCLUSION STUDY

The Central Vein Occlusion Study (CVOS) was organized to better understand the natural course of perfused (nonischemic) central retinal vein occlusion (CRVO) and to evaluate the role of grid laser photocoagulation in eyes with a perfused CRVO and macular edema. It also was designed to assess the issue of timing of scatter laser photocoagulation in eyes with a nonperfused CRVO, that is, with greater than 10 disc areas of capillary nonperfusion, as seen on fluorescein angiography.

Study Objectives

The CVOS was designed to answer the following four questions:

- What is the natural course of eyes with perfused CRVO, defined as less than 10 disc areas of retinal capillary nonperfusion on fluorescein angiography?

- Does macular grid-pattern laser photocoagulation improve visual acuity in eyes with reduced vision caused by perfused macular edema associated with CRVO?

- In eyes with nonperfused CRVO, defined as at least 10 disc areas of retinal capillary nonperfusion on fluorescein angiography, does early panretinal laser photocoagulation prevent iris neovascularization (INV)?

- In eyes with nonperfused CRVO, is early panretinal photocoagulation more effective than panretinal photocoagulation delayed until the identification of INV in preventing additional ocular consequences caused by progressive neovascular glaucoma?

Treatment Groups/Trial Design

Eyes were categorized into four study groups: Group P (perfused), Group N (nonperfused), Group I (indeterminate perfusion), and Group M (macular edema).

Eyes were initially entered into their respective groups and then placed into other groups if their retinal capillary perfusion status warranted. All patients were followed up at least every 4 months for 3 years after entry into their final study group or until February 28, 1994, whichever came first.

- Group P: Eyes had less than 10 disc areas of retinal capillary nonperfusion on fluorescein angiography. These eyes served as a source for possible later entry into Group M. Eyes in Group P were observed for progression into Group N or I. The primary outcome variable for Group P eyes was perfusion status.

- Group N: Eyes showed 10 or more disc areas of retinal capillary nonperfusion on fluorescein angiography. Group N eyes were randomly assigned to either observation or panretinal laser photocoagulation. Eyes were followed up monthly. The primary outcome variable was the development of 2 clock hours of INV (TC-INV), any neovascularization of the angle (ANV), or progressive neovascular glaucoma.

- Group I: Eyes showed sufficient intraretinal hemorrhage to obscure the determination of the perfusion status by fluorescein angiography. These eyes were initially enrolled into Group I and were followed up monthly. Clearing of the hemorrhage permitted determination of the perfusion status, allowing such eyes to be transferred to either Group P or N.

- Group M: Eyes had a visual acuity between 20/50 and 5/200 due to perfused macular edema involving the foveal center visible on fluorescein angiography. These eyes were randomized to either observation or grid-pattern argon green laser photocoagulation. The primary outcome measure was visual acuity. Secondary outcome measures included the total area of macular edema, in disc areas, as well as change in fluorescein staining intensity over successive angiograms. After treatment, if the visual acuity improved by nine or fewer letters and perfused macular edema persisted angiographically, treatment was repeated.

Summary of Results and Implications for Clinical Practice

The CVOS was not designed to test whether panretinal photocoagulation should be performed in a CRVO eye complicated by INV/ANV. No investigator was willing to withhold panretinal photocoagulation for an eye with early INV because of the risk of progression to neovascular glaucoma. Instead, the study compared prophylactic panretinal photocoagulation with deferral of such photocoagulation until the first sign of INV/ANV was noted. The CVOS was a prospective study with long-term follow-up of more than 700 eyes with CRVO and no neovascularization at presentation. The following recommendations and conclusions could be gleaned from the study:

- One third of eyes with initially perfused CRVO progress to the nonperfused category by 3 years.

- Macular grid-pattern laser photocoagulation for eyes with perfused macular edema is not supported by the CVOS. Such treatment led to a significant reduction in angiographic macular edema but did not result in significant visual improvement. There was a tendency for visual improvement in treated patients under age 65 years but there were too few such patients to draw any definite conclusions.

- The majority of eyes that are classified with indeterminate perfusion are nonperfused.

- Prophylactic panretinal photocoagulation performed prior to the development of INV/ANV does not prevent the development of INV/ANV in all eyes and is not recommended. Prompt regression of neovascularization, in response to panretinal photocoagulation, is more likely to occur in eyes that have not previously received panretinal photocoagulation.

- Although the visual prognosis is guarded and depends on the presenting status, careful monitoring for INV/ANV and prompt panretinal photocoagulation treatment when early INV/ANV appears should diminish the development of neovascular glaucoma.

- Patients presenting with a CRVO should be followed up monthly for the development of INV/ANV for the first 6 months. Any patient whose visual acuity changes abruptly in the follow-up period should begin a schedule of monthly follow-up visits for the ensuing 6 months.

- Every patient examination should begin with slit lamp examination with high magnification of an undilated pupil to scrutinize the pupillary border and gonioscopy before pupillary dilation. If INV/ANV is observed, panretinal photocoagulation should be initiated promptly.

THE MULTICENTER TRIAL OF CRYOTHERAPY FOR RETINOPATHY OF PREMATURITY

Retinopathy of prematurity (ROP) was first recognized in the early 1940s by Terry. Hyperoxia, among other events, was thought to cause ROP, but the most prevalent and consistent risk factor has always been severe prematurity. Japanese investigators were the first to use transscleral cryotherapy to treat the anterior avascular retina to prevent progression to retinal detachment. This treatment, however, was not widely adopted or accepted until the results of the Multicenter Trial of Cryotherapy for Retinopathy of Prematurity (Cryo-ROP study) were published.

The Cryo-ROP study would not have been possible without the development of the uniform system of classification of the disease. The International Classification of Retinopathy of Prematurity (ICROP) was devised by 23 ophthalmologists from 11 different countries. It was published and widely accepted in 1984. The ICROP defined the location (zone) of the disease in the retina and the extent (stage) of the developing vasculature involved.

ICROP Stages

- Stage 1 (demarcation line) is defined as a thin, flat structure that separates avascular retina anteriorly from vascularized retina posteriorly.

- Stage 2 (ridge) is present when the line of stage 1 has grown, has height and width, and occupies a volume extending out of the plane of the retina.

- Stage 3 (ridge with extraretinal fibrovascular proliferation) exists when vessels leave the plane of the stage 2 ridge into the vitreous. Stage 3 is further subdivided into mild, moderate, and severe.

- Stage 4 (retinal detachment) is present when a subtotal retinal detachment is seen.

- Stage 5 (total retinal detachment) defines a total traction retinal detachment.

Plus Disease

Progressive vascular incompetence occurring along with the changes at the edge of the abnormally developing retinal vasculature is noted by increasing

- dilation and tortuosity of peripheral retinal vessels;

- iris vascular engorgement;

- pupillary rigidity;

- vitreous haze; or

- dilation and tortuosity of the posterior retinal vessels.

Study Objectives

The Cryo-ROP study was designed primarily to test whether cryotherapy to the anterior avascular retina of one eye with severe ROP would reduce the risk of cicatricial ROP (stage 4 or above) in the treated eye. The secondary goal of the study was to determine the incidence and natural course of ROP through prospective data analysis during the prethreshold monitoring phase of the study.

Treatment Groups/Trial Design

Eligible patients were those whose birth weight was less than 1251 g. Serial examinations were begun at 4 to 6 weeks of age and repeated every 2 weeks, unless the ROP reached a prethreshold level of disease, in which case examinations were done weekly. Prethreshold disease was defined as follows:

- Zone 1, any stage;

- Zone 2, stage 2 (ridge) with plus disease; and

- Zone 2, stage 3 (ridge with extraretinal fibrovascular proliferation).

Eyes either regressed spontaneously or progressed to threshold disease, a level of severity with a risk of blindness approaching 50%. Threshold disease was defined as

- 5 contiguous or;

- 8 non-contiguous cumulative clock hours of stage 3 ROP in zone 1 or 2, in the presence of plus disease.

If both eyes reached threshold ROP (symmetrical case), one eye was randomized to receive cryotherapy and the other eye was left untreated. If only one eye was at threshold (asymmetric case), then only that eye would be randomized to cryotherapy or no treatment. Cryotherapy was done within 72 hours of determination of threshold disease to limit the risk of progression to retinal detachment. Treatment was applied contiguously to the entire anterior avascular retinal periphery for 360° under indirect ophthalmoscopic guidance.

Outcome Measures

Detailed fundus examinations were performed independently by two separate investigators at the 3- and 12-month examinations. Photographs of the posterior pole and anterior segments of each eye were taken and sent to a central reading center. Objective evidence was sought for the presence or absence of the following:

- a retinal fold involving the macula;

- a retinal detachment involving zone 1 of the posterior pole; or

- retrolental tissue or "mass."

Eyes with any of these findings were classified as having had "unfavorable outcome." Functional outcomes were assessed at 12 to 16 months after randomization using monocular grading acuity assessments.

At 3.5 years after randomization, the HOTV crowded letter was used to assess functional outcome, and at 5.5 years after randomization, the ETDRS chart was used. Favorable visual outcome was defined as a Snellen visual acuity of better than 20/200; an unfavorable outcome was 20/200 or worse.

Summary of Results and Implications for Clinical Practice

The data and safety monitoring committee for the study recommended early termination because of the overwhelming beneficial effect of cryotherapy for eyes reaching threshold ROP. The Cryo-ROP study showed definitively that cryotherapy to the avascular retina significantly reduced the risk of an unfavorable structural outcome. These results persisted at 1 year and at the 5.5-year follow-up visits. Observed were a 45.8% reduction in an unfavorable outcome in treated eyes at 1 year and a 41% reduction at 5.5 years, as compared to untreated eyes.

Visual acuity outcomes, however, declined from the 1-year to the 5.5-year visits. A positive reduction in unfavorable functional outcome for treated compared to untreated eyes was 37.8% at 1 year and 24% at 5.5 years. This difference in structural vs functional outcomes showed that cryotherapy, while having a clearly beneficial effect on structural outcome, does not always lead to normal function. In fact, fewer treated eyes (13%) were in the best visual acuity group at 5.5 years compared to control eyes (17%). This finding was not anticipated and cannot be easily explained. By using cryotherapy, the surgeon may be sacrificing the best visual outcome in an effort to prevent blindness from retinal detachment. This risk underscores the need to avoid treating at levels of ROP less than threshold. This may also be less of an issue now that laser photocoagulation has largely supplanted cryotherapy in the management of threshold ROP.

Natural Course Information

The Cryo-ROP study has provided a wealth of information about the natural course of the disease. It is natural to question whether or not "threshold" disease represents the optimal benchmark for treatment, and to wonder whether treatment should be considered for ROP of lesser severity. It was found that untreated eyes with zone 2 ROP without plus disease and eyes with any zone 3 ROP had less than a 1% risk of an unfavorable outcome. Treatment of these eyes would generally mean treating an eye that had an acceptable natural outcome. Eyes with stages 1 and 2 ROP in zone 1 have an 8% to 11% risk of an unfavorable outcome. These eyes may progress rapidly to more severe disease, and careful follow-up is warranted. Zone 1 eyes present a special case, and earlier intervention may be indicated. Zone 2, stage 3 eyes with fewer than 5 clock hours of stage 3 disease had an 8.6% incidence of an unfavorable outcome. These latter groups have a somewhat higher risk of an unfavorable outcome, but the risk is still low compared to that of threshold ROP (greater than 22%). The answers to these questions may be better elucidated with longer follow-up, and as more information about other tests of visual function, such as peripheral visual fields, is gathered and assessed.

THE MACULAR PHOTOCOAGULATION STUDY

Although photocoagulation was recognized as being potentially beneficial for the treatment of choroidal neovascularization in the 1970s, many questions remained. The results of the Macular Photocoagulation Study (MPS) in dozens of publications have provided ophthalmologists with invaluable information relating to the clear benefits of laser ablation of subretinal neovascular lesions, with respect to their location to the fovea in the underlying disease process. The MPS, moreover, examined the influence of laser wavelength on treatment benefit and helped ophthalmologists understand the prognostic value of specific fundus features.

Study Objectives

The MPS set out initially to examine the utility of laser photocoagulation to leaking subretinal new vessel growth outside the fovea in preventing significant loss of visual acuity. This question was addressed for eyes with neovascular age-related macular degeneration (AMD), neovascular ocular histoplasmosis syndrome (OHS), and neovascular idiopathic choroidal neovascular membranes. Subsequent reports examined the incidence and risk factors for neovascular membrane persistence or recurrence and evaluated the benefit of photocoagulation of persistent and recurrent choroidal neovascularization (CNV). The visual outcomes in eyes receiving photocoagulation of extrafoveal and juxtafoveal CNV were compared with untreated control eyes in each group (AMD, OHS, or idiopathic CNV). The treatment benefit for laser photocoagulation of new and recurrent subfoveal CNV was evaluated for AMD only. In addition, the influence of laser wavelength on treatment benefit and the interpretation and prognostic value of specific fundus features was evaluated.

Treatment Groups/Trial Design

The Extrafoveal Study

For inclusion in the extrafoveal study, the major eligibility criteria were as follows:

- angiographic evidence of a well-demarcated choroidal neovascular membrane 200 μm to 2500 μm from the center of the foveal avascular zone (FAZ);

- best-corrected visual acuity ≥20/100;

- symptoms attributable to the neovascular membrane;

- drusen in eyes eligible for the AMD arms;

- at least one characteristic "histo-spot" in eyes eligible for the OHS arm;

- the absence of atrophic scars, drusen, or other retinal findings that could account for the neovascular membrane in eyes eligible for the idiopathic arms;

- a minimum age of 18 years for the OHS and idiopathic arms; and

- a minimum age of 50 years at the time of randomization in the AMD arm.

Patients were excluded if they had a history of prior laser photocoagulation or coexisting ocular disease that may otherwise affect visual acuity.

The Juxtafoveal (Krypton) Study

Eligible eyes had the following characteristics:

- well-demarcated neovascular AMD, neovascular OHS, or idiopathic CNV;

- the edge of the CNV was 1 μm to 199 μm from the center of the FAZ;

- CNV greater than 200 μm from the FAZ with adjacent blood or pigment (blocked fluorescence) extending within 200 μm; and

- best corrected visual acuity ≥20/400.

Other inclusion criteria were identical to those of the extrafoveal studies.

The Subfoveal New CNV AMD Study

Eligible patients had a fluorescein angiogram obtained less than 96 hours before randomization that demonstrated CNV with well-demarcated boundaries showing new vessel growth underneath the center of the FAZ covering a total area less than 3.5 MPS standard disc areas and a visual acuity between 20/40 and 20/320.

The Subfoveal Recurrent CNV Study

Major eligibility criteria included the following:

- a fluorescein angiogram obtained less than 96 hours before randomization demonstrating either:

  1. CNV under the center of the FAZ contiguous with a prior treatment scar or
  2. CNV within 150 μm from the center of the FAZ contiguous with a scar that had expanded under the fovea;

- visual acuity at entrance of 20/40 to 20/320;

- following proposed laser photocoagulation, some portion of the retina within 1.5 mm from the center of the FAZ would remain untreated;

■ the total area occupied by prior new treatment areas would be less than 6 MPS disc area;

■ apart from the scar, the majority of the lesion was composed of CNV; and

■ patients 50 years or older without other ocular disease potentially affecting visual acuity.

Eligible eyes of consenting patients were randomized to either laser treatment or no treatment. Eyes enrolled in the subfoveal studies that were randomized to laser photocoagulation were further randomized to treatment with argon green laser or krypton red laser photocoagulation.

Outcome Measures

The primary MPS outcome measure was "severe visual loss" defined as a loss of six or more lines of visual acuity as measured on the ETDRS chart. The subfoveal studies evaluated reading speed and contrast threshold as secondary outcome measures. The rates of recurrent and persistent CNV in treated eyes and the incidence of CNV in previously unaffected eyes were also recorded.

Summary of Results and Implications for Clinical Practice

Patient Monitoring and Examination

Patients at risk for developing CNV should be examined periodically to evaluate eligibility for treatment. These patients should monitor their central vision in each eye daily with alternate monocular cover tests. A symptomatic disturbance of reading vision, distance vision, or Amsler grid testing should be followed by prompt examination to identify a treatable lesion at the earliest possible time.

Extrafoveal and Juxtafoveal Lesions (Tables 1 and 2)

The results of the MPS are particularly compelling and unambiguous for extrafoveal and juxtafoveal CNV lesions, including peripapillary and nasal macular lesions.

■ For AMD, OHS, and idiopathic groups, laser-treated eyes lost less vision than untreated eyes.

■ Although hypertensive AMD patients did not appear to benefit from laser treatment for juxtafoveal lesions, laser treatment is recommended for all eyes with extrafoveal and juxtafoveal CNV meeting eligibility criteria for AMD, OHS, and idiopathic studies.

■ Retrobulbar or peribulbar anesthesia is recommended, but successful treatment can be accomplished with topical anesthesia in selected patients.

■ Careful comparison of pre- and post-treatment photographs enhance efforts to apply complete and adequate coverage of the CNV complex.

■ Because of high persistence and recurrence rates, the improved visual outcome in patients without recurrence, and the expected poor visual outcome following subfoveal extension of a previously extrafoveal or juxtafoveal lesion, close monitoring after treatment are recommended.

■ Evaluation with fluorescein angiography at 2-week intervals after treatment is recommended.

Subfoveal Lesions (Tables 3 and 4)

Only eyes with AMD and subfoveal CNV lesion complexes received laser treatment in the subfoveal arm of the MPS.

■ Laser treatment should be considered for neovascular lesions that meet eligibility criteria for the Subfoveal New CNV Study or the Subfoveal Recurrent CNV Study.

■ Because there may be an initial drop in visual acuity (particularly in eyes with visual acuity better than 20/100 or lesions greater than 2 MPS disc areas), a frank discussion with the patient regarding the visual expectations and long-term treatment benefit is critical.

■ Although data supporting the treatment of recurrences in eyes previously treated for subfoveal CNV are lacking, close follow-up is recommended to limit the size of the laser scar should persistence or recurrence be detected and treated.

TABLE 1

Five-Year Outcome of Eyes with Extrafoveal Choroidal Neovascularization Assigned to Laser or No Treatment*

Patient Groups	SVL, %	Lost Lines	Median VA	Persistence/Recurrence, %
AMD (Treated)	46	5.2	20/125	54
AMD (Untreated)	64	7.1	20/200	...
OHS (Treated)	12	0.9	20/40	26
OHS (Untreated)	42	4.4	20/80	...
INV (Treated)	23	2.7	20/64	34
INV (Untreated)	48	4.4	20/80	...

SVL indicates severe visual loss; AMD, age-related macular degeneration; OHS, ocular histoplasmosis syndrome; INV, idiopathic choroidal neovascularization; VA, visual acuity.

* Shown are 5-year rates for SVL, mean decrease in VA by lost lines, median final VA, and cumulative 5-year recurrence rate for AMD, OHS, and INV. (Derived from Macular Photocoagulation Study Group. Argon laser photocoagulation for neovascular maculopathy: five-year results from randomized clinical trials. *Arch Ophthalmol.* 1991;109:1109–1114.)

TABLE 2

Five-Year Outcome of Eyes with Juxtafoveal Neovascularization Assigned to Laser or No Treatment*

Patient Groups	SVL, %	Lost Lines	Median VA	Persistence/Recurrence, %
AMD (Treated)	55	5.0	20/200	78
AMD (Untreated)	65	6.2	20/250	...
OHS (Treated)	12	0.2	20/40	33
OHS (Untreated)	28	2.1	20/64	...
INV (Treated)	21	0.9	20/50	22
INV (Untreated)	34	2.6	20/80	...

SVL indicates severe visual loss; AMD, age-related macular degeneration; OHS, ocular histoplasmosis syndrome; INV, idiopathic choroidal neovascularization; VA, visual acuity.

* Shown are 5-year rates for SVL, mean decrease in VA by lost lines, median final VA, and cumulative 5-year recurrence rate for AMD, OHS, and INV. (Derived from Macular Photocoagulation Study Group. Laser photocoagulation for juxtafoveal choroidal neovascularization: five-year results from randomized clinical trials. *Arch Ophthalmol.* 1994;112:500–509.)

TABLE 3

Three-Year Outcome of Eyes with AMD, Subfoveal Recurrent Choroidal Neovascularization Assigned to Laser or No Treatment*

Patient Groups	SVL, %	Lost Lines	Median VA	Reading Speed
Treated	17	2.6	20/250	35 wpm
Untreated	39	3.9	20/320	15 wpm

SVL indicates severe visual loss; AMD, age-related macular degeneration; VA, visual acuity.
* The rates at 36 months for SVL, mean decrease in VA by lost lines, median reading speed (words per minute), and median final VA are shown. (Derived from Macular Photocoagulation Study Group. Laser photocoagulation of subfoveal neovascular lesions of age-related macular degeneration: updated findings from two clinical trials. *Arch Ophthalmol.* 1993;111:1200–1209.)

TABLE 4

Four-Year Outcome of Eyes with AMD, New Subfoveal Choroidal Neovascularization Assigned to Laser or No Treatment*

Patient Groups	SVL, %	Lost Lines	Median VA	Reading Speed
Treated	23	3.5	20/320	22 wpm
Untreated	45	5.0	20/500	13 wpm

SVL indicates severe visual loss; AMD, age-related macular degeneration; VA, visual acuity.
* The rates at 48 months for severe visual loss SVL, mean decrease in VA by lost lines, median final VA, and median reading speed (words per minute) are shown. (Derived from Macular Photocoagulation Study Group. Laser photocoagulation of subfoveal neovascular lesions of age-related macular degeneration: updated findings from two clinical trials. *Arch Ophthalmol.* 1993;111:1200–1209.)

THE TREATMENT OF AGE-RELATED MACULAR DEGENERATION WITH PHOTODYNAMIC THERAPY (TAP) STUDY

Age-related macular degeneration (AMD) is the leading cause of blindness in the western world. The severe visual loss that is seen in this disease process is largely secondary to the ingrowth of new vessels from the choriocapillaris. These new vessels are accompanied by eventual cicatricial changes that can destroy central vision over a period of months to years. Conventional thermal laser photocoagulation is a viable treatment option for very few of these patients. In the setting of subfoveal choroidal neovascularization (CNV), such treatment is accompanied by an immediate and significant loss of central vision. While this loss of vision is more likely to remain stable and unchanging over time, as compared to the natural course of the disease, such treatment has never gained widespread acceptance despite the clear recommendations of the Macular Photocoagulation Study (MPS).

The goal of photodynamic therapy is to selectively destroy the abnormal subretinal vessels while limiting the destruction to the overlying retina. It involves giving the patient an intravenous injection of verteporfin, a photosensitizer or light-activated drug. After infusion, the photosensitizer is activated by the light of a low-energy laser source at a wavelength that corresponds to the absorption peak of the drug. The Treatment of Age-Related Macular Degeneration with Photodynamic Therapy (TAP) investigation was initiated in North America and Europe to determine whether verteporfin therapy could reduce the risk of visual loss compared with placebo in people with subfoveal CNV caused by AMD.

Study Design/Treatment Groups

Eligible patients had subfoveal CNV lesions secondary to AMD ≤ 5400 μm in size with some evidence of classic CNV, and a best corrected visual acuity of approximately 20/40 to 20/200.

A total of 609 patients were randomized (2:1) to intravenous infusion of verteporfin or placebo. Fifteen minutes following the infusion, all patients were subjected to laser light at 689 nm delivered over 83 seconds, using a spot size with a diameter 1000 μm larger than the greatest linear dimension of the CNV lesions. Subjects were followed up at 3 monthly intervals and retreatment was given with the same treatment regimen if the fluorescein angiogram demonstrated fluorescein leakage.

The primary outcome measure was the proportion of eyes with a loss of fewer than 15 letters (approximately <3 lines of visual acuity) compared with the baseline examination at 1 year after study entry. Secondary out-

come measures included the proportion of eyes that lost fewer than 30 letters (approximately <6 lines of visual acuity) compared with the baseline examination, mean changes in visual acuity, mean changes in contrast threshold, and angiographic outcomes.

Summary of Results and Implications for Clinical Practice

There were 351 (87%) of 402 patients in the verteporfin group compared with 178 (86%) of 207 patients in the placebo group who completed the examination at month 24. Visual acuity and contrast sensitivity outcomes were better in the verteporfin-treated eyes than in the placebo-treated eyes at every follow-up examination through the 24-month examination. These visual results were supported by the findings on fluorescein angiography, namely, that verteporfin reduced lesion growth, was associated with cessation of leakage from classic CNV, and decreased the progression of classic CNV.

At the 12-month examination, 246 (61%) of 402 eyes assigned to verteporfin compared to 96 (46%) of 207 eyes assigned the placebo had lost fewer than 15 letters of visual acuity from baseline. At the 24-month examination, 213 (53%) of 402 verteporfin-treated patients compared with 78 (38%) of 207 placebo-treated patients lost fewer than 15 letters. Verteporfin-treated patients received an average of 5.6 treatments over the 24 months of their involvement in the study.

Subgroup analysis suggested that the visual acuity benefit of verteporfin therapy was present in only those eyes that demonstrated an area of classic CNV occupying 50% or more of the area of the entire lesion (predominantly classic CNV lesions). Among this group, 94 (59%) of 159 verteporfin-treated patients compared with 26 (31%) of 83 placebo-treated patients lost fewer than 15 letters at the 24-month examination. This finding was especially true when the lesions treated were entirely classic CNV lesions. In this group, 65 (70%) of 93 verteporfin-treated patients lost fewer than 15 letters compared with 14 (29%) of 49 placebo-treated patients at the 24-month examination. No statistically significant differences in visual acuity were noted when the area of classic CNV was less than 50% of the area of the entire lesion. Very few ocular or other systemic adverse events were associated with verteporfin infusion.

The benefits of verteporfin therapy for AMD patients with predominantly classic subfoveal CNV are clear, compelling, and safely sustained for 2 years. The TAP study group recommends treatment with verteporfin in this patient population.

SELECTED REFERENCES

The Diabetic Retinopathy Study

1. Quillen DA, Gardner TW, Blankenship GW. The Diabetic Retinopathy Study. In: Kertes PJ, Conway MD, eds. *Clinical Trials in Ophthalmology: A Summary and Practice Guide*. Baltimore, Md: Lippincott Williams & Wilkins; 1998:1–13.

2. The Diabetic Retinopathy Study Research Group. Photocoagulation treatment of proliferative diabetic retinopathy: the second report of Diabetic Retinopathy Study findings. *Ophthalmology*. 1978;85:82–106.

3. The Diabetic Retinopathy Study Research Group. Photocoagulation treatment of proliferative diabetic retinopathy: clinical applications of Diabetic Retinopathy Study (DRS) findings. DRS Report No. 8. *Ophthalmology*. 1981;88:583–600.

4. The Diabetic Retinopathy Study Research Group. Indications for photocoagulation treatment of diabetic retinopathy: Diabetic Retinopathy Study No. 14. *Int Ophthalmol Clin*. 1987;27:239–252.

The Early Treatment Diabetic Retinopathy Study

1. Akduman L, Olk RJ. The Early Treatment Diabetic Retinopathy Study. In: Kertes PJ, Conway MD, eds. *Clinical Trial in Ophthalmology: A Summary and Practice Guide*. Baltimore, Md: Lippincott Williams & Wilkins; 1998:15–35.

2. Early Treatment of Diabetic Retinopathy Study. Photocoagulation for diabetic macular edema: Early Treatment Diabetic Retinopathy Study Report No. 4. *Int Ophthalmol Clin*. 1987;27:265–272.

3. Early Treatment of Diabetic Retinopathy Study. Early photocoagulation for diabetic retinopathy. ETDRS Report Number 9. *Ophthalmology*. 1991;98:766–785.

4. Ferris F. Early photocoagulation in patients with either type I or type II diabetes. Early Treatment Diabetic Retinopathy Study Report 23. *Trans Am Ophthalmol Soc*. 1996;94:505–537.

The Diabetic Retinopathy Vitrectomy Study

1. Meredith TA. The Diabetic Retinopathy Vitrectomy Study. In: Kertes PJ, Conway MD, eds. *Clinical Trials in Ophthalmology: A Summary and Practice Guide*. Baltimore, Md: Lippincott Williams & Wilkins; 1998:37–48.

2. The Diabetic Retinopathy Vitrectomy Study Research Group. Two-year course of visual acuity in severe proliferative diabetic retinopathy with conventional management. Diabetic Retinopathy Vitrectomy Study (DRVS) Report 1. *Ophthalmology*. 1985;92:492–502.

3. The Diabetic Retinopathy Vitrectomy Study Research Group. Early vitrectomy for severe vitreous hemorrhage in diabetic retinopathy: two-year results of a randomized trial. Diabetic Retinopathy Vitrectomy Study Report 2. *Arch Ophthalmol*. 1985;103:1644–1652.

4. The Diabetic Retinopathy Vitrectomy Study Research Group. Early vitrectomy for severe proliferative diabetic retinopathy in eyes with useful vision: results of a randomized trial. Diabetic Vitrectomy Study Report 3. *Ophthalmology*. 1988;945:1307–1320.

5. The Diabetic Retinopathy Vitrectomy Study Research Group. Early vitrectomy for severe proliferative diabetic retinopathy in eyes with useful vision: clinical application of results of a randomized trial. Diabetic Retinopathy Vitrectomy Study Report 4. *Ophthalmology*. 1988;95:1307–1320.

6. The Diabetic Retinopathy Vitrectomy Study Research Group. Early vitrectomy for severe vitreous hemorrhage in diabetic retinopathy: four-year results of a randomized trial. Diabetic Retinopathy Vitrectomy Study Report 5. *Arch Ophthalmol*. 1990;108:958–964.

The Diabetes Control and Complications Trial

1. Klein R. The Diabetes Control and Complications Trial. In: Kertes PJ, Conway MD, eds. *Clinical Trials in Ophthalmology: A Summary and Practice Guide*. Baltimore, Md: Lippincott Williams & Wilkins; 1998:49–69.

2. The Diabetes Control and Complications Trial Research Group. The effect of intensive treatment of diabetes on the development and progression of long-term complications in insulin-dependent diabetes mellitus. *N Engl J Med*. 1993;329:977–986.

3. The Diabetes Control and Complications Trial Research Group. The effect of intensive diabetes treatment on the progression of diabetic retinopathy in insulin-dependent diabetes mellitus: the Diabetes Control and Complications Trial. *Arch Ophthalmol*. 1995;113:36–51.

4. The Diabetes Control and Complications Trial Research Group. Lifetime benefits and costs of intensive therapy as practiced in the Diabetes Control and Complications Trial. The Diabetic Control and Complications Trial. *JAMA*. 1996;276:1409–1415.

The Branch Vein Occlusion Study

1. Orth DH. The Branch Vein Occlusion Study. In: Kertes PJ, Conway MD, eds. *Clinical Trials in Ophthalmology: A Summary and Practice Guide*. Baltimore, Md: Lippincott Williams & Wilkins; 1998:113–127.

2. The Branch Vein Occlusion Study Group. Argon laser photocoagulation for macular edema in branch vein occlusion. *Am J Ophthalmol*. 1984;98:271–282.

3. The Branch Vein Occlusion Study Group. Argon laser scatter photocoagulation for prevention of neovascularization and vitreous hemorrhage in branch vein occlusion: a randomized clinical trial. *Arch Ophthalmol*. 1986;104:34–41.

The Central Vein Occlusion Study

1. Fekrat S, Finkelstein D. The Branch Vein Occlusion Study. In: Kertes PJ, Conway MD, eds. *Clinical Trials in Ophthalmology: A Summary and Practice Guide.* Baltimore, Md: Lippincott Williams & Wilkins; 1998:129–143.

2. The Central Vein Occlusion Study Group. Evaluation of grid pattern photocoagulation for macular edema in central vein occlusion. The Central Vein Occlusion Group M Report. *Ophthalmology.* 1995;102:1425–1433.

3. The Central Vein Occlusion Study Group. A randomized clinical trial of early panretinal photocoagulation for ischemic central vein occlusion. The Central Vein Occlusion Study Group N Report. *Ophthalmology.* 1995;102:1434–1444.

4. The Central Vein Occlusion Study Group. Natural history and clinical management of central retinal vein occlusion. *Arch Ophthalmol.* 1997;115:486–491.

The Multicenter Trial of Cryotherapy for Retinopathy of Prematurity

1. McNamara JA. The Multicenter Trial of Cryotherapy for Retinopathy of Prematurity. In: Kertes PJ, Conway MD, eds. *Clinical Trials in Ophthalmology: A Summary and Practice Guide.* Baltimore, Md: Lippincott Williams & Wilkins; 1998:145–162.

2. Schaffer DB, Palmer EA, Plotsky DF, Metz HS, Flynn JT, Tung B, Hardy RJ, for the Cryotherapy for Retinopathy of Prematurity Cooperative Group. Prognostic features in the natural course of retinopathy of prematurity. *Ophthalmology.* 1993;100:230–237.

3. The Cryotherapy for Retinopathy of Prematurity Cooperative Group. Multicenter trial of cryotherapy for retinopathy of prematurity: 3½-year outcome: structure and function. *Arch Ophthalmol.* 1993;111:339–344.

4. The Cryotherapy for Retinopathy of Prematurity Cooperative Group. Multicenter trial of cryotherapy for retinopathy of prematurity: Snellen visual acuity and structural outcome at 5½ years after randomization. *Arch Ophthalmol.* 1996;114:417–424.

The Macular Photocoagulation Study

1. Berger JW, Maguire MG, Fine SL. The Macular Photocoagulation Study. In: Kertes PJ, Conway MD, eds. *Clinical Trials in Ophthalmology: A Summary and Practice Guide.* Baltimore, Md: Lippincott Williams & Wilkins; 1998:71–92.

2. The Macular Photocoagulation Study Group. Argon laser photocoagulation for neovascular maculopathy: five-year results from randomized clinical trials. *Arch Ophthalmol.* 1991;109:1109–1114.

3. The Macular Photocoagulation Study Group. Laser photocoagulation of subfoveal neovascular lesions in age-related macular degeneration: results of a randomized clinical trial. *Arch Ophthalmol.* 1991;109:1220–1231.

4. The Macular Photocoagulation Study Group. Laser photocoagulation for juxtafoveal choroidal neovascularization: five-year results from randomized clinical trials. *Arch Ophthalmol.* 1994;112:500–509.

5. The Macular Photocoagulation Study Group. Risk factors for choroidal neovascularization in the second eye of patients with juxtafoveal or subfoveal choroidal neovascularization secondary to age-related macular degeneration. *Arch Ophthalmol.* 1997;115:741–747.

The Treatment of Age-Related Macular Degeneration with Photodynamic Therapy (TAP) Study

1. Fine SL. Photodynamic therapy with verteporfin is effective for selected patients with neovascular age-related macular degeneration. *Arch Ophthalmol.* 1999;117:1400–1402.

2. Miller JW, Schmidt-Erfurth U, Sickenberg M, Pournaras CJ, Laqua H, Barbazetto I, et al. Photodynamic therapy with verteporfin for choroidal neovascularization caused by age-related macular degeneration: results of a single treatment in a phase 1 and 2 study. *Arch Ophthalmol.* 1999;117:1161–1173.

3. Schmidt-Erfurth U, Miller JW, Sickenberg M, Laqua H, Barbazetto I, Gragoudas ES, et al. Photodynamic therapy with verteporfin for choroidal neovascularization caused by age-related macular degeneration: results of retreatments in a phase 1 and 2 study. *Arch Ophthalmol.* 1999;117:1177–1187.

4. The Treatment of Age-Related Macular Degeneration with Photodynamic Therapy (TAP) Study Group. Photodynamic therapy of subfoveal choroidal neovascularization in age-related macular degeneration with verteporfin: One-year results of 2 randomized clinical trials. TAP Report 1. *Arch Ophthalmol.* 1999;117:1329–1345.

5. The Treatment of Age-Related Macular Degeneration with Photodynamic Therapy (TAP) Study Group. Photodynamic therapy of subfoveal choroidal neovascularization in age-related macular degeneration with verteporfin: two-year results of 2 randomized clinical trials. TAP Report 2. *Arch Ophthalmol.* 2001;119:198–207.

Laser Photocoagulation and
Photodynamic Therapy
for Retinal and Choroidal Disease

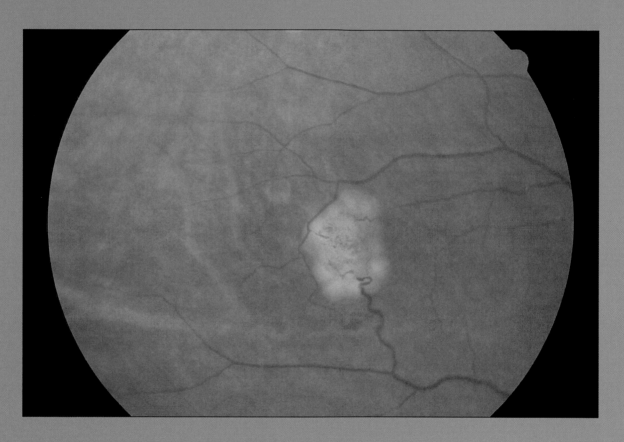

Peter J. Kertes, MD

David A. Quillen, MD

BRANCH RETINAL VEIN OCCLUSION: MACULAR EDEMA

Laser photocoagulation is indicated for the treatment of branch retinal vein occlusion (BRVO) that is complicated by visual loss related to macular edema. The BRVO Study established the following eligibility criteria: (1) recent onset of BRVO (within 3–18 months); (2) visual acuity of 20/40 or worse; (3) sufficient clearing of intraretinal hemorrhage and no foveal hemorrhage; (4) fluorescein angiogram demonstrating macular edema involving the fovea with good perfusion; and (5) no other ocular disorder contributing to visual loss.

Technique

Most ophthalmologists observe patients with acute BRVOs for 3 months to allow for spontaneous resolution. If after that time vision remains 20/40 or worse and there has been sufficient clearing of the intraretinal hemorrhage, a fluorescein angiogram is obtained to assess macular perfusion and the extent and location of leakage. If macular edema accounts for the visual loss (rather than macular ischemia), macular laser treatment is recommended.

Patients must provide informed consent before undergoing laser photocoagulation. Photocoagulation is performed using a slit lamp delivery system with a fundus contact lens and topical anesthesia. Several commercially available lenses are designed to optimize viewing of the macula. Laser settings are as follows: 100-μm to 200-μm spot size; 0.1- to 0.15-second duration; and intensity to achieve a light to medium retinal burn. Treatment involves a grid pattern of laser energy over the area of capillary leakage, extending no closer to the fovea than the edge of the foveal avascular zone. Treatment should not extend beyond the major vascular arcades (unless there is associated neovascularization/vitreous hemorrhage). Burns are placed approximately one burn width apart throughout the involved area.

Complications

Complications of macular laser treatment for BRVO are uncommon, but they include loss of vision, central and paracentral scotomas, choroidal neovascularization, and subretinal fibrosis. Surgeons must identify the center of the macula to avoid inadvertent foveal burns. Having the patient fixate on the laser-aiming beam, while the laser is in the standby setting, may identify the center of the macula. Areas of retinal hemorrhage should be avoided to reduce the risk of retinal damage and epiretinal membrane formation.

Follow-up Considerations

Patients are evaluated 3 months after laser photocoagulation. Additional laser treatment may be considered in those whose condition does not respond to the initial treatment.

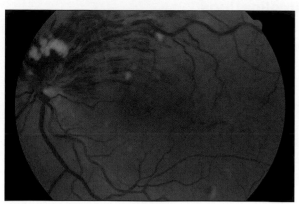

A 56-year-old man presented with acute visual loss in his left eye. He was diagnosed with a superotemporal branch retinal vein occlusion. His blood pressure was 160/94 mm Hg, and he was referred to his primary care doctor for evaluation and treatment of hypertension.

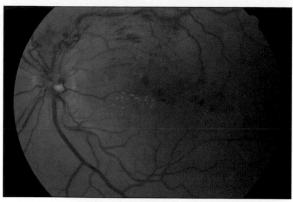

During the subsequent 3 months, visual acuity in the left eye remained 20/50. His examination revealed reduction of the intraretinal hemorrhage but more prominent macular edema and lipid exudate.

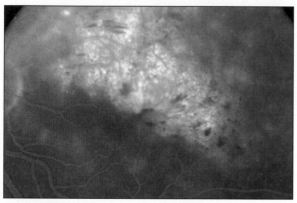

Fluorescein angiogram of the left eye of the same patient in at 3-month follow-up reveals significant leakage throughout the superior macula with relatively good vascular perfusion.

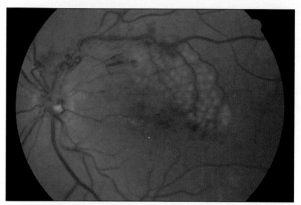

Laser photocoagulation was performed. A grid pattern of laser energy was applied to the area of retinal thickening using the following parameters: 100-μm spot size burns placed one burn width apart; 0.1-second duration; and power intensity to achieve a moderately white burn (100 mW).

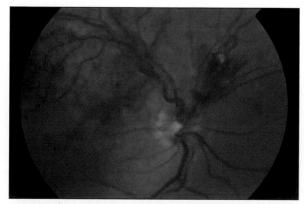

This example of branch retinal vein occlusion is associated with macular edema. Laser photocoagulation was performed.

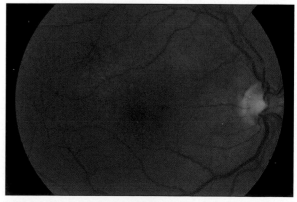

This fundus photograph of the same eye was taken approximately 6 months following laser treatment. The macular edema has resolved. Note the hyperpigmented spots at the level of the retinal pigment epithelium corresponding to the laser burns.

BRANCH RETINAL VEIN OCCLUSION: NEOVASCULARIZATION

Scatter laser photocoagulation is indicated for the treatment of branch retinal vein occlusion (BRVO) that is complicated by the development of neovascularization and/or vitreous hemorrhage. The risk of neovascularization and/or vitreous hemorrhage is associated with the extent of retinal ischemia in the distribution of the BRVO. Neovascularization usually occurs at the junction of the perfused and nonperfused retina but may be found at the optic disc or a distant site.

Technique

The mechanism for the development of neovascularization presumably involves the release of vasogenic substances from the ischemic retina. Scatter laser photocoagulation is applied to the peripheral retina in the distribution of the BRVO to reduce the stimulus for neovascularization and induce regression of the new vessels. It is important to distinguish peripheral scatter laser photocoagulation in the distribution of the BRVO from panretinal photocoagulation, which involves scatter laser photocoagulation of the entire peripheral fundus.

Informed consent must be obtained from the patient before scatter laser photocoagulation is performed. Laser therapy usually is completed in one session using topical anesthesia. Both slit lamp and binocular indirect ophthalmoscopic laser photocoagulation delivery systems may be used. A variety of wide-field fundus contact lenses is available to facilitate peripheral scatter laser application. The green wavelength is preferred for most patients; however, the red wavelength may be used in cases of significant cataract or vitreous hemorrhage. Typical laser parameters include 200-μm to 500-μm spot size; 0.1-second duration; and intensity to obtain a moderately white retinal burn. Spots are placed one-half to one burn width apart in a scatter pattern throughout the involved quadrant or region. The posterior portion of the BRVO should be demarcated with two or three rows of laser burns. Treatment is then extended in a posterior to anterior direction to reduce the risk of extension into the macula.

Complications

Complications of peripheral scatter laser photocoagulation are uncommon. Care must be taken to avoid inadvertent laser treatment of the macula.

Follow-up Considerations

Patients are reexamined 6 to 8 weeks following completion of the scatter laser photocoagulation. Additional laser photocoagulation may be applied in eyes that fail to respond to initial treatment.

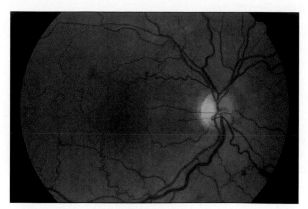

A 68-year-old man presented with complaints of floaters and mild visual loss in the right eye. He had a history of "broken blood vessels." The fundus photograph reveals a chronic superior branch retinal vein occlusion with venous sheathing and telangiectatic capillaries.

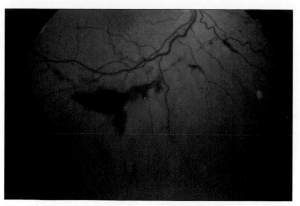

The same patient has preretinal hemorrhage along the inferotemporal vascular arcade in the right eye.

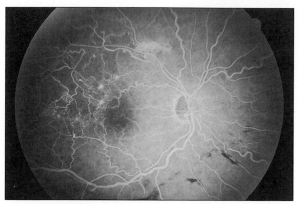

Fluorescein angiogram of the same patient reveals an ischemic branch retinal vein occlusion. The hyperfluorescence is consistent with neovascularization along the superotemporal vascular arcade at the site of the vein occlusion.

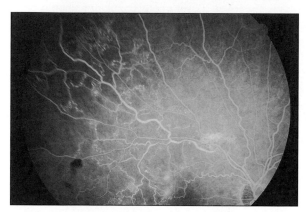

A peripheral view of the same eye demonstrates diffuse hypofluorescence consistent with widespread nonperfusion in the distribution of the occlusion. Note the neovascularization at the junction of the perfused and nonperfused retina.

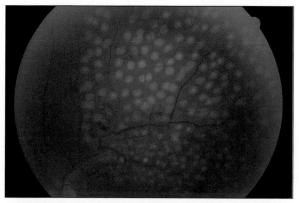

This fundus photograph was taken immediately following laser photocoagulation of a patient with ischemic branch retinal vein occlusion complicated by neovascularization and macular edema. Macular grid and peripheral scatter patterns of laser photocoagulation were performed.

CENTRAL SEROUS CHORIORETINOPATHY

Most cases of central serous chorioretinopathy resolve spontaneously without the need for treatment. However, laser photocoagulation may be indicated for patients with the following features: duration greater than 4 months; history of visual loss in the same or fellow eye from previous episodes of central serous chorioretinopathy; the need for rapid recovery of vision; atypical central serous chorioretinopathy with large bullous retinal detachment; and central serous chorioretinopathy associated with corticosteroid use.

Technique

Informed consent must be obtained from the patient prior to performing laser photocoagulation for central serous chorioretinopathy. A fluorescein angiogram should be completed to identify the leakage site and ensure that laser burns can be applied safely without involving the fovea. Laser photocoagulation should be performed with a slit lamp delivery system. Central serous chorioretinopathy has been successfully treated with all available wavelengths of laser (yellow, green, and red). A variety of fundus contact lenses is available to improve visualization and treatment of the macula. Laser is applied directly to the leakage site. Common laser parameters include 100-μm spot size; 0.1- to 0.2-second duration; and laser intensity enough to produce a moderately white burn.

Complications

Laser photocoagulation is safe and effective for central serous chorioretinopathy, with little risk of significant adverse effects. Special care must be exercised to avoid inadvertent laser burns on the fovea. Initially, laser intensity should be low and carefully increased to avoid the risk of choroidal rupture and secondary choroidal neovascularization.

Follow-up Considerations

The subretinal fluid usually resorbs within 6 to 8 weeks following laser photocoagulation. Retroretinal protein precipitates may be more prominent during the resolution phase of central serous chorioretinopathy. Recovery of vision may lag behind resorption of the subretinal fluid.

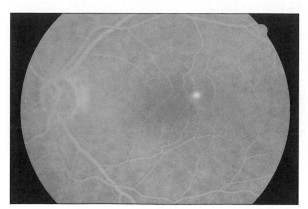

A 53-year-old woman developed central serous chorioretinopathy following a corticosteroid injection for joint disease. Her fluorescein angiogram revealed a hyperfluorescent spot that continued to leak throughout the study.

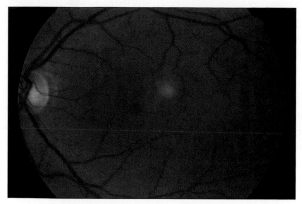

The same patient elected to have laser photocoagulation. This fundus photograph, taken immediately after laser treatment, demonstrates a moderately white burn applied directly to the leakage site. The subretinal fluid resolved during 6 weeks after laser therapy.

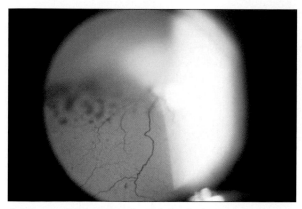

A 26-year-old man developed atypical central serous chorioretinopathy characterized by a bullous serous retinal detachment. This slit lamp photograph shows the retina located just behind the lens. Note the large subretinal protein deposits.

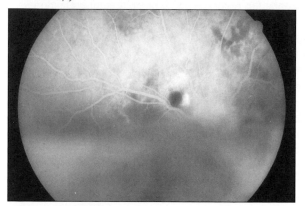

Fluorescein angiogram reveals a hyperfluorescent spot located above the superotemporal vascular arcade. Leakage was significant throughout the fluorescein study.

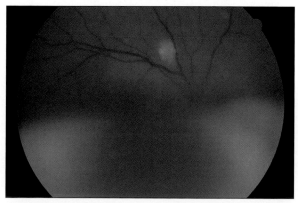

Laser photocoagulation was performed on the same patient. A moderately intense burn was placed at the leakage site. The laser parameters were 100-μm spot size; 0.2-second duration; and intensity to produce a moderately white burn (150 mW).

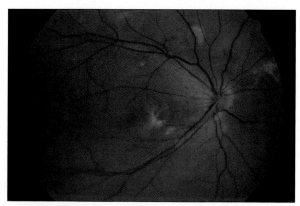

The subretinal fluid resorbed during 6 weeks after laser treatment. Extensive retinal pigment epithelial abnormalities and subretinal fibrosis are seen.

CENTRAL RETINAL VEIN OCCLUSION

Panretinal laser photocoagulation (PRP) is indicated for the treatment of central retinal vein occlusion (CRVO) complicated by the development of iris or angle neovascularization/neovascular glaucoma. Iris or angle neovascularization/neovascular glaucoma develops in response to widespread retinal ischemia. Panretinal laser photocoagulation is applied to the ischemic peripheral retina to reduce the stimulus for neovascularization and induce regression of the new vessels. Laser photocoagulation for macular edema secondary to CRVO may help to reduce the macular edema but does not appear to have a significant impact on visual acuity.

Technique

Eyes with CRVO are followed up closely for the development of iris (NVI) or angle (NVA) neovascularization. Once NVI and/or NVA is detected, prompt PRP is recommended to reduce the risk of neovascular glaucoma.

Informed consent must be obtained from the patient prior to performing PRP. Because of the devastating effects of neovascular glaucoma, PRP usually is performed in a single session with use of retrobulbar anesthesia. Both binocular indirect ophthalmoscopic and slit lamp laser photocoagulation delivery systems may be used. A variety of wide-field contact lenses are available for standard PRP. Many of the commercially available lenses magnify the spot size by 1.5 to two times and provide an inverted and reversed image of the fundus. The green wavelength is most commonly employed; red may be used in patients with significant cataract or vitreous hemorrhage. Common laser parameters are 200-μm to 500-μm spot size; 0.1- to 0.2-second duration; and intensity to produce a moderately white burn. The average number of 500-μm spots needed to complete PRP is approximately 1600. Laser burns are spaced one-half to one spot width apart.

The placement of laser therapy in a posterior to anterior direction helps to reduce the risk of inadvertent extension into the macula. The posterior fundus is demarcated with two to three rows of laser burns. The posterior border should be placed approximately 1 disc diameter from the optic disc nasally and from the major retinal vascular arcades superiorly and inferiorly. The temporal border is placed at an imaginary line located approximately 2 disc-to-fovea diameters from the optic disc.

In addition to medications to lower intraocular pressure, some ophthalmologists recommend using topical corticosteroid and cycloplegic eyedrops to enhance patient comfort and reduce the risk of postlaser choroidal effusions.

Complications

Complications of PRP include blurred vision, nyctalopia, visual field constriction, poor color discrimination, transient myopia, accommodation defects, corneal burns, narrow-angle glaucoma, iris burns, lens opacities, inadvertent macular burns, macular edema, exudative macular detachment, ciliochoroidal effusion, choroidal/choriovitreal neovascularization, optic neuropathy, and complications of local anesthesia (globe trauma, retrobulbar hemorrhage).

Follow-up Considerations

Patients are reexamined 1 week following PRP to assess the response to laser therapy and measure the intraocular pressure. Additional laser photocoagulation may be necessary, unless the new vessels have significantly regressed. Supplemental laser burns may be placed between previous burn sites and to the far peripheral retina using a three-mirror lens or a binocular indirect ophthalmoscopic laser delivery system. Gonioscopy is performed to assess regression of NVA and the extent of peripheral anterior synechiae.

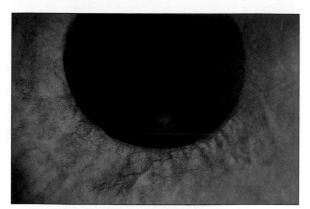

Laser photocoagulation is indicated for the treatment of central retinal vein occlusions complicated by iris or angle neovascularization/neovascular glaucoma. Iris neovascularization may be seen along the pupillary margin, the iris face, or anterior chamber angle.

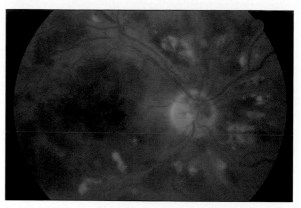

Laser photocoagulation may reduce macular edema but does not have a significant impact on visual acuity. As a result, macular laser is generally not considered unless the patient is younger than 65 years.

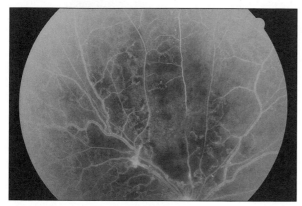

Iris neovascularization/neovascular glaucoma develops in patients with ischemic central retinal vein occlusion. This fluorescein angiogram shows widespread capillary nonperfusion in a patient with neovascular glaucoma.

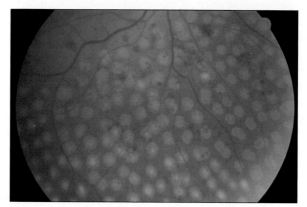

Prompt panretinal photocoagulation treatment when early iris or angle neovascularization appears should diminish the development of neovascular glaucoma. This fundus photograph demonstrates a typical laser photocoagulation pattern.

CHOROIDAL NEOVASCULARIZATION

In the era of photodynamic therapy, thermal laser photocoagulation should probably be limited to treating patients with clearly defined choroidal neovascular membranes (CNV) that do not involve the foveal center. Treatment should largely be confined to those patients with CNV secondary to age-related macular degeneration (AMD), the presumed ocular histoplasmosis syndrome (POHS), or idiopathic causes. Choroidal neovascular membranes secondary to conditions such as high myopia, angioid streaks, choroidal ruptures, and others can be considered by the treating surgeon.

Technique

High-quality color photography and fluorescein angiography transiting the eye to be treated are mandatory to determine the need for treatment and to help guide the treatment. Ideally, these images should be obtained within 72 hours of treatment. A decision to offer treatment is made only after the angiogram is thoroughly scrutinized under magnification and a careful stereoscopic evaluation of the macula has been done. When providing an informed consent, patients must understand that this kind of laser photocoagulation will result in a dense paracentral scotoma. Patients also need to understand that recurrence, especially in the setting of AMD, is frequent if not universal given enough time.

Treatment may be done with use of a high-magnification fundus contact lens and topical anesthesia, if the patient can reliably fixate with the fellow eye. If the patient cannot reliably keep from moving the eye during laser treatment, then retrobulbar or peribulbar anesthesia is preferred. A high-magnification copy of a midphase frame of the angiogram needs to be close at hand to help identify landmarks and guide treatment. The slit lamp delivery system is used, and argon green or krypton red laser wavelengths are preferred. Red may be advantageous in treating lesions with associated subretinal hemorrhage or those within the papillomacular bundle. The treatment needs to be carefully planned ahead of time, as all areas of both occult and classic choroidal neovascularization need to be completely ablated. If proximity to the fovea permits, an effort should be made to overlap the edges of the CNV so that 100 µm of normal retina is also treated to reduce the risk of recurrence.

The desired end point is a chalky white burn. To achieve this and minimize the risk of perforation of Bruch's membrane and/or hemorrhage, a long-duration, large, and low-intensity burn is preferred to a high-power, short-duration, smaller burn. Test burns with a 200-µm spot size and at least 0.2-second duration are placed within the neovascular complex away from the fovea. The power is titrated up from 100 mW to achieve a chalky white burn and to observe the spread of the laser burn. Once the desired power has been determined, the foveal edge is treated first with overlapping 200-µm spots. If 100-µm overlap of the CNV is desired, the 200-µm burn is centered on the edge of the CNV. If less overlap is needed, the burn is centered inward. A second and third contiguous row of laser burns is then applied inside this foveal edge. Burns are placed in an overlapping

fashion to ensure complete coverage. Once this foveal edge has been treated, the lesion can then be outlined with overlapping 200-µm burns of adequate intensity. The non-foveal edges are overlapped by 100 µm. The lesion can then be filled in with larger, longer-duration burns. The desired end point is a uniform chalky whiteness of the entire neovascular complex. Once treatment has been finished, a careful comparison should be undertaken between the high-magnification mid-phase angiogram and the eye, so that additional treatment can be done at the same sitting, if necessary.

Complications

A common complication of this type of intense laser treatment is hemorrhage, generally from bleeding CNV or perforating Bruch's membrane. A bubble may be seen if this occurs. Bleeding is best controlled with increasing the pressure on the contact lens to raise intraocular pressure and control oozing. This pressure should continue for at least 30 seconds after the bleeding has stopped to allow it to clot. While such bleeding can be alarming, it is not an indication to discontinue treatment. Treatment should continue but at a lower laser power. It is important to remember that a break in Bruch's membrane is itself a risk factor for the development of CNV. Special care should be taken during the follow-up period to monitor for this complication.

The most dreaded complication of this type of thermal laser photocoagulation is inadvertently burning the fovea. This adverse event should be avoidable with careful prelaser planning, identification of important landmarks on fluorescein angiography, and careful discussion with the patient to ensure proper fixation or, failing that, adequate anesthesia.

Persistence (less than 6 weeks following treatment) or recurrence of CNV is a frequent problem. This likely occurs universally given enough follow-up in patients with CNV secondary to AMD. Patients need to be counseled to return if they notice any new distortion or other significant visual changes. Recurrences that do not involve the foveal center may be re-treated with thermal laser photocoagulation. It is useful to take an immediate posttreatment photograph to help the clinician identify potential areas of inadequate treatment and to help guide any potential future treatment.

Follow-up Considerations

Patients should be seen 2 to 3 weeks following laser treatment and undergo fluorescein angiography. At this first postlaser visit, much of the subretinal fluid that may have been present may have resorbed, although some swelling may persist within the laser scar. Fluorescein angiography usually shows central hypofluorescence surrounded by a rim of hyperfluorescence. The presence of any leakage almost certainly indicates persistence/recurrence and, after correlation with the clinical examination, additional treatment is undertaken as necessary. These patients do need to be followed up closely with clinical examination and fluorescein angiography. An interval of every 2 to 4 weeks for the first 3 to 4 months is quite reasonable.

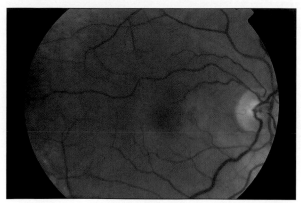

This 65-year-old woman presented with visual loss in her right eye. Her examination revealed a yellowish gray lesion associated with subretinal fluid located nasal to the fovea.

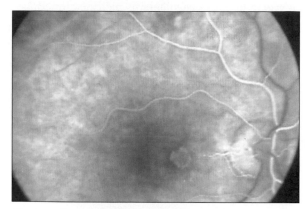

Fluorescein angiography of the same patient demonstrates a classic, well-defined extrafoveal choroidal neovascular membrane.

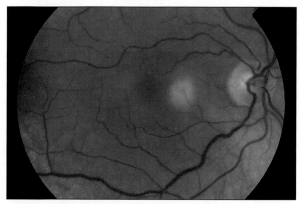

The same patient elected to undergo laser photocoagulation. This fundus photograph was taken immediately following treatment. Intense laser burns cover the entire neovascular complex.

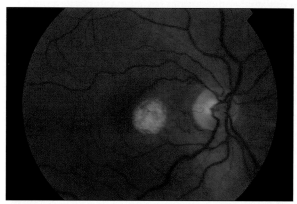

One year after treatment, the patient has a well-defined chorioretinal scar corresponding to laser photocoagulation. No recurrence is evident.

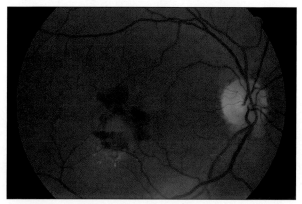

This 62-year-old woman with presumed ocular histoplasmosis syndrome presented with distortion and reduced vision in her right eye. She had a history of visual loss in her left eye related to choroidal neovascularization. Note the subretinal blood, fluid, and lipid.

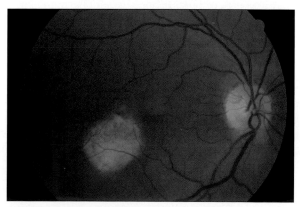

Fluorescein angiography of the same patient demonstrated a classic extrafoveal choroidal neovascular membrane, and laser photocoagulation was performed. This fundus photograph taken almost 2 years after treatment reveals an atrophic scar with no evidence of recurrence.

DIABETIC RETINOPATHY: CLINICALLY SIGNIFICANT MACULAR EDEMA

Focal grid laser photocoagulation is indicated for clinically significant macular edema defined as any one of the following: (1) retinal thickening within 500 μm of the center of the macula; (2) lipid exudates within 500 μm of the center of the macula associated with retinal thickening; or (3) retinal thickening greater than 1 disc area within 1 disc diameter of the center of the macula.

Technique

Clinically significant macular edema is diagnosed with use of a fundus contact lens. Once this diagnosis is established by clinical examination, a fluorescein angiogram is obtained to identify treatable lesions. Treatable lesions include discrete points of hyperfluorescence or focal leakage (eg, microaneurysms), areas of diffuse leakage (eg, intraretinal microvascular abnormalities, capillary bed leakage), and areas of capillary nonperfusion (except for the normal foveal avascular zone).

After obtaining the patient's informed consent, laser photocoagulation is performed using a slit lamp delivery system with a fundus contact lens. There are several lenses designed to optimize viewing of the macula. Many physicians prefer to use yellow-wavelength energy, if available, for the treatment of microaneurysms (preferential absorption by hemoglobin). Since the yellow wavelength can be absorbed by intraretinal hemorrhage, these areas should be avoided to reduce the risk of severe retinal damage. Laser settings are 50-μm to 100-μm spot size, 0.1- to 0.15-second duration, and intensity to achieve mild retinal whitening.

Direct treatment is applied to areas of focal leakage. Sufficient intensity should be used to obtain definite whitening around the microaneurysm or site of leakage. For larger microaneurysms, the surgeon should attempt to obtain whitening (or darkening) of the microaneurysm itself. A grid pattern of laser burns should be applied to areas of diffuse leakage or capillary nonperfusion.

Complications

Great care must be taken to avoid treatment of the fovea. In eyes with central macular edema, the normal foveal landmarks may be unrecognizable. Having the patient fixate on the laser-aiming beam while the laser is in the standby setting may facilitate identification of the center of the macula. In addition to inadvertent foveal burns, complications of macular photocoagulation include reduced vision, paracentral and central scotomas (temporary or permanent), choroidal neovascularization, and subretinal fibrosis.

Follow-up Considerations

Patients are reexamined within 6 to 8 weeks to evaluate the response to laser treatment. It is not unusual to see a temporary increase in the amount of lipid exudate as the macular edema resorbs. Three to 4 months following the laser session, additional macular laser photocoagulation may be performed in eyes with residual clinically significant macular edema. Treatment of lesions up to 300 μm from the center of the macula may be performed, unless there is perifoveal capillary dropout.

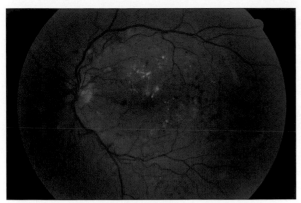

This 34-year-old man presented with high-risk proliferative diabetic retinopathy and clinically significant macular edema. He met all three criteria for clinically significant macular edema.

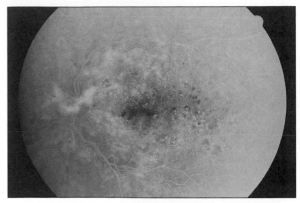

A fluorescein angiogram was obtained to identify treatable lesions. Numerous hyperfluorescent spots are consistent with microaneurysms scattered throughout the macula. Also present is hyperfluorescence of the optic disc consistent with neovascularization.

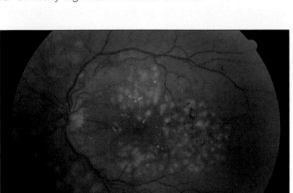

Macular laser was applied to the microaneurysms; care was taken to avoid the fovea. Laser parameters were 50-μm spot size; 0.1-second duration; and intensity to obtain whitening (or darkening) of the microaneurysm. Nasal panretinal photocoagulation was initiated at the same time.

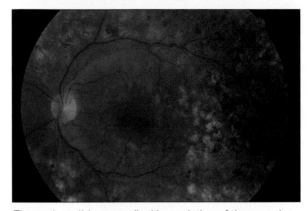

The patient did very well with resolution of the macular edema and regression of the neovascularization.

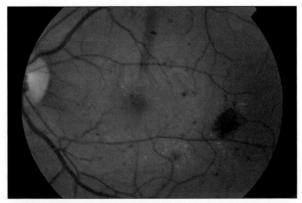

Fundus photograph of the left eye in a patient with diabetes and clinically significant macular edema.

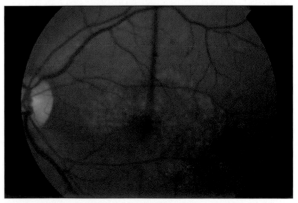

Fundus photograph of the same patient following grid laser photocoagulation to the area of retinal thickening.

DIABETIC RETINOPATHY: HIGH-RISK PROLIFERATIVE DIABETIC RETINOPATHY

Panretinal photocoagulation (PRP) is indicated for the treatment of high-risk proliferative diabetic retinopathy (PDR). High-risk PDR is defined as three or four of the following risk factors: (1) new vessels present; (2) new vessels on or within 1 disc diameter (DD) of the optic disc (NVD); (3) severe new vessels (NVD greater than one-third disc area or in the absence of NVD, neovascularization elsewhere [NVE] greater than one-half disc area); or (4) preretinal and/or vitreous hemorrhage.

The presence of these conditions translates into three clinical scenarios: NVD greater than one-third disc area; any NVD associated with preretinal or vitreous hemorrhage; and NVE greater than one-half disc area associated with preretinal or vitreous hemorrhage. Iris neovascularization and neovascular glaucoma also require prompt PRP. In eyes with less severe PDR or severe nonproliferative diabetic retinopathy, the treating ophthalmologist must weigh the benefits of early PRP with the potential adverse effects.

Technique

Informed consent must be obtained from the patient before PRP is performed. Treatment with PRP may be performed with topical or retrobulbar anesthesia, and it may be conducted in one or multiple sessions. Most surgeons complete PRP in two treatment sessions. Both binocular indirect ophthalmoscopic and slit lamp laser photocoagulation delivery systems may be used. A variety of wide-field contact lenses are available for standard PRP. Many of the commercially available lenses magnify the spot size 1.5 to two times at the retina and provide an inverted and reversed image of the fundus. Yellow and/or green wavelengths are most commonly employed; red may be used in patients with significant cataract or vitreous hemorrhage. Common laser parameters are 200-μm to 500-μm spot size; 0.1- to 0.2-second duration; and intensity to produce a moderately white burn. The average number of 500-μm spots needed to complete PRP is approximately 1500. Laser burns are spaced one-half to one spot width apart.

The placement of laser burns in a posterior to anterior direction helps to reduce the risk of inadvertent extension into the macula. The posterior fundus is demarcated with two to three rows of laser burns. The posterior border should be placed approximately one-half to 1 DD from the optic disc nasally and the major retinal vascular arcades superiorly and inferiorly. The temporal border is at an imaginary line located approximately 2 disc-to-fovea diameters from the optic disc.

Complications

Complications of PRP include blurred vision, nyctalopia, visual field constriction, poor color discrimination, transient myopia, accommodation defects, corneal burns, narrow-angle glaucoma, iris burns, lens opacities, inadvertent macular burns, macular edema, exudative macular detachment, ciliochoroidal effusion, choroidal/choriovitreal neovascularization, optic neuropathy, and complications of local anesthesia (globe trauma, retrobulbar hemorrhage).

Follow-up Considerations

A follow-up visit is scheduled 2 or 3 weeks after the photocoagulation for additional laser treatment if divided sessions are used or in 1 month following completion of PRP. In eyes that fail to regress despite standard PRP, supplemental PRP may be helpful.

Supplemental laser therapy is indicated for the failure of neovascularization to regress, increasing neovascularization or new areas of neovascularization, or vitreous hemorrhage associated with active neovascularization.

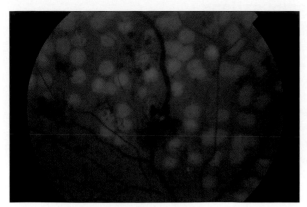

Panretinal photocoagulation is usually divided into 2 sessions. On average, a total of 1200 to 1600 burns of 500-μm spot size are necessary to complete the laser treatment.

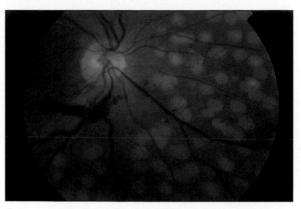

Burns are placed one burn width apart, and care is taken to avoid treatment of the major vessels.

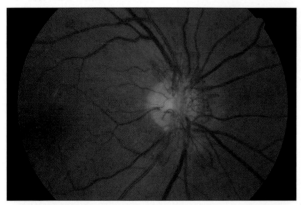

The efficacy of panretinal photocoagulation is related to the regression of retinopathy risk factors. This patient had high-risk proliferative diabetic retinopathy with greater than one-third disc area of neovascularization of the disc.

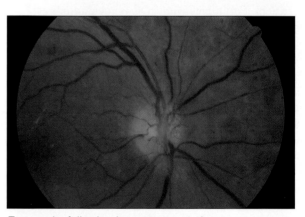

Two weeks following laser treatment, the neovascularization of the disc is significantly regressed.

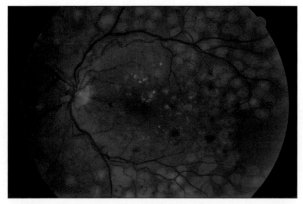

Fundus photograph of a man with high-risk proliferative diabetic retinopathy immediately following panretinal photocoagulation.

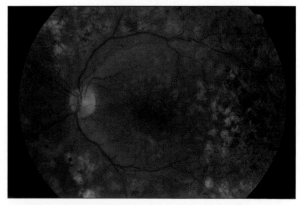

Fundus photograph of the same patient, two years following his initial laser treatment. The old laser scars demonstrate variable levels of atrophy and hyperpigmentation. Successful laser therapy results in regression of the neovascularization and reduction of the venous caliber. The results are long lasting.

PERIPHERAL RETINAL NEOVASCULARIZATION

A variety of conditions are associated with peripheral retinal neovascularization. These include retinopathy of prematurity (ROP), sickle cell retinopathy, peripheral branch retinal vein occlusions (BRVO), familial exudative vitreoretinopathy (FEVR), Eales' disease, pars planitis, and sarcoidosis. The unifying feature of all of these conditions is peripheral retinal ischemia. Laser photocoagulation is applied to the peripheral ischemic retina to reduce the stimulus for new vessel formation.

Technique

Informed consent must be obtained from the patient before laser photocoagulation is performed. Fluorescein angiography may be helpful in identifying the areas of retinal capillary nonperfusion. Peripheral scatter laser photocoagulation may be performed with either a slit lamp or binocular indirect ophthalmoscopic laser delivery system. For infants with ROP, binocular indirect ophthalmoscopic laser photocoagulation has been proved to be as effective as peripheral retinal cryotherapy for threshold ROP and has become the treatment of choice among those caring for these premature infants. Treatment parameters for binocular indirect ophthalmoscopic laser photocoagulation include a duration between 0.2 and 0.5 second and power intensity to obtain moderate retinal whitening. The spot size is determined by the power of the indirect condensing lens, the refractive state of the patient's eye, and the distance between the patient and the surgeon. The average spot size achieved with a 20-diopter lens is approximately 400-μm. Scatter laser burns are placed one-half to one burn width apart in the region of the ischemic retina. For threshold ROP, a more confluent pattern of laser burns is generally necessary to induce regression of the neovascularization.

Complications

Complications of peripheral scatter laser treatment include blurred vision, nyctalopia, visual field constriction, poor color discrimination, transient myopia, accommodation defects, corneal burns, narrow-angle glaucoma, iris burns, lens opacities, inadvertent macular burns, macular edema, exudative macular detachment, ciliochoroidal effusion, choroidal/ choriovitreal neovascularization, optic neuropathy, and complications of local anesthesia (globe trauma, retrobulbar hemorrhage).

Follow-up Considerations

Patients should be reexamined approximately 2 to 4 weeks after laser photocoagulation to ensure regression of the neovascularization. Neonates with ROP are usually examined 1 week following laser photocoagulation. Supplemental laser therapy is recommended for eyes in which regression of the neovascularization fails.

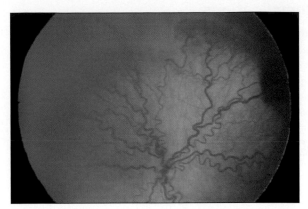

Fundus photograph of a baby with threshold retinopathy of prematurity. Note the fibrovascular proliferation with preretinal hemorrhage in the upper right aspect of the photograph. Plus disease is present with vascular dilation and tortuosity.

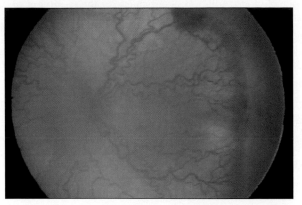

This fundus photograph of the same baby demonstrates the extent of the stage 3 retinopathy of prematurity as it involves the entire temporal retina.

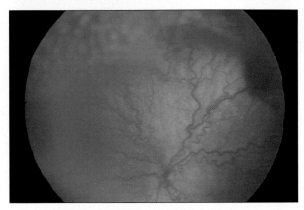

Fundus photograph of the same baby taken immediately following laser photocoagulation. Laser spots are visible in the upper left side of the photograph.

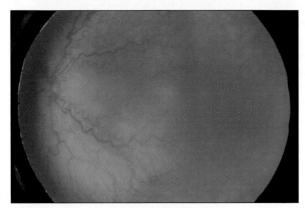

The laser burns are placed in the peripheral avascular retina to reduce the stimulus for neovascularization. A binocular indirect ophthalmoscopic laser delivery system is used. The intensity is adjusted to obtain a moderately white burn in a confluent pattern.

RETINAL ARTERIAL MACROANEURYSM

Laser photocoagulation is indicated for the treatment of retinal arterial macroaneurysms complicated by exudative macular edema involving the fovea. Ruptured macroaneurysms characterized by subretinal, intraretinal, and preretinal hemorrhage often resolve spontaneously without the need for laser treatment.

Technique

Informed consent from the patient must be obtained before performing laser photocoagulation. A fluorescein angiogram is helpful in delineating the size and location of the macroaneurysm. Retinal arterial macroaneurysms are treated at the slit lamp with use of a fundus contact lens. Topical anesthesia is used for most patients. Yellow and/or green wavelengths are used because of the preferential absorption by hemoglobin. A lower-intensity, longer-duration (0.2- to 0.5-second) burn is recommended to reduce the risk of aneurysm rupture during the treatment session. A spot size of 200-μm to 500-μm is sufficient. The outside margin of the macroaneurysm is treated to obtain mild whitening. The body of the aneurysm may be treated directly following successful treatment of the peripheral margin. Again, the end point is mild to moderate retinal whitening.

Complications

Complications of laser photocoagulation for retinal arterial macroaneurysms include loss of vision, aneurysm rupture, and branch retinal artery occlusion. It is not unusual to see an increase in the amount of lipid exudate initially as the edema resorbs; this may be the cause of temporary visual loss following laser photocoagulation.

Follow-up Considerations

Patients should be reexamined approximately 1 month following laser photocoagulation. Multiple treatment sessions may be necessary to achieve closure of the macroaneurysm.

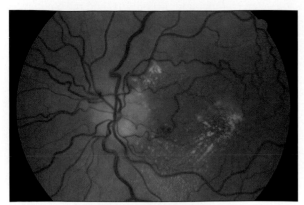

This 68-year-old woman had visual loss in her left eye as a result of macular edema. She had a macroaneurysm along a small inferior branch retinal arteriole. Associated lipid exudation extends through the fovea.

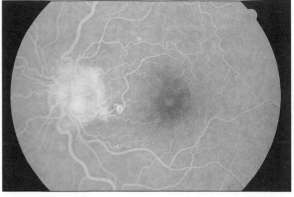

Fluorescein angiogram of the same patient identifies the aneurysm site along an anomalous retinal arteriole. Laser photocoagulation was applied to the margins of the macroaneurysm to reduce the risk of retinal arterial occlusion.

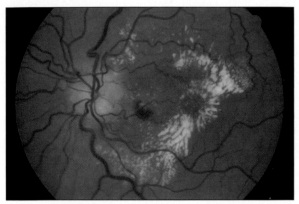

This fundus photograph of the same patient, taken 1 month following laser treatment, reveals intraretinal hemorrhage at the macroaneurysm site and more prominent lipid exudate throughout the macula. The patient's vision declined from 20/60 to 20/100.

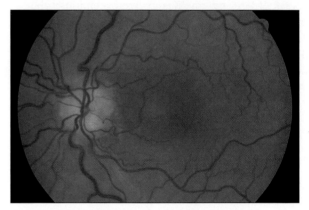

Approximately 6 months following laser treatment, the macular edema and lipid exudate resolved, and the patient's vision improved to 20/25.

RETINAL TEARS AND RETINAL DETACHMENT

The goal of laser retinopexy is to prevent retinal detachment or to prevent progression of a limited retinal detachment. It is, therefore, essential to detect retinal breaks that are at risk for causing a retinal detachment. Certainly treatment is indicated for most horseshoe-shaped retinal tears in patients who are acutely symptomatic and, while convincing evidence may be lacking, probably also for any break associated with subretinal fluid or a retinal dialysis. Lattice degeneration without breaks or with round atrophic holes, operculated retinal holes, and retinoschisis without detachment generally do not need to be treated. A history of retinal detachment in the fellow eye or a strong family history of retinal detachment or other planned intraocular surgery may lower one's threshold to treatment in selected cases.

Technique

The goal of laser treatment is to create a chorioretinal scar or adhesion to prevent the accumulation of liquid vitreous in the subretinal space. To achieve this, typically three rows of closely spaced laser burns are used to encircle the retinal break or retinal detachment. Laser photocoagulation must be applied to attached retina and, in situations where subretinal fluid extends to the ora serrata and the lesion cannot be adequately surrounded by laser, the laser retinopexy should go from the ora serrata on one side to the ora serrata on the other side.

Most patients can tolerate treatment with topical anesthesia alone. However, if the patient cannot tolerate the required treatment with only topical anesthesia, it is better to proceed with peribulbar or retrobulbar anesthesia than risk leaving the patient with inadequate treatment. Either the slit lamp or indirect laser delivery systems can be used. Argon green laser is the wavelength of choice except in the setting of a significant vitreous hemorrhage where krypton red laser may be preferable. For the slit lamp delivery system, the Goldmann three-mirror contact lens or a wide-angle biconcave lens can be used. A spot size of 200-μm or greater, a duration of 0.1 to 0.2 second, and a power titrated up from 150 mW to achieve a gray-white burn are the starting parameters of choice. For the three rows of laser burns surrounding the retinal break, spots are placed approximately one-half spot width apart.

The indirect laser delivery system allows treatment of more peripheral retina. A 20- or 28-diopter condensing lens is used with the patient in a supine position. A green or red wavelength may be used with the following starting parameters: duration of 0.1 to 0.2 second and a power titrated up from 200 mW to achieve a gray-white burn. While most patients can tolerate indirect laser treatment with a topical anesthetic, this type of laser delivery often causes more discomfort, and retrobulbar or peribulbar anesthesia may be necessary.

Complications

Although the goal of laser treatment is to prevent retinal detachment, it is unfortunately not always achievable. With an inadequate laser barrier, or even in the presence of a satisfactory laser barrier, ongoing vitreous traction can result in an extension of the tear and progression of subretinal fluid beyond the laser barrier. It should also be noted that 15% to 20% of patients who have an acutely symptomatic posterior vitreous detachment in association with a retinal tear may develop new tears in the first 4 weeks of their acute symptoms. Patients need to be carefully counseled that a posterior vitreous detachment is a dynamic process and that they should return immediately for an examination if they experience any new visual symptoms. Patients should also be made aware of the fact that the purpose of laser treatment is to prevent retinal detachment; the laser therapy will have no effect on their floaters and or flashes.

Both retinal tears and laser retinopexy are risk factors for the development of epiretinal membranes. It is hard to separate the contribution of each, but in patients who require extensive laser retinopexy, it may be reasonable to discuss the possible late development of premacular gliosis.

Follow-up Considerations

Following laser retinopexy, patients are typically asked to return in 1 week's time or sooner should any new symptoms develop. Careful examination of the retinal periphery should be undertaken with indirect ophthalmoscopy with 360° of scleral depression to monitor for new retinal breaks and to ensure adequacy of the original laser treatment. Patients are then asked to return 3 to 4 weeks after that, when a similar careful and thorough examination of the retinal periphery is undertaken.

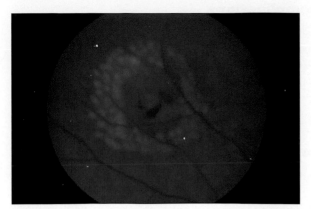

Fundus photograph taken immediately following laser photocoagulation for an acute, symptomatic horseshoe-shaped retinal tear. Approximately three rows of laser burns are placed around the retinal tear to reduce the risk of retinal detachment.

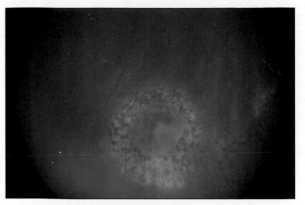

This fundus photograph demonstrates a well-treated retinal flap tear. The chorioretinal scarring generated by laser photocoagulation prevents the passage of fluid through the retinal tear.

RETINAL TELANGIECTASIS AND RETINAL ANGIOMAS

Laser photocoagulation is indicated for the treatment of Coats' disease, idiopathic juxtafoveal retinal telangiectasis group 1, and occasional cases of idiopathic juxtafoveal retinal telangiectasis group 2 complicated by subretinal neovascularization. Isolated retinal angiomas and retinal angiomas associated with von Hippel-Lindau disease may be successfully treated with laser photocoagulation.

Technique

Informed consent must be obtained from the patient prior to laser photocoagulation. Laser photocoagulation may be performed with a slit lamp or binocular indirect ophthalmoscopic laser delivery system. Yellow and/or green wavelengths are most effective because of their preferential absorption by hemoglobin. Fluorescein angiography is helpful in identifying retinal telangiectasis as well as areas of peripheral capillary nonperfusion. Telangiectatic vessels are treated directly with moderately intense, confluent laser burns; peripheral scatter laser photocoagulation is applied to areas of capillary nonperfusion. Multiple sessions may be required to achieve successful closure of the telangiectatic vessels.

Laser photocoagulation for subretinal neovascularization in patients with idiopathic juxtafoveal retinal telangietasis is similar to that described in patients with choroidal neovascularization. (See "Choroidal Neovascularization" earlier in this chapter.)

Retinal angiomas may require multiple treatment sessions to achieve closure. Again, yellow and/or green wavelengths are most effective because of their preferential absorption by hemoglobin. Treatment is applied directly to the tumor with sufficient intensity to obtain a moderately intense white burn. The typical spot size is 200-μm to 500-μm with a 0.2- to 0.5-second duration.

Complications

Complications of laser photocoagulation for retinal telangiectasis and retinal angiomas include loss of vision. It is not unusual to see an increase in the amount of lipid exudate initially as the edema resorbs; this may be the cause of temporary visual loss following laser photocoagulation.

Follow-up Considerations

Multiple treatment sessions may be necessary to successfully treat retinal telangiectasis. Treatment may be applied at 8- to 12-week intervals. Patients with extensive Coats' disease must be treated aggressively because of the risk of exudative retinal detachment, neovascular glaucoma, and phthisis bulbi.

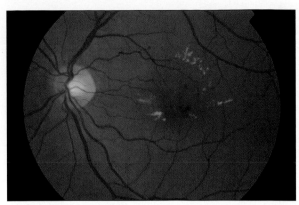

Fundus photograph of a patient with idiopathic juxtafoveal retinal telangiectasis group 1, demonstrating visible microaneurysms, lipid exudate, and macular edema in his left eye.

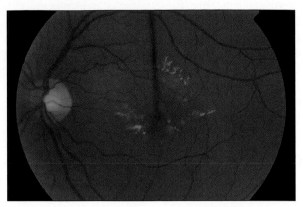

Fundus photograph of the left eye of the same patient immediately after focal laser treatment to the leaking retinal vascular abnormalities.

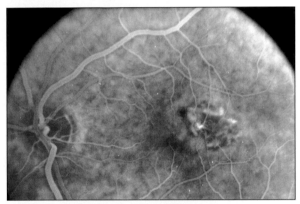

This man with idiopathic juxtafoveal retinal telangiectasis group 2 developed an extrafoveal subretinal neovascular membrane in his left eye. Fluorescein angiography demonstrates a well-defined extrafoveal neovascular complex.

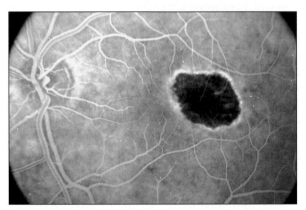

Laser photocoagulation was performed on the same patient. Fluorescein angiography demonstrates prominent hypofluorescence of the laser-treated area, with no evidence of persistent or recurrent neovascularization.

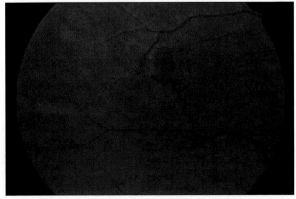

Von Hippel-Lindau disease is characterized by the presence of retinal capillary hemangiomas. This woman had a small angioma with a prominent draining vessel. There was no significant fluid or lipid exudation.

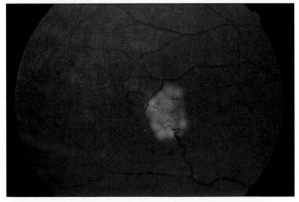

Laser photocoagulation was performed on the same patient. The retinal capillary angioma was treated directly with intense laser photocoagulation to achieve closure. Some individuals experience exacerbation of fluid and lipid exudation following treatment.

PHOTODYNAMIC THERAPY WITH VERTEPORFIN

Photodynamic therapy (PDT) with verteporfin is indicated for the treatment of predominantly classic, subfoveal choroidal neovascular membranes associated with age-related macular degeneration (AMD), presumed ocular histoplasmosis syndrome, and pathologic myopia. The role of PDT in other conditions associated with choroidal neovascularization (eg, choroidal rupture, angioid streaks, multifocal choroiditis) is being investigated.

Contraindications for PDT with verteporfin include pregnancy, liver disease, porphyria, or known hypersensitivity to verteporfin.

Technique

Informed consent must be obtained from the patient to conduct PDT. Fluorescein angiography is necessary to identify the location and type of choroidal neovascularization. Photodynamic therapy is most effective for subfoveal new vessels that are predominantly classic (classic component occupies at least 50% of the entire choroidal neovascular complex). Classic choroidal neovascularization is characterized by a well-defined, lacy pattern of vessels early in the fluorescein angiogram followed by late leakage. The size of the treatment area is usually limited to 5400 μm or smaller.

The dosage of verteporfin is based on the patient's total body surface area calculated using the patient's height and weight. According to the patient's body surface area, a verteporfin dosage of 6 mg/m^2 is prepared. To form a total volume of 30 mL, 5% dextrose is added.

The medication is infused through an arm vein over 10 minutes (using an infusion pump set to deliver 3 mL of solution per minute). Following a 5-minute waiting period, the medication is activated with a 689-nm wavelength of light for 83 seconds. The light dose is 50 J/cm^2 or 600 mW/cm^2, which is automatically set by the photoactivator.

The size of the treatment area is determined by adding 1000 μm to the greatest linear diameter of the choroidal neovascular complex. The greatest linear diameter can be calculated manually or measured with commercially available computer software. There are no visible funduscopic changes during or immediately following treatment.

Complications

The patient must be observed closely during the infusion process. In the event of extravasation, the infusion must be stopped immediately. Complications of PDT include visual disturbance (blurred vision, scotoma), infusion-related complications (rash, extravasation of medication), photosensitivity, headache, back pain, and allergic reaction. Severe visual loss may occur in 1% to 4% of patients. This may be related to macular infarction or optic nerve damage. Patients must avoid exposure to direct sunlight for 5 days following the infusion to reduce the risk of skin damage.

Follow-up Considerations

Patients are reevaluated every 3 months. Fluorescein angiography is performed to determine if leakage persists from the choroidal neovascular complex. If leakage is detected, additional PDT is recommended. Most individuals require 5 to 6 treatments over the course of 2 years.

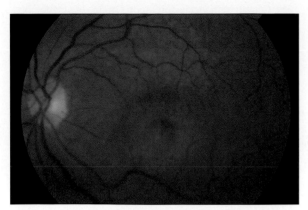

Fundus photograph of a patient's left eye with a subfoveal choroidal neovascular membrane secondary to age-related macular degeneration and 20/400 vision.

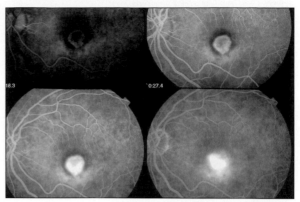

Early (upper left), midphase (upper right and lower left), and late-phase (lower right) fluorescein angiograms demonstrate an entirely classic subfoveal choroidal neovascular membrane secondary to age-related macular degeneration. Such classic small lesions with poor vision did especially well with photodynamic therapy as compared to controls in the Treatment of Age-Related Macular Degeneration with Photodynamic Therapy (TAP) study.

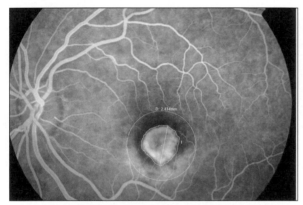

Top-Con Imagenet software is used to help calculate the spot size to be used for photodynamic therapy. The spot size is set to cover a diameter of 1000 μm larger than the greatest linear dimension of the choroidal neovascular membrane.

SELECTED REFERENCES

Branch Retinal Vein Occlusion: Macular Edema

1. Branch Vein Occlusion Study Group. Argon laser photocoagulation for macular edema in branch vein occlusion. *Am J Ophthalmol.* 1984;98:271–282.

2. Folk JC, Pulido JS. *Laser Photocoagulation of the Retina and Choroid.* Ophthalmology Monographs 11. San Francisco, Calif: American Academy of Ophthalmology; 1997:110–121.

3. Orth DH. The Branch Vein Occlusion Study. In: Kertes PJ, Conway MD, eds. *Clinical Trials in Ophthalmology: A Summary and Practice Guide.* Baltimore, Md: Lippincott Williams & Wilkins; 1998:113–127.

Branch Retinal Vein Occlusion: Neovascularization

1. Branch Vein Occlusion Study Group. Argon laser scatter photocoagulation for prevention of neovascularization and vitreous hemorrhage in branch vein occlusion: a randomized clinical trial. *Arch Ophthalmol.* 1986;104:34–41.

2. Folk JC, Pulido JS. *Laser Photocoagulation of the Retina and Choroid.* Ophthalmology Monographs 11. San Francisco, Calif: American Academy of Ophthalmology; 1997:110–121.

3. Orth DH. The Branch Vein Occlusion Study. In: Kertes PJ, Conway MD, eds. *Clinical Trials in Ophthalmology: A Summary and Practice Guide.* Baltimore, Md: Lippincott Williams & Wilkins; 1998:113–127.

Central Serous Chorioretinopathy

1. Folk JC, Pulido JS. *Laser Photocoagulation of the Retina and Choroid.* Ophthalmology Monographs 11. San Francisco, Calif: American Academy of Ophthalmology; 1997:237–240.

Central Retinal Vein Occlusion

1. Fekrat S, Finkelstein D. The Branch Vein Occlusion Study. In: Kertes PJ, Conway MD, eds. *Clinical Trials in Ophthalmology: A Summary and Practice Guide.* Baltimore, Md: Williams and Wilkins; 1998:129–143.

2. Folk JC, Pulido JS. *Laser Photocoagulation of the Retina and Choroid.* Ophthalmology Monographs 11. San Francisco, Calif: American Academy of Ophthalmology; 1997:97–109.

3. The Central Vein Occlusion Study Group. A randomized clinical trial of early panretinal photocoagulation for ischemic central vein occlusion. The Central Vein Occlusion Study Group N Report. *Ophthalmology.* 1995;102:1434–1444.

4. The Central Vein Occlusion Study Group. Evaluation of grid pattern photocoagulation for macular edema in central vein occlusion. The Central Vein Occlusion Group M Report. *Ophthalmology.* 1995;102:1425–1433.

5. The Central Vein Occlusion Study Group. Natural history and clinical management of central retinal vein occlusion. *Arch Ophthalmol.* 1997;115:486–491.

Choroidal Neovascularization

1. Folk JC, Pulido JS. *Laser Photocoagulation of the Retina and Choroid.* Ophthalmology Monographs 11. San Francisco, Calif: American Academy of Ophthalmology; 1997:149–209.

2. Macular Photocoagulation Study Group. Argon laser photocoagulation for neovascular maculopathy after five years: results from randomized clinical trials. *Arch Ophthalmol.* 1991;109:1109–1114.

3. Macular Photocoagulation Study Group. Laser photocoagulation for juxtafoveal choroidal neovascularization: five-year results from randomized clinical trials. *Arch Ophthalmol.* 1994;112:500–509.

4. Macular Photocoagulation Study Group. Persistent and recurrent neovascularization after krypton laser photocoagulation for neovascular lesions of ocular histoplasmosis. *Arch Ophthalmol.* 1989;107:344–352.

Diabetic Retinopathy: Clinically Significant Macular Edema

1. Akduman L, Olk RJ. The Early Treatment Diabetic Retinopathy Study. In: Kertes PJ, Conway MD, eds. *Clinical Trial in Ophthalmology: A Summary and Practice Guide.* Baltimore, Md: Lippincott Williams & Wilkins; 1998:15–35.

2. Early Treatment of Diabetic Retinopathy Study. Photocoagulation for diabetic macular edema. Early Treatment Diabetic Retinopathy Study Report No. 4. *Int Ophthalmol Clin.* 1987;27:265–272.

3. Folk JC, Pulido JS. *Laser Photocoagulation of the Retina and Choroid.* Ophthalmology Monographs 11. San Francisco, Calif: American Academy of Ophthalmology; 1997:25–61.

Diabetic Retinopathy: High-Risk Proliferative Diabetic Retinopathy

1. Folk JC, Pulido JS. *Laser Photocoagulation of the Retina and Choroid.* Ophthalmology Monographs 11. San Francisco, Calif: American Academy of Ophthalmology; 1997:63–95.

2. Quillen DA, Gardner TW, Blankenship GW. The Diabetic Retinopathy Study. In: Kertes PJ, Conway MD, eds. *Clinical Trials in Ophthalmology: A Summary and Practice Guide*. Baltimore, Md: Lippincott Williams & Wilkins; 1998:1–13.

3. The Diabetic Retinopathy Study Research Group. Indications for photocoagulation treatment of diabetic retinopathy. Diabetic Retinopathy Study No. 14. *Int Ophthalmol Clin*. 1987;27:239–252.

4. The Diabetic Retinopathy Study Research Group. Photocoagulation treatment of proliferative diabetic retinopathy: clinical applications of Diabetic Retinopathy Study (DRS) findings. DRS Report No. 8. *Ophthalmology*. 1981;88:583–600.

5. The Diabetic Retinopathy Study Research Group. Photocoagulation treatment of proliferative diabetic retinopathy: the second report of Diabetic Retinopathy Study findings. *Ophthalmology*. 1978:85:82–106.

Peripheral Retinal Neovascularization

1. Cryotherapy for Retinopathy of Prematurity Cooperative Group. Multicenter trial of cryotherapy for retinopathy of prematurity: 3½-year outcome: structure and function. *Arch Ophthalmol*. 1993;111:339–344.

2. Cryotherapy for Retinopathy of Prematurity Cooperative Group. Multicenter trial of cryotherapy for retinopathy of prematurity: snellen visual acuity and structural outcome at 5½ years after randomization. *Arch Ophthalmol*. 1996;114:417–424.

3. Folk JC, Pulido JS. *Laser Photocoagulation of the Retina and Choroid*. Ophthalmology Monographs 11. San Francisco, Calif: American Academy of Ophthalmology, 1997:123–147.

4. McNamara JA. The multicenter trial of cryotherapy for retinopathy of prematurity. In: Kertes PJ, Conway MD, eds. *Clinical Trials in Ophthalmology: A Summary and Practice Guide*. Baltimore, Md: Lippincott Williams & Wilkins; 1998:145–162.

Retinal Arterial Macroaneurysm

1. Folk JC, Pulido JS. *Laser Photocoagulation of the Retina and Choroid*. Ophthalmology Monographs 11. San Francisco, Calif: American Academy of Ophthalmology; 1997:219–221.

Retinal Tears and Retinal Detachment

1. Folk JC, Pulido JS. *Laser Photocoagulation of the Retina and Choroid*. Ophthalmology Monographs 11. San Francisco, Calif: American Academy of Ophthalmology; 1997:211–219.

2. Wilkinson CP. Evidence-based analysis of prophylactic treatment of asymptomatic retinal breaks and lattice degeneration. *Ophthalmology*. 2000;107:12–5.

3. Wilkinson CP. Evidence-based medicine regarding the prevention of retinal detachment. *Trans Am Ophthalmol Soc*. 1999;97:397–404.

Retinal Telangiectasis and Retinal Angiomas

1. Folk JC, Pulido JS. *Laser Photocoagulation of the Retina and Choroid*. Ophthalmology Monographs 11. San Francisco, Calif: American Academy of Ophthalmology; 1997:221–231.

Photodynamic Therapy with Verteporfin

1. Fine SL. Photodynamic therapy with verteporfin is effective for selected patients with neovascular age-related macular degeneration. *Arch Ophthalmol*. 1999;117:1400–1402.

2. Miller JW, Schmidt-Erfurth U, Sickenberg M, et al. Photodynamic therapy with verteporfin for choroidal neovascularization caused by age-related macular degeneration: results of a single treatment in a phase 1 and 2 study. *Arch Ophthalmol*. 1999;117:1161–1173.

3. Puliafito CA, Rogers AH, Martidis A, Greenberg PA. *Ocular Photodynamic Therapy*. Thorofare, NJ: Slack, Inc; 2002.

4. Schmidt-Erfurth U, Miller JW, Sickenberg M, et al. Photodynamic therapy with verteporfin for choroidal neovascularization caused by age-related macular degeneration: results of retreatments in a phase 1 and 2 study. *Arch Ophthalmol*. 1999;117:1177–1187.

5. Treatment of Age-Related Macular Degeneration with Photodynamic Therapy (TAP) Study Group. Photodynamic therapy of subfoveal choroidal neovascularization in age-related macular degeneration with verteporfin: one-year results of 2 randomized clinical trials—TAP Report 1. *Arch Ophthalmol*. 1999;117:1329–1345.

6. Treatment of Age-Related Macular Degeneration with Photodynamic Therapy (TAP) Study Group. Photodynamic therapy of subfoveal choroidal neovascularization in age-related macular degeneration with verteporfin: two-year results of 2 randomized clinical trials—TAP Report 2. *Arch Ophthalmol*. 2001;119:198–207.

INDEX

Proliferative diabetic retinopathy, see Retinopathy, diabetic, proliferative
Proliferative vitreoretinopathy, see Vitreoretinopathy
Propionibacterium acnes, bacterial endophthalmitis, 248, *249*
Protozoal infections (toxoplasmosis), 274, *275*
Pseudo-retinitis pigmentosa, *342*
Pseudohypopyon, *161*
Pseudophakia, cystoid macular edema-associated toxicities, *197*
Pseudorosette, *338*
Pseudovasculitis, diabetic retinopathy, *129*
Pseudoxanthoma elasticum, angioid streaks, *12, 95*
Punctate inner choroiditis, 254
Pupil size, 2
Purtcher's retinopathy
    cotton wool spot, *46*
    clinical features, treatment, etc, 292, *293*
    selected references, 300

Radiation retinopathy, 146, *147*, 155
Radiography, foreign body (iron toxicity), 198
Research, 345-366
    The Branch Vein Occlusion Study, 354, 364
    The Central Vein Occlusion Study, 355-356, 365
    Course of Visual Acuity in Severe PDR with Conventional Management (study), 349-350
    The Diabetes Control and Complications Trial, 352-353, 364
    The Diabetic Retinopathy Study, 346, 364
    The Diabetic Retinopathy Vitrectomy Study, 349-351, 364
    The Early Treatment Diabetic Retinopathy Study, 347-348, 364
    Early Vitrectomy for Severe PDR in Eyes with Useful Vision (study), 350
    Early Vitrectomy for Severe Vitreous Hemorrhage (study), 351
    The Macular Photocoagulation Study, 359-362, 365
    The Multicenter Trial of Cryotherapy for Retinopathy of Prematurity, 357-358, 365
    selected references, 364-365
    The Treatment of Age-Related Macular Degeneration with Photodynamic Therapy (TAP) Study, 363, 365
Reticular pattern dystrophy, *109*
Reticulum cell sarcoma, see Lymphoma, intraocular
Retina, see also Hemorrhage, retinal (intraretinal); Telangiectasis; headings beginning with Retinal, Retinopathy, below;
    adherence, normal, 6
    adhesion, by RPE, 4
    albinism, 158, *159*
    anatomy, 1-7
    bear tracks pigmentation, *57*
    blunt trauma injury (commotio retinae), *10*
    "candlewax drippings," *265*
    commotio retinae, 288, *289*, 300
    cystoid degeneration with focal retinoschisis, histopathology, *343*
    degenerative diseases, use of electroretinography, 28
    disease chart (specific clinical features related to conditions and diagnoses), *71-81*
    diseases, clinical features, 41-84
    drug toxicities, 189-202
    electroretinography, 28
    flecked, syndromes, 49, *49, 73, 82*
    hamartoma, histopathology, *338*
    hereditary disorders, 28, 157-187
    histopathology, 329-344
    hypoperfusion, 22
    idiopathic juxtafoveal telangiectasis, 388, *389, 393*
    ischemia, 382, *383*
    lattice degeneration, histopathology, *343*
    neurosensory, 2, 4, *5*
    peripheral diseases, *71-81*, 301-312, *343*
    peripheral neovascularization, 382, *383*, 393
    photographs (clinical correlation), *10-13*
    physiology, 8-13
    pregnancy-related disease, 144, *145*
    "salt-and-pepper" stippling, *173*

Stargardt disease, 180, *181*
telangiectasia; Coats' disease, *125*
tumors, clinical features, etc, 64, *64*
unilateral wipeout syndrome, 246
whitening, in Behçet's disease, *241*
Retinal adhesion, see Retinal detachment
Retinal angioma, 388, *389*, 393
Retinal artery, see also Retinal vascular system;
    branch, occlusion, 116, *117*
    branch, occlusion, selected references, 154
    central, occlusion, 120, *121*
    central, occlusion, histopathology, *332*
    central, occlusion, selected references, 154
    description, 4
    macroaneurysm, lipid exudates, *52*
    macroaneurysm; preretinal hemorrhage, *58*
    macroaneurysms, 148, 155, *149, 384, 385, 393*
    occlusion, *10*
    occlusion, arteritis; in acute retinal necrosis *239*
    occlusion; cherry red spot, *43*
    occlusion; rubeosis, *62*
Retinal breaks, 306, 307, 312
Retinal capillaries, see Retinal vascular system
Retinal cavernous hemangioma, *336*
Retinal crystals
    clinical features, etc, 59, *59*
    idiopathic juxtafoveolar retinal telangiectasis, *139*
    retinal diseases exhibiting (chart), *77*
    selected references, 83
Retinal detachment
    acute retinal necrosis, *239*
    adherence, normal, 6
    adhesion, by RPE, 4
    bullous, *309*
    chronic, demarcation line; peripheral pigmentation, *55*
    cystic retinal tufts, 302, *303*
    cytomegalovirus retinitis, *245*
    exudative; posterior scleritis, *261*
    funnel (echography) *35*
    laser retinopexy, 386, *387*, 393
    lattice degeneration, *305*
    photographs, *13*
    proliferative diabetic retinopathy, 133
    proliferative vitreoretinopathy, 324, *325*
    proliferative vitreoretinopathy with, histopathology, *343*
    retinal breaks, 306, 307
    rhegmatogenous, 308, *309*
    selected references, 312
    toxemia of pregnancy, *21*
    Vogt-Koyanagi-Harada syndrome, *279*
    wrinkled surface, *309*
    X-linked juvenile retinoschisis, *183*
Retinal diseases, clinical features, 41-84
Retinal fold
    persistent hyperplastic primary vitreous, *321*
    proliferative vitreoretinopathy, *325*
    shaken baby syndrome, *295*
Retinal hemorrhage, see Hemorrhage, retinal (intraretinal)
Retinal hole
    proliferative diabetic retinopathy, *133*
    retinal breaks, *307*
    X-linked juvenile retinoschisis, *183*
Retinal ischemic whitening
    aminoglycoside toxicity, *191*
    branch retinal artery occlusion, 116, *117*
    central retinal artery occlusion, *121*
Retinal necrosis, 238, *239*
    acute (retinitis), *61*
    AIDS, HIV retinopathy, *251*
    selected references, 282
Retinal neovascularization
    branch retinal vein occlusion, selected references, 392
    clinical features, etc, 60, *60*
    histopathology, *334, 335*
    peripheral, 382, *383*, 393
    retinal diseases exhibiting (chart), *78*
    selected references, 83
    sickle cell retinopathy, *153*

Retinal pigment epithelial cells, see Pigment epithelial cells
Retinal pigment epithelium, see Pigment epithelium
Retinal tear
    cystic retinal tufts, *303*
    laser retinopexy, 386, *387*, 393
    operculated, histopathology, *343*
    posterior vitreous detachment, *323*
    retinal breaks, 307
Retinal telangiectasis, see Telangiectasis
Retinal tufts, cystic, 302, *303*, 312
Retinal tumors, 64, *64*
Retinal vascular system, see also Hemorrhage, retinal (intraretinal); Retinal artery; Retinal neovascularization; Retinal vein; Telangiectasis; Vasculitis;
    aneurysms, histopathology, *336*
    arteriovenous malformations (Wyburn-Mason syndrome), 228, *229*
    attenuation in retinitis pigmentosa, *177*
    blood flow, 4
    capillaries, nonperfusion, *25*
    capillary hemangiomas (Von Hippel-Lindau disease), 227
    clinical features and conditions (chart), *71-81*
    Coats' disease, 124, *125*
    diabetic retinopathy (nonproliferative), 126, *127-129*
    diabetic retinopathy (proliferative), 130, *131-133*
    diseases, *71-81*, 115-156
    Eales' disease, 134, *135*
    endothelial cells, 4, *5*
    fluorescein angiography, 16-25
    hamartoma, histopathology, *336*
    histopathology, *332-335*
    hypertensive retinopathy, 136, *137*
    hypoperfusion, 22
    idiopathic juxtafoveolar retinal telangiectasis, 138, *139*
    leukemic retinopathy, 140, *141*
    microaneurysms, histopathology, *334*
    ocular ischemic syndrome, 142, *143*
    sheathing in inflammatory disease, histopathology, *341*
    Valsalva retinopathy, 298, *299*
Retinal vasculitis, see Vasculitis
Retinal vein, see also Retinal vascular system;
    beading; diabetic retinopathy, *127*
Retinal vein, branch, occlusion, 118, *119*
    The Branch Vein Occlusion Study, 354, 364
    histopathology, *332*
    neovascularization; scatter photocoagulation, 370, *371*
    peripheral retinal neovascularization, 382
    photocoagulation, 368, *369*
    selected references, 154, 392
Retinal vein, central, occlusion, 122, *123*
    The Central Vein Occlusion Study, 355-356, 365
    panretinal laser photocoagulation, 374, *375*
    selected references, 154, 392
Retinal vein occlusion, *10, 24, 25*
    cotton wool spot, *46*
    fluorescein angiography, *19*
    intraretinal hemorrhages, *51*
    ischemia (electroretinogram), *31*
    lipid exudates, *52*
    rubeosis, *62*
11-cis-retinaldehyde, 8
All-trans-retinaldehyde, 8
Retinitis
    acute retinal necrosis, 238, *239*
    clinical features, etc, 61, *61*
    cytomegalovirus, 244, *245, 251, 282, 340*
    HIV, selected references, 282-283
    punctata albescens, *167*
    retinal diseases exhibiting (chart), *78*
    selected references, 83
    toxoplasmosis, 274, *275*
Retinitis pigmentosa
    clinical features, treatment, etc, 176, *177*
    cystoid macular edema, *47*
    electroretinogram, *29*
    intraretinal pigment migration, *11*